D0207590

MISCARRIAGE

This book is dedicated to my twin daughters
Clare and Jenny.
They have been a source of joy and inspiration to me
and I am very privileged to be their mother.

MISCARRIAGE

WHAT EVERY WOMAN NEEDS TO KNOW

A Positive New Approach

PROFESSOR LESLEY REGAN

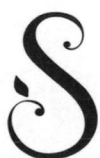

First published in Great Britain in 1997 by Bloomsbury
This revised and updated edition published in 2018 by Orion Spring
an imprint of The Orion Publishing Group Ltd
Carmelite House, 50 Victoria Embankment
London EC4Y 0DZ

An Hachette UK Company

1 3 5 7 9 10 8 6 4 2

Copyright © Lesley Regan, 1997, 2001, 2018

The moral right of Lesley Regan to be identified as
the author of this work has been asserted in accordance
with the Copyright, Designs and Patents Act of 1988.

All rights reserved. No part of this publication may be reproduced,
stored in a retrieval system, or transmitted in any form or by any means,
electronic, mechanical, photocopying, recording, or otherwise, without
the prior permission of both the copyright owner and the
above publisher of this book.

Every effort has been made to ensure that the information in the book
is accurate. The information in this book may not be applicable in each
individual case so it is advised that professional medical advice is obtained
for specific health matters and before changing any medication or dosage.
Neither the publisher nor author accepts any legal responsibility for any
personal injury or other damage or loss arising from the use of the
information in this book. In addition, if you are concerned about
your diet or exercise regime and wish to change them, you
should consult a health practitioner first.

A CIP catalogue record for this book is
available from the British Library.

ISBN (Trade Paperback): 978 1 4091 7568 1
ISBN (Ebook): 978 1 4091 7569 8

Printed in Great Britain by CPI Group (UK) Ltd,
Croydon, CR0 4YY

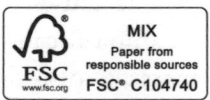

MIX
Paper from
responsible sources
FSC® C104740

www.orionbooks.co.uk

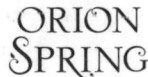

ORION
SPRING

CONTENTS

PART THREE: PRACTICAL ISSUES AND ANSWERS TO YOUR QUESTIONS

PART FOUR: THE NEXT STEP

INTRODUCTION

If you are reading this book it is because you have probably experienced a miscarriage or maybe more than one and my heart goes out to you.

This book will help you, because knowledge is power – it will help you to understand the possible causes, identify the limits of our current scientific knowledge, explain the tests and treatments, and what options are open to you to ensure you get the best possible care from the NHS.

Professor Lesley Regan is uniquely qualified to advise you; she runs the recurrent miscarriage clinic at St Mary's Hospital in Paddington, London, and has pioneered good care for parents experiencing miscarriages. Her clinics have become famous for their approach; ensuring parents have all the relevant tests and treatments and importantly avoiding those that don't make any difference, and making sure that people are treated with kindness and compassion. She has helped many families to have the much-wanted baby they have been striving for. Professor Regan has also been conducting medical research in this area for many years and so she knows all the latest discoveries and treatments available to parents. You are in good hands.

Many hospitals in the UK take part in medical research to find out how we can help parents experiencing miscarriage, by recruiting patients onto clinical trials. I want to encourage you to consider taking part; you will be helping the next generation of parents to get better treatments and care and we know that people who take part in clinical trials tend to have better outcomes than people not in clinical trials so it makes sense to get involved if you are able to.

It's important that you know the truth; there are still many things that are unknown and theories and tests have been developed which don't have a good evidence base and often prey on vulnerable people who are desperate to have a baby. Medical science has not found all the answers and for some people they may never know the reason why they miscarried. Professor Lesley Regan will be honest with you and that is one of the many merits about this book.

It's also true that care, testing and treatment options vary around the NHS from hospital to hospital and I hope this book will help you to assertively navigate your way around the NHS and ensure that you receive the care that you need.

Your physical health as well as your mental health can have an impact on a successful pregnancy; please don't ignore the advice to maintain a healthy weight, eat a healthy diet, take regular exercise, take folic acid and ensure your vitamin D levels are optimal – for some this makes all the difference and this book will explain why and help you to be in control.

I often say that for some parents getting pregnant and having a healthy baby is easy but others, like you, need huge determination and resilience to have that happy ending – I want to encourage you, because for most people, whatever the journey, they do become parents. Never give up hope.

I know you will find this book useful and I want to wish you all the very best for the journey ahead.

Jane Brewin
Tommy's Chief Executive

UPDATED FOREWORD
TO THE FIRST EDITION

The experience of miscarriage can be devastating. While some women and their partners may see it as a 'blip' in their pregnancy history and move on quite quickly and positively, for many others it is a bereavement, a time of loss and grief for their baby-to-be and the plans they had for this new life.

Frequently there is a sense of shock and bewilderment. We may know that miscarriages happen, but we don't expect them to happen to us. We look at the wonderful advances in medical research and treatment and we expect things to go well or, at the very least, to know why they go wrong and how to put things right next time. We look for explanations and for answers and for certainty.

This new edition of Professor Lesley Regan's book helps enormously. It contains a wealth of meticulously researched information about miscarriage causes, management and treatment and more besides, but this internationally acknowledged expert is unafraid to remind us how much yet remains unknown, uncertain. She provides clarity, information and hope – but never false hope.

In the book, Professor Regan draws on her extensive experience at St Mary's Hospital in London, together with research from across the world, to remove much of the mystery, fear and confusion surrounding pregnancy loss. She explains the often unexplained, encouraging the reader to learn more about the processes of conception and pregnancy as a tool to understanding what happens when things go wrong. She examines both popular myths and diverse medical opinion, explaining her own conclusions and practice. Types of loss, causes and treatments are set out clearly and medical terminology interpreted.

Along with the important and detailed information, the reader will find understanding and empathy. Professor Regan sees at close hand patients' pain, anxiety, grief, anger and sometimes despair. She also sees their hope and determination, whether that results in them trying again, taking part in research trials or making the decision to stop trying and find another way forward.

Above all, what shines through these pages is Professor Regan's passion both for driving research and for sharing the knowledge gained with as wide an audience as possible. With the publication of this new edition of her much-recommended book, we all benefit.

Ruth Bender Atik
National Director of the Miscarriage Association

FOREWORD
TO THE THIRD EDITION

Miscarriage is a shattering experience for most women and it is very often an unexpected event. Typically, it occurs early in gestation, just as the woman is celebrating the news of her pregnancy. Sadly, this unwelcome outcome is extremely common.

For far too long health professionals have given insufficient scientific attention to this important problem and the resources to address the causes and solutions have been woefully lacking. Added to which most miscarriage sufferers have received very little in terms of emotional support and insufficient information on their condition. These realities have led to many well-meaning recommendations, with very little evidence base and are often based on personal opinions and not on the results of well-designed scientific studies. At the same time, there is an understandable tendency for the patient to blame herself or her partner for the pregnancy loss. Yet rarely do lifestyle habits or exposures provide a robust explanation.

Fortunately, considerable knowledge has been gained in this field since the last edition of *Miscarriage: What Every Woman Needs To Know* was published in 2001. The readers are provided with a welcome cutting-edge volume from Professor Lesley Regan based on her considerable practical experience as a clinician. It is unusual to have a medical problem like miscarriage and its treatments addressed by an international authority who has not only performed the sentinel studies underpinning investigation and treatment, but has for decades provided the frontline care for patients experiencing miscarriages.

A great strength of this volume is that it covers literally all of the many explanations for miscarriages proposed – and as the reader will discover – there are many. We are told just which 'causes' are valid and for which there are recommended and efficacious treatments. Distress over lack of an explanation is understandable; however, undergoing treatment lacking a scientific basis is fruitless, as well as delaying identification of warranted treatment.

We should be grateful for Professor Regan and her colleagues for updating this volume. Professor Regan shows her practicality and passion for communicating her knowledge and experience to other healthcare providers, the patients attending her own clinic at St Mary's and the general public. Her contributions to the field of miscarriage have had a global impact, benefiting women across the world and emphasising the importance of them receiving high-quality evidence-based care and access to their reproductive rights. She is the 2016–19 president of the Royal College Obstetricians and Gynaecologists, the first female president in over 65 years and only the second in history. She is recipient of many prestigious awards and honorary international fellowships. In 2017 she was elected as one of the very rare foreign associates to the United States National Academy of Medicine.

In short, the reader of this third edition of *Miscarriage: What Every Woman Needs To Know* should expect much and will not be disappointed, since much is delivered.

Professor Joe Leigh Simpson
President of the International Federation of Fertility Societies

PREFACE
TO THE THIRD EDITION

Why do we need a third edition of this book?

The answer is simple and also very exciting. Since the last edition was published, some very important advances have been made into our understanding of the causes of miscarriage. Armed with this new knowledge we have been able to develop new investigative tests that are helping us to identify a further group of women with previously unexplained miscarriages. It will only be a short time before these women can also be offered treatments that will help them achieve their goal – a live take-home baby.

There are too many examples of the progress that has been made to mention them all in this brief introduction, but I think you will be heartened to hear that every chapter of this book has needed amending to reflect our improved knowledge and understanding. Technical advances in molecular biology mean that we are now better able to identify genetic abnormalities in the embryo or fetus. Advances in fertility therapy have provided more couples with the possibility of conceiving and maintaining their pregnancy. Indeed, entirely new sections on implantation and uterine receptivity and the role that inflammatory responses make in establishing an early pregnancy are now included. These are accompanied by much clearer explanations of the complex interplay that occurs in early pregnancy between our immune systems and haemostatic or blood-clotting pathways.

The realisation that so much of what goes on in our bodies is determined by microbes or bugs has allowed us to appreciate that infective organisms not only cause diseases but they also play a key role in maintaining our health and, in particular, our reproductive health. It will not be long before we are able to offer women an accurate prediction of the outcome of her pregnancy and alert us to the potential complications that may occur, by studying her personal profile or microbiome in easily accessible body fluids. Indeed, in some cases we will soon be able to intervene and offer preventative treatments for miscarriage.

The other reason for this third edition is that my patients keep asking me for further information and updates on the medical advances that they hear and read about in the media and the outcome of the research projects that they have contributed to. They quiz me (and so they should!) about the details and want to ensure that they have the most up-to-date information. Over the last few years the type of questions that my patients ask about have changed quite considerably. I welcome this change and I am sure that it reflects the fact that much medical information is now so easily available via the Internet and other sources such as social media. However, there are times when the sheer volume of information can cause confusion, leaving women desperate to know what is fact and what is not. This is where I hope that this book will provide you with the most help and reassurance.

So, in this edition I have tried to provide answers to some of these newer questions. There are further sections on maternal and paternal age, the impact that obesity has on miscarriage and our reproductive health generally, sperm quality, vitamin supplements, environmental hazards, exercise and air travel in pregnancy, the different types of immune tests and the power of the new types of molecular testing that we can now access – to name but a few. I have also provided much detail about the different types of treatments currently available and what we have learnt about their benefits and their safety profile.

Sometimes the questions cannot be answered with facts alone because they are dependent on the individual situation and the woman's personal views and circumstances. Here I have tried to offer advice based on my previous experience or my personal opinion without being too directive. I hope that you enjoy the new edition and that it provides you with the information, reassurance and determination you need to embark on another pregnancy.

THE NEED FOR THIS BOOK

A quarter of all women who become pregnant will experience at least one miscarriage – it is the most common complication of pregnancy. The aim of this book is to take the mystery out of the subject. I want to make this difficult and confusing topic understandable to the millions of people it affects by providing clear, comprehensive, up-to-date information about the known causes and treatments of miscarriage. I hope that, by reading my book, you will be able to approach the subject without fear or confusion.

Women frequently arrive at my clinic having been shunted from one doctor to another, not fully aware of what has happened to them and what is likely to happen in the future. Some have miscarried on several occasions, yet have never been able to find out why. Others have been given different advice, diagnoses and treatments from every doctor they have consulted. Often patients who have plucked up the courage to ask questions about their miscarriages have been ignored by doctors too busy and overworked, or sometimes, regrettably, too superior to spend time explaining to them the nature of their problem. Every day I meet women who have come to believe that they will never experience the joy of a successful pregnancy, women who blame themselves for the loss of their babies.

The clinic where I work, St Mary's Hospital in London, is the largest referral unit in Europe. We see over 800 new patients every year and continue to look after several thousand more. Few of their cases are straightforward. By their nature they have come to the clinic because of a recurring problem for which no answer or solution has been provided. I am constantly amazed and inspired by their fortitude, courage and tenacity. Some of the stories they tell are heartbreaking. As a mother, I am regularly filled with admiration and humility for their ability to put bitter disappointments behind them and their determination to carry on and reach their goal.

This book is, in part, a tribute to those patients and their partners, whose desire to bring life into this world has been unswayed by loss, and undaunted by the often perplexing advice and treatments of modern medicine.

I have set out to describe the causes and treatments of miscarriage which, from experience, I have found most easily understood by the women who attend our clinic. The emphasis is on understanding what doctors know already and what they are trying to find out. As a practising consultant gynaecologist and obstetrician who is also engaged in research, I have seen the distress and confusion that may be caused by differing medical viewpoints. Often this is simply a reflection of the clinician's particular expertise – or even bias – and I hope that, with accurate information at your fingertips, you will be able to identify and get around this problem.

I also stress the importance of entering clinical trials. This is a positive way in which you can help yourself to understand and receive the dedicated care needed to solve your particular problem. I have found that women who join clinical trials are more likely to succeed next time – even if they are in the control group!

This book is for everyone who has a question to ask about miscarriage. I do not pretend that I know all the answers but I hope that you will feel encouraged by the knowledge that doctors and scientists all over the world are trying to find out more about this problem. Above all, this book reinforces the fact that, given time, luck and a little medical help, you are more than likely to enjoy a successful pregnancy.

ACKNOWLEDGEMENTS

The writing of the original version of this book was a challenge, and I want to thank the people who helped me. Without doubt, the most important contributors have been my patients, and my thanks go to every one of them. The problems, fears, courage and honesty they have shared with me over the many years that I have been working in the recurrent miscarriage clinic at St Mary's are a continuing source of inspiration. I hope that I have done justice to their repeated requests for more information. Their baby photographs are now displayed in our 'Rogues' Gallery', which brightens up many of the walls of the clinic office.

I am deeply grateful to Maggie Pearlstine for her long-standing friendship and encouragement. Her certainty that I could and would 'write it all down on paper' was a driving force to complete the first edition. I was also lucky to have the practical help and skills of Matthew Baylis for which I remain enormously grateful. Maggie has continued to encourage me to produce this extensively updated third edition. It is a pleasure for me to be able to express my thanks to her here for all her advice and enthusiastic interest in my subject.

Thank you also to Andrew Mukherjee and other recent trainees at St Mary's who have identified areas of the second edition book that were most in need of updating.

The readers of this book will quickly recognise how much I rate the importance of both clinical and laboratory research. I consider myself lucky to have had such excellent research fellows over the years and would like to take this opportunity of thanking them all for their hard work and dedicated contributions to the clinic and its patients.

My twin daughters and closest friends have also made a significant contribution to this book. Although they know how much I value their love and support, I welcome the opportunity of paying them a special tribute. When I wrote the first edition of *Miscarriage*, Jenny and Clare were still toddlers and now they are grown women with lives and careers of their own. Being their mother has taught me some very important lessons and also given me enormous happiness – thank you, girls.

PART ONE
THE BASIC FACTS

1

WHAT IS A MISCARRIAGE?

The readers of this book may wonder why I have chosen to devote the first chapter of a book about miscarriage to the definition of medical terms. At first glance, it must seem a very cold and clinical way to start writing about one of the most emotional topics in medicine – losing a baby. There is no doubt in my mind that miscarriage is one of the most devastating blows that nature can deliver. However, experience has taught me that clear explanations of the terminology used by doctors and nurses are very important. Many of the couples I meet in the miscarriage clinic are both distressed and confused by the words they have heard to describe their problem. I believe that once you understand the medical terminology, your miscarriage problems will become much less frightening and, most importantly, more understandable.

A miscarriage is a pregnancy which ends naturally before the baby (fetus) can possibly survive outside the mother's womb. The medical term used to describe a baby's potential ability to survive outside the womb is 'viability'. Viability may be defined in terms of the gestational age of the pregnancy (the length of time since the last missed period) or the size and weight of the baby.

The reason for including two definitions of viability within the definition of miscarriage is an important one. Most babies will have reached an average size or weight which corresponds to the gestational age (measured in weeks) of pregnancy. Some babies will be smaller (weigh less) and a few babies will be larger (weigh more) than is expected by the dates from the woman's last menstrual period. However, the weight of the baby at the time of delivery is a crucial factor in determining whether it can survive outside the womb, irrespective of how long it has been in the womb. The bigger the baby, the better the chances of survival.

Many of the women who come to my clinic are uncertain about the difference between a miscarriage and a stillbirth. Essentially, it is a difference of timing, but the terms used can make a lot of difference for the women who have had to go through the experience. Miscarriage may occur at any stage in a pregnancy from the time of the positive pregnancy test until 24 weeks of gestation. After this date, the delivery of a baby which then dies is called a stillbirth. A baby which dies in the womb after 24 weeks is called an intrauterine death. These definitions are described in more detail later in this chapter.

Early deliveries

The survival of a baby delivered very early depends upon whether the baby is healthy and upon the medical expertise (neonatal services) available to nurture the baby after it leaves the womb. Neonatal services have improved dramatically over the last twenty years in the United Kingdom. As a result, we are now able to offer the hope of survival to much younger and smaller babies, as long as they do not suffer from severe abnormalities at the time of their birth.

When I started my training in obstetrics and gynaecology, babies born before 28 weeks of gestation (or weighing less than 1000g) were rarely capable of surviving, despite the efforts of the neonatal doctors (paediatricians specialising in newborn babies). Nowadays, babies born between 24 and 28 weeks of gestation have a much better chance of survival, as long as they are delivered in hospitals that have special care facilities for tiny babies. This fact is so well recognised that obstetric units now operate a policy of 'in utero transfer' for women in established premature labour. This means that pregnant women who are considered to be at risk of premature delivery are transferred to hospitals with the appropriate neonatal facilities before they deliver. This policy ensures that every baby born very early has the best chance of survival because the neonatal doctors are on hand at the time of delivery. The treatment that the baby receives during the first 24 hours of his or her life is crucial.

Miscarriage versus abortion

I am very conscious of the fact that many of the patients I see in the miscarriage clinic have felt distressed and angry with doctors and nurses who have referred to their miscarriage as an 'abortion'. Medical terms used by doctors are designed to be a precise way of describing the medical problem to other doctors and nurses. Unfortunately, for a patient who has suffered a miscarriage, this medical description may seem an insensitive way of describing the facts.

The words are not meant to be deliberately hurtful or insensitive. I think that most of the misunderstandings and distress stem from the fact that many people in our society use the word 'abortion' to describe a pregnancy that is deliberately ended. For a woman who is miscarrying a much-wanted pregnancy, hearing the word 'abortion' will always be distressing if she is unaware of the correct meaning of the words used.

'Abortion' is the correct medical word for any pregnancy that ends before its time. A spontaneous abortion is a pregnancy that ends before the baby is viable – in other words, a miscarriage. A termination of pregnancy is a pregnancy that is deliberately halted. The term 'induced abortion' may also be used to describe termination of pregnancy. The termination may be performed for social reasons (an unwanted pregnancy) or it may be performed for medical reasons. There are many medical reasons for performing a termination of pregnancy – to protect the life of the mother, because the baby has an abnormality which is incompatible with a healthy life, or because the baby has died in the womb – another type of miscarriage – which we refer to as an 'intrauterine death' or IUD.

There has been a definite move by doctors and nurses over the last ten years to manage miscarriage problems with greater sensitivity and understanding. When I first started seeing patients with a history of recurrent miscarriage, the referral letter from the general practitioner or hospital doctor almost always started with, 'Thank you for seeing this unfortunate woman who has suffered recurrent abortions . . .' I am glad to report that 'recurrent abortion' is rarely used now. Most referral letters now refer to 'recurrent miscarriage'. Similarly, when I am invited to give a lecture, I no longer have to change the wording of the title from abortion to miscarriage. There have been numerous media articles in newspapers, magazines and websites about the importance of using more sensitive words when talking to a woman who has miscarried.

But if you do meet a doctor or nurse who refers to your lost baby as an abortion, I suggest you explain to them, calmly and firmly, that you find the word distressing – I suspect that they will respond positively to your feelings and will also wish to apologise to you for being insensitive.

Miscarriage and stillbirth: legal definitions

The legal definition of a miscarriage in the United Kingdom at the present time is the spontaneous loss of a baby with a gestational age of 24 weeks or less. This definition (made by an amendment to an Act of Parliament in 1991) takes into account that the neonatal services currently available offer a baby born at 24 weeks the chance of survival. Before 1991, the legal definition of miscarriage (which had been in force since 1929) was the spontaneous loss of a baby with a gestational age of 28 weeks or less and corresponding to a birth weight of 1000g.

The World Health Organisation (WHO) uses a different definition of miscarriage – the loss of a baby weighing 500g or less, which corresponds to a gestational age of 20 to 22 weeks of gestation. The problem with the WHO definition is that it leaves any baby who is miscarried between 20 and 24 weeks in a sort of no-man's land. Fortunately, the legal definition in the UK has prevented the WHO recommendations from causing confusion.

After 24 weeks of gestation, the spontaneous loss of a baby is called a stillbirth. If the baby dies in the womb but is not miscarried spontaneously, it is called an intrauterine death. The physical process of miscarriage has to be induced artificially, but the baby, when delivered, is a stillbirth and not a termination. A baby of any gestational age or birth weight who demonstrates signs of life at the delivery is defined as a liveborn infant. The death of a liveborn baby during the first seven days of life is called an early neonatal death.

Having explained some of the terminology that you are likely to come across when talking to doctors about your lost baby, the following chapters of this book are aimed at helping you to understand why the miscarriage happened and what you can do to minimise your chances of it happening again. Above all, what I want to draw the reader's attention to is that miscarriage is very common, that doctors do not understand all the reasons why miscarriages occur and that the only way to improve this situation is to support and contribute to future research in this important field of medicine.

2

THE SIZE OF THE PROBLEM

Miscarriage – the loss of a pregnancy before the baby can possibly survive – is extremely common. It has been estimated that one in four of all women suffer a miscarriage at some stage in their reproductive life. This means that miscarriage is the commonest complication of pregnancy. As you walk down the street, visit the supermarket, catch a bus or go about your work today, every fourth woman you see will have experienced a recognised miscarriage. Many women look at me in disbelief when I tell them this fact. You may have no idea that your friend or neighbour has had to cope with the problem of miscarriage until you too experience one. This is because miscarriage is still a taboo subject for many people. It is almost always accompanied by sadness and distress and it can be very difficult to discuss these feelings or to offer words of comfort to a woman who is experiencing them. I hope that this chapter will help you to understand just how common miscarriage is.

Recognising a pregnancy

I know that many women find it surprising when I tell them that doctors still do not know exactly how many pregnancies end in miscarriage. It may seem a very straightforward question, but the answer is difficult to obtain. This is because it is only possible to be accurate about the outcome of pregnancies that are recognised clinically.

By clinically recognised, I mean those pregnancies in which the patient and her doctor know that she is pregnant. This may be as a result of a pregnancy test or an early ultrasound scan. Of course, after the woman has missed a few periods and has obvious symptoms of pregnancy such as nausea, tender breasts, weight gain and tiredness, the diagnosis is much simpler. And when an ultrasound scan has visualised a pregnancy sac in the uterus, the diagnosis of pregnancy is clinically confirmed.

Gathering statistics – the problems

Doctors generally accept that 15% – or one in six of all clinically recognised pregnancies – end in miscarriage. It is useful to remember that this figure may be higher or lower depending upon how the numbers are collected. For example, if the number of miscarriages is calculated from those women who show up at an emergency department with bleeding in early pregnancy, the figure rises. On the other hand, when the number of miscarriages are counted by looking at women who are already booked into an antenatal clinic for pregnancy care, the figure will be lower, because any miscarriages that have occurred before the woman attends the antenatal clinic will be missed.

Some groups of women have a higher risk of clinically recognised miscarriage. That maternal age is one of the most important factors in establishing the size of the risk of miscarriage has been known for many years. However, it was only after a large population study carried out in Scandinavia and published in 2000, that we fully understood how significantly the age of the mother influences the risk of miscarriage. This study showed that women aged between 20 and 29 years have a miscarriage risk in the region of 12%. Between 30 and 34 years this figure rises to 15% and reaches 25% between 35 and 39 years. Alarmingly, by the age of 40 years the risk has increased to just over 50%. After the age of 45 years the risk of miscarriage exceeds 80% – a figure that many women that are attending my clinics find particularly distressing.

Unseen pregnancies

However, we now realise that a large number of pregnancies are lost at such an early stage in development that the woman has no specific symptoms and physical signs of being pregnant. These very early miscarriages are called subclinical or 'occult' miscarriages. The reason for using these words is that the miscarriages are occurring during the period of time between fertilisation of the egg by the sperm, the implantation of the tiny embryo into the womb lining and the clinical identification of the pregnancy. These events are usually hidden from our view (hence 'occult') and so it is difficult to realise that they are happening, let alone that they may go wrong.

Before we had access to the very sensitive pregnancy tests and the even more sophisticated imaging techniques that are now available, the vast majority of these very early losses went unrecognised. Indeed, for some women they still go unrecognised, but the ready availability of fertility tracking apps on websites and smart phones means that many women I see have a very clear understanding of their reproductive cycles. I can no longer say that it is usually only those women who have had problems becoming pregnant or have suffered previous miscarriages, who perform a pregnancy test before they have even missed a period and certainly well before 5 weeks have elapsed since their last period. When a pregnancy test is positive, but the menstrual period occurs a few days later, we call the pregnancy a 'biochemical' one. The tiny embryo has started to make some HCG (human chorionic gonadotrophin, or pregnancy hormone) which can be detected in the mother's urine or blood, but because the embryo does not implant properly in the womb lining, the pregnancy cannot continue, and the pregnancy test becomes negative again. Some women might notice that their menstrual period has been delayed for a few days, or may detect a slightly increased blood loss. It is just as likely, however, that they consider the period to be entirely normal.

I think you will be interested to hear the results of an important study performed by a group of well-respected researchers in this field. They recruited normal fertile women who were trying to become pregnant and followed them carefully over a period of 6 months. With the help of hormonal blood tests these researchers identified the day on which the woman ovulated and, by taking repeated urine samples and measuring the level of HCG hormone, were able to pinpoint the day of implantation for each of the pregnancies that these women went on to conceive. When they analysed the outcome of these pregnancies they were able to show that in most successful pregnancies the tiny embryo implants 8 to 10 days after ovulation (which corresponds to day 22 to 24 of a normal menstrual cycle). The risk of very early miscarriage (before 6 weeks) increased dramatically when the day of implantation was delayed. For example, when implantation occurred before the ninth post-ovulatory day the early loss rate was 13%. But after day 11 the early miscarriage rate was a staggering 82%. This elegant study helps to remind us that there is a very specific window of implantation during which the endometrial (womb) lining is receptive to the tiny embryo.

Theoretically there are several reasons why pregnancies that follow the late implantation of the embryo fail to develop successfully. Unhealthy embryos may develop more slowly or the actual implantation process may be defective, resulting in later or weaker production of HCG. Whichever, it is likely that a tight window of implantation is a special human design feature which helps to ensure that damaged embryos do not progress very far.

Even if we were able to document every biochemical pregnancy that occurs, this would still not be an accurate estimate of the wastage involved in human reproduction. The fate of a fertilised egg is an unhappy one. As many as 15% of the eggs from healthy fertile women are lost before they are fertilised. A further 15% of fertilised eggs degenerate (fall apart) before they are able to implant in the womb lining. Of those embryos that do implant, at least 30% are unable to progress into a recognisable pregnancy. If we collect all these figures together, we come up with the amazing figure that 60% (nearly two-thirds) of all conceptions or potential pregnancies are lost.

Furthermore, the majority of these losses are so early that we usually do not know about them. Unless the woman is undergoing special monitoring to see whether she has become pregnant as a result of infertility treatment, we will not know how many tiny embryos fail to implant successfully in the womb lining or whether they start to implant and produce HCG pregnancy hormone but then miscarry. So when we study the number of miscarriages that occur in any population or in any group of women, it is important to start off by trying to distinguish between the separate contributions that are made by both clinical and subclinical pregnancy losses.

I hope that the reader is now in a position to realise the true size of the problem of miscarriage. Although we talk most frequently about the 15% of clinically recognised pregnancies that we actually see being miscarried, these are just the 'tip of the iceberg' of pregnancy losses. Underneath the surface of the water, a much larger number of pregnancies are miscarried, often without the woman or her doctor realising that she has been pregnant. Most doctors working in this field believe that 1 in 2 conceptions never develop far enough to be recognised.

3

DIFFERENT TYPES OF MISCARRIAGE AND PREGNANCY LOSS

We have already seen that a miscarriage can occur at any stage in pregnancy from the time of the first missed menstrual period until 24 weeks of gestation. Not surprisingly, such a wide time span means that there are many types of miscarriage with many different causes, and many women feel confused by the variety of terms used to describe the miscarriages. The different causes are discussed in later chapters. In this chapter, we will look at the terminology used to describe the various types of miscarriage and the methods that are used to identify them.

Early miscarriage

A miscarriage is called 'early' if it occurs before the 13th week of pregnancy. The 13th week marks the end of the first trimester (the first three months) of pregnancy. Long before ultrasound was available, doctors were aware that the majority of miscarriages occurred in this early stage – after this date miscarriage is fairly uncommon.

Now that an early pregnancy can be so clearly visualised on the ultrasound scan, we know that most early miscarriages have occurred by eight weeks of gestation, well before the 13-week point. Many of the miscarriages which were thought to have occurred between eight and 13 weeks in the past, can now be identified as having occurred at an earlier date. The pregnancy has ended but the physical process of miscarriage and expulsion from the uterus has been delayed (see over, 'missed miscarriage'). As we will see in this chapter, most of the terms used to describe pregnancy loss actually represent different stages in the physical process of early miscarriage.

Late miscarriage

The miscarriage is termed 'late' if it involves the loss of a baby of 13 weeks' size or more. This is an important point to recognise, because in some cases of pregnancy loss, the physical process of miscarriage may not happen until the second trimester, for example at 16 weeks. Ultrasound scans are very important in these cases, because they enable the doctor to determine the size of the fetus, and hence the probable causes of the loss. Without an US scan, it is possible to mistakenly conclude that a woman has had a late miscarriage, when in actual fact her pregnancy could have been 'lost' at an earlier stage. The causes of late miscarriage are quite different from the causes of early miscarriage. In addition the symptoms and signs that accompany late miscarriage are usually different. For example, a late miscarriage may be heralded by ruptured membranes (breaking of the waters) which is not usually noticed in early miscarriages, and the pain experienced may resemble labour contractions because the baby being miscarried is so much larger. All cases of late miscarriage should be carefully investigated in an attempt to find an underlying cause. True late miscarriages are relatively rare. It has been estimated that only 1–2 % of pregnancies miscarry after 13 weeks of gestation.

Sporadic miscarriage

When a pregnancy miscarries due to an occasional or isolated occurrence, it is called a sporadic miscarriage. These are pregnancies that are lost because of a 'one-off' genetic abnormality in the baby, or because the mother has caught a severe viral infection during the early weeks of pregnancy. It is unlikely, though not impossible, that the cause of the miscarriage will recur. This is why sporadic miscarriages are sometimes referred to as bad luck or chance episodes of pregnancy loss. I always try to avoid these descriptions in the clinic because they sound so insensitive to someone who has just lost her baby.

Sporadic miscarriage is the commonest complication of pregnancy. It has been estimated that 25% of women experience a sporadic miscarriage.

Recurrent miscarriage

In contrast to sporadic miscarriage, recurrent miscarriage is uncommon, affecting no more than 1% of women. Various definitions are in use, but the one that I consider to be the most useful is the loss of three or more consecutive pregnancies. Although three miscarriages in a row can be due to bad luck or chance (as we will discuss in more detail in Chapter 6), it is also possible that an underlying cause may be responsible for the repeated miscarriages which, if identified, may be treatable (see Chapters 7–13).

It is useful for the reader to understand that over recent years, some doctors have chosen to define recurrent miscarriage as two or more miscarriages. Indeed both the European and American Colleges of Obstetrics and Gynaecology have adopted this definition and many of the women that I hear from who have experienced two or more losses very much want to be referred to the recurrent miscarriage clinic at St Mary's. Although there is nothing wrong with using this definition it is important to appreciate that it changes the scale of the problem of recurrent miscarriage to include not 1% but nearly 5% of all couples who are trying to achieve a live take-home baby. It also means that many of the evidence-based research studies and treatment trials become difficult to interpret meaningfully.

Threatened miscarriage

A threatened miscarriage can occur at any stage in pregnancy until 24 weeks. However, the problem is much more common during the first three months of pregnancy. The first symptoms are usually vaginal bleeding and/or mild stomach pain. On physical examination, the doctor may identify some tenderness in the lower abdomen, usually just above the pubic bone, but this is not always present. Gentle examination often reveals some blood in the vagina, but no tissues (products of pregnancy) are seen. Most importantly, the neck of the womb (cervix) remains closed and the size of the womb (uterus) is consistent with that expected from the date of the last period.

The diagnosis of threatened miscarriage is made with the help of an ultrasound scan. In very early pregnancies (before six weeks) the scan will probably only be able to visualise the presence of an intact pregnancy sac containing amniotic fluid and a small 'fetal pole' – a nubbin of embryo tissue which, as it grows, will become recognisable as the tiny baby. After six weeks the scan can usually show a heartbeat, particularly if a vaginal scan is performed. Sometimes the scan may show up a small blood clot at the edge of the placenta, which identifies the source of the bleeding, but more often nothing abnormal is seen.

Miscarriage is a process, not a single event, and the loss of the baby is by no means inevitable in all cases. Once bleeding has started there are several possible outcomes. The bleeding may resolve spontaneously in a few days and not recur again. The bleeding may continue, or stop and start over several days or weeks. It is only when abdominal pains follow that the process moves in the direction of inevitability. Even then, the process can still stop and the pregnancy continue safely. Threatened miscarriage is very common. It has been estimated that an episode of bleeding occurs in as many as half of all pregnancies. Happily, in the majority of cases the pregnancy continues normally, but if you notice any bleeding, you should contact your doctor straightaway.

Inevitable miscarriage

In some cases of threatened miscarriage, the process continues and unfortunately becomes what we call an 'inevitable miscarriage'. The important difference is that the cervix starts to open or dilate. Once this happens, the miscarriage is 'inevitable' because the cervix cannot close up again. In these cases, the vaginal bleeding is usually accompanied by pain, caused by the opening of the cervix and the passage of the pregnancy sac, containing the baby, into the canal of the cervix. The pain is cramping in nature, which reflects the fact that the muscles of the uterus are contracting in an attempt to expel the pregnancy. The bleeding usually becomes more severe and the pregnancy sac may break, releasing the amniotic fluid or 'waters' surrounding the baby.

The diagnosis is obvious when a vaginal examination is performed and the cervix is found to be opening. In this situation, an ultrasound scan is not useful because even if a live baby can be visualised, the process of miscarriage cannot be halted. The inevitable miscarriage may be incomplete or complete.

Incomplete miscarriage

If some of the pregnancy tissues are retained in the uterus, the miscarriage is described as 'incomplete'. The findings on examination depend upon when the miscarriage became inevitable. If this was recently, then the cervix may still be open and tissues seen in the cervical canal or in the vagina. If the miscarriage process became inevitable some time ago, the cervix may have started to close again. An ultrasound scan is useful if there is concern that the miscarriage is incomplete and pieces of placenta and membranes from the pregnancy sac have been left behind in the uterine cavity, which in some cases may lead to heavy bleeding. Current NICE guidance suggests that a period of conservative management should be allowed initially to allow spontaneous passage of the products. This could be anything from 1–4 weeks. If this is unsuccessful, and a scan subsequently shows that pieces of tissue remain, then it is likely that you will be advised to have the tissues removed by vacuum aspiration (MVA) using some local anaesthetic or after being given some pain relief or a mild sedative. Alternatively, you may be offered a 'D & C' (dilatation and curettage) or an 'ERPC' (evacuation of retained products of conception) to remove the tissues under a light general anaesthetic. This is a quick procedure lasting only a few minutes and your recovery will be swift.

Complete miscarriage

If the fetus and all the placental tissues are expelled spontaneously by the uterus, the miscarriage is called 'complete'. The symptoms of this are heavy bleeding and the passing of blood clots and tissue. Some women may even be able to recognise a pregnancy sac or fetus. As soon as the uterus is empty, the bleeding usually subsides as the uterus contracts down to its normal size and the cervix closes up again. If there is any doubt that the miscarriage is truly complete, an ultrasound scan is useful to see whether any pieces of tissue have been left behind. The doctors will usually wait some time before carrying this out, because if the scan is performed too soon after the miscarriage, small blood clots in the uterus might be mistaken for tissue, but they will be passed without complication if left alone for a short while.

It is difficult to estimate the true numbers of complete early miscarriages that occur. This is because they usually do not require medical intervention and quite often people do not report them if they happen in very early pregnancy. Of course, if you have any cause for concern, you should consult your doctor – even if the pregnancy is progressing safely, being worried will do you no good.

Septic miscarriage

Any type of miscarriage that is complicated by infection is called a septic miscarriage. Fortunately, this is a rare complication these days because incomplete early miscarriages are usually dealt with proactively to prevent infection of any retained tissues. Furthermore the introduction of legal termination of pregnancy in this country greatly reduced the risk of infection, which used to be a common sequel to 'back-street' abortions.

However, if you have miscarried recently, and experience a recurrence of bleeding, develop a smelly discharge, a temperature or fever, or constant abdominal pain, it is likely that you have some endometritis (inflammation of the womb lining). This can be swiftly treated with antibiotics and, if necessary, the removal of retained tissues from the uterus, to prevent infection in the pelvis and the risk of secondary infertility.

There is no evidence to suggest that infection is more common after a complete late miscarriage. Because some late miscarriages may be caused by infection (see Chapters 4 and 10), your doctor will look carefully for any signs of infection at the time of the miscarriage, particularly when the late miscarriage occurs after the waters around the baby have broken. In this situation, organisms normally present in the vagina can travel up into the uterus and cause inflammation of the placeta, membranes and womb lining followed by infection which is called chorioamnionitis or endometritis.

If this happens to you, make sure that you are checked for ascending infection and treated swiftly if need be.

Anembryonic miscarriage

This is the term used to describe a pregnancy which appears to consist of a pregnancy sac containing placental tissue but no embryo (fetal pole). Obviously it is only possible to make this diagnosis with accuracy after an ultrasound scan has been performed (or after a pathologist has examined the complete pregnancy sac under a microscope, which is rarely possible). Anembryonic miscarriages are one of the most common types of early miscarriage, a fact that doctors were unaware of until ultrasound was routinely available.

The old-fashioned name for anembryonic pregnancy was 'blighted ovum'. This name reflected previous thinking that the cells required for the embryo to develop were either absent, rudimentary or grossly deformed from the beginning of the pregnancy, usually because of a major genetic abnormality in the embryo. More recent research studies suggest that the apparently empty pregnancy sacs did contain an embryo at one time, but that the embryo was reabsorbed very early in its development.

Since anembryonic miscarriage occurs at a very early stage, it is unusual for a woman to suspect that there is any problem until she has had an ultrasound scan. Having identified that the pregnancy cannot continue, the doctors may suggest you undergo an MVA or an ERPC to clean out the uterus, although some women prefer to let the tissues pass away of their own accord (see 'Expectant management of miscarriage', later in this chapter).

Embryonic miscarriage

An embryonic miscarriage is the term used to describe a pregnancy that fails after an embryo with an active fetal heartbeat has developed. From a practical point of view this means that the embryo must be larger than 5mm in length when seen on the ultrasound scan, which approximates to a six-week pregnancy. The reason for this definition is that we can be confident that an embryo of six weeks' size has developed heart activity in order to reach this size. The importance of distinguishing between embryonic and anembryonic miscarriage is that the underlying cause may be different. Embryonic miscarriage is much less common and suggests that some event has occurred to stop the progress of the pregnancy after the embryo has developed fetal heart activity. In anembryonic miscarriage, the development of the pregnancy is halted at a very early stage.

Missed miscarriage

A missed miscarriage or missed abortion are the terms used to describe the situation in which the fetus/embryo dies in the womb but no clinical signs of miscarriage follow. These words are not very helpful to the uninitiated patient and hence a scientific study group held at the Royal College of Obstetricians and Gynaecologists some years ago, recommended that the terms missed miscarriage and blighted ovum be replaced by early embryonic death or early fetal demise. It is not understood why the uterus fails to expel some failed pregnancies. In some cases women do recall a brief episode of light vaginal bleeding and sometimes mild cramping pain, which are then resolved. In retrospect, some women can then pinpoint the time at which subjective symptoms of pregnancy, such as nausea and breast tenderness, disappeared. However, this is not always the case and some women may be unaware that they are no longer pregnant. This situation, as you can imagine, can be quite distressing. 'How could I not have realised that my baby had died?' is a question I am asked frequently. I always try to remind the woman that there is no reason why she should have realised that her baby had died at this early stage in the pregnancy and that blaming herself is going to make a difficult situation harder for herself to deal with.

If a vaginal examination reveals that the uterus is much smaller than would be expected from the menstrual dates, then a missed miscarriage is likely. This is confirmed if the ultrasound scan demonstrates a baby of greater than six weeks' size, with no heart activity. If the pregnancy died some time ago, the scan may also show that the fetus and membranes are being resorbed and cannot be visualised clearly. If no action is taken, the uterus will eventually expel the pregnancy or the tissues will be resorbed completely. However, some women may prefer to speed up the process and finally end the pregnancy by taking medical treatment to empty the uterus or undergo a surgical removal of the retained tissue.

Ectopic pregnancy

A pregnancy which starts to develop outside the uterine cavity is called an ectopic pregnancy. The vast majority of ectopic pregnancies occur in the fallopian tubes, but occasionally may be found on the ovary or in the abdominal cavity. The ectopic pregnancy dies because there is not enough room for the pregnancy to grow (i.e. in the wall of the fallopian tube) or because the placenta cannot implant properly (i.e. on the surface of the ovary). Although some ectopics undoubtedly 'miscarry' completely without complication (tubal miscarriage or abortion), there is a risk that the pregnancy might continue to grow and even rupture through the walls of the fallopian tube. This is why your doctors will take immediate action if they suspect an ectopic pregnancy.

Since an ectopic pregnancy may mimic a 'normal' miscarriage – that is, one which takes place in the uterus (intrauterine miscarriage) – and because prompt action is important if one should occur, a few points need mentioning here. The general symptoms of an ectopic pregnancy are the same as of early pregnancy, accompanied by a positive pregnancy test and lower abdominal pain, which almost always starts before any vaginal bleeding has occurred. This pain may become severe, suggesting that the fallopian tube is being stretched and/or internal bleeding has started. Sometimes these symptoms appear to settle down and then restart a few days later as the ectopic enlarges in size.

If you notice any of these symptoms, you should contact your doctor immediately. The first step will usually be to send you for an ultrasound scan. This will demonstrate that there is no pregnancy sac within the uterine cavity, although the lining of the uterus may be thickened. Sometimes it is possible to see fluid in the bottom of the pelvis, behind the uterus, if bleeding has already occurred. The scan may suggest that there is a poorly defined mass outside the uterus (the ectopic) but it is often very difficult to visualise the pregnancy clearly or see a fetal heartbeat. If there is any doubt about the diagnosis, the doctor may carry out a laparoscopy – which is carried out under anaesthetic, and involves the insertion of a microscopic 'camera' into the abdomen, just below the navel. Once a diagnosis has been made, the ectopic will be removed by surgery. Most gynaecology departments now have the facilities and expertise required to deal with an ectopic pregnancy using keyhole surgical techniques or laparoscopy, which avoids the need for an open operation. This has significant advantages to offer: less trauma to the tissues, a shorter stay in hospital and quicker long-term recovery. A laparoscopic procedure may also help to preserve your future fertility, since it usually means that there is less chance of the second fallopian tube being damaged and of adhesions developing in the pelvis at a later date after an open laparotomy procedure.

However, it may be possible to avoid surgery altogether if the ectopic is small, has not ruptured, and the HCG levels are low (less than 2000IU), by giving the woman an injection of methotrexate. This is a cytotoxic drug which destroys very actively dividing cells, such as those in the early placenta. When successful, the methotrexate causes the pregnancy to stop developing and gradually it shrivels away. However, this treatment is not always successful – we usually quote an 8% failure rate – so it is very important that any woman who is treated in this way agrees to undergo regular HCG blood tests for a few weeks to ensure that the levels have fallen satisfactorily. Longer term studies have shown that following methotrexate treatment for an ectopic pregnancy that subsequent conception rates and repeat ectopic rates are very similar to the figures achieved after keyhole surgery.

Ectopic pregnancies are quite common. In this country it is estimated that one in 80 pregnancies implants outside the uterine cavity. Although the reasons why some pregnancies are ectopic are not fully understood, it is well recognised that there are several groups of women who are at greater risk. For example, recent studies have reported that the risk of ectopic pregnancy is more than doubled in women with endometriosis from 1 in 80 to 1 in 40. Damage to the fallopian tubes caused by infection or previous abdominal surgery increases the chances of the fertilised egg implanting in the scarred portion of the tube. Hence, if you have had any infertility problems, there is an increased risk of an ectopic, since you may also have damaged tubes. For similar reasons the risk is increased if you have had a previous ectopic pregnancy or used an intrauterine contraceptive device, which can lead to low-grade infection of the uterine cavity and fallopian tubes.

It is not entirely clear to me why the incidence of ectopic pregnancy is higher in women with recurrent miscarriages. However, when we looked at the women attending the recurrent miscarriage clinic at St Mary's Hospital, we noticed that nearly 3% of the women had experienced an ectopic pregnancy in the past, compared to the 1% incidence expected in the general population. Some recurrent miscarriage sufferers have also had problems becoming pregnant, which accounts for a certain number of cases, but this is not the whole story, since most of the fertility problems in this group of women are due to disordered ovulation, and not to damage of the uterus or fallopian tubes.

Hydatidiform moles

Hydatidiform moles are the most common type of placental tumour. There are complete moles and partial moles. Complete moles are rare in Caucasian women, occurring no more frequently than one in 1500–2000 pregnancies, although they are very much more common in women in South-East Asia. Complete moles are derived entirely from the cells of the father, due to an accident that occurs at the time of fertilisation. No embryo is present in the pregnancy sac, but the placental tissues develop rapidly in an uncontrolled fashion. On the ultrasound scan these placental cells resemble bunches of grapes because they became swollen with fluid.

Persistent bleeding and severe nausea are usually associated with the presence of these moles, and the size of the uterus is usually larger than would be expected for the menstrual dates.

The important difference between complete and partial moles is that a complete mole may develop into an invasive cancer in a small percentage of cases. Specialist treatment and follow-up is needed, which in this country is concentrated in a few specialist centres with extensive experience in the management of this rare condition.

Partial moles are much more common and usually mimic the appearance of an inevitable or incomplete miscarriage. The partial mole contains a fetus/embryo which has three sets of chromosomes instead of the usual two. The placental cells do swell and proliferate but not to the same degree as occurs in a complete mole. It can be difficult to distinguish between a partial mole and a normal miscarriage on the basis of the ultrasound findings alone. Quite often, women with partial moles experience no unusual symptoms, and the diagnosis is only made by the pathologist after removal of all the tissues from the uterus (ERPC), which emphasises the importance of always trying to send evacuated pregnancy tissues for laboratory analysis when available. Very rarely a partial mole may develop into an invasive mole, but no cases of actual cancer have ever been reported. Nonetheless, any woman who has a partial mole is carefully followed up at special hospitals with experience in managing these unusual types of early pregnancy loss.

Medical management of miscarriage

For the last 50 years the standard method of emptying the uterus after the diagnosis of a failed pregnancy has usually been surgical – involving a local or light general anaesthetic and a brief operation (either an MVA or ERPC). The successful development of medical (drug) treatments to terminate pregnancies has meant that we can now use these methods to empty the uterus for women who have suffered a miscarriage and avoid the need for a surgical procedure. In brief, the woman is first given a drug that blocks the effect of progesterone (the hormone that is essential for the continuation of pregnancy) and after 36–48 hours she then takes a second drug (a prostaglandin) that encourages the uterus to contract and expel its contents.

The success rates of this treatment were intially very varied, ranging from 13–100%. However, most units would agree that when the women are selected carefully, medical treatment will be successful in more than 85–90% of cases. It is important that the woman returns for a follow-up visit to ensure that the medical evacuation is complete. A few women will need to have a subsequent operation for heavy bleeding, or an incomplete miscarriage. This method appears to be acceptable to many women and in some cases preferable to the surgical alternative, although it must be noted here that if the pregnancy tissues need to be sent for genetic analysis the testing is less likely to be successful. Only pregnancies that have not progressed beyond nine weeks of gestation are suitable for this type of treatment and there are several contraindications to using it, such as women with heart, kidney and severe chest disease.

Expectant management of miscarriage

Over the last few years many doctors have questioned the need to surgically or medically empty the uterus after the diagnosis of a failed pregnancy. Historically, it was believed to be risky to leave the mother with retained tissues in her uterus. Junior doctors were all instructed about the potential dangers of life-threatening uterine bleeding and severe pelvic infection. However, these complications of infection and haemorrhage are actually quite common after surgical evacuation has been performed. Indeed, some experts in this field argue that infection is more common after surgical evacuation because dilating the cervix may interfere with the normal cervical barrier against infective organisms, allowing them to ascend into the uterine cavity. Further, that the curettage, or scrape, then contaminates the whole of the uterine cavity and may also increase the chances of the infection reaching the woman's bloodstream and causing a generalised illness. Added to these potential risks are the need for an anaesthetic and the possibility of surgical complications such as perforation of the uterus during the procedure.

These issues have led many doctors to reassess the situation and reconsider the option of expectant management – and just leave the miscarried tissues to come away of their own accord. Several studies have looked at the feasibility of this and the results so far have been encouraging. Not surprisingly, the success of expectant management appears to depend on the quantity of tissue in the uterine cavity, and ultrasound measurements of the retained products are important in the assessment of which pregnancies are most suitable. Experience to date suggests that the highest success rates are achieved when the miscarriage is incomplete and that over 85–90% of these women will have an empty uterus on US scan within three days. However, the figure may be as low as 50% for women who present with a missed miscarriage. I think it is reassuring to note that although women who have chosen expectant management continue to have vaginal bleeding for a few days longer than women who have a surgical or medical evacuation, their blood counts do not appear to be lower. The extensive studies that have now been completed also suggest that there is no difference in the time taken for the woman to return to having normal menstrual periods or to become pregnant again. Current guidance from NICE encourages the use of expectant management as the large treatment trials have concluded that there is no increase in the risk of miscarriage complications for women undergoing expectant management and, most importantly, it avoids exposing the woman to any anaesthetic or surgical complications.

The role of the pathologist

Throughout this book I will keep referring to the importance of involving a pathologist in the investigation of miscarriage. Even if the quantity of miscarried tissue is very small it is always worth trying to obtain a genetic analysis and asking the histopathologist to look at the structure of the placental tissues and membranes under the microscope. The pathologist can confirm that the pregnancy was intrauterine and that no signs of an ectopic or molar pregnancy are present. It may also be possible to identify the gestational age at which the pregnancy failed which is particularly useful when US scan reports are not available. Specialist pathologists can also make an assessment of the degree of placental development and give us an idea of how well (or otherwise) the placenta was attached to the uterine lining. In some cases of infection, histology will be able to accurately determine whether the underlying infection was the cause or the consequence of the miscarriage. In women with prothrombotic disorders (see Chapter 13) it may also be possible to tell whether the placenta was fibrosed (shrunken) or contains any areas of infarction due to lack of blood flow.

Even more useful is the fact that the microscope slides can be stored for many years, if required, and this is potentially very valuable for future research. The tissue samples which have been used for diagnosis go through a process of 'fixing' in formalin solution and are then embedded in blocks of paraffin wax. The blocks are now ready for thin slices to be cut from them and can be examined under the microscope (formalin fixed paraffin embedded (FFPE) tissue blocks). As well as being used for immediate diagnostic purposes at the time of the miscarriage, these blocks can be safely stored for many years and later used for research projects which may help to shed new light on the causes of miscarriage. For example, our understanding of how antiphospholipid antibodies might be linked to miscarriage through impairing placental implant-ation was largely determined through this type of review by my talented pathology colleagues Harold Fox and Neil Sebire.

Recent advances in laboratory techniques now mean that it is possible to extract DNA, RNA, proteins and other components from these FFPE blocks. These are very exciting developments which open the door to important discoveries into the role that genetic factors, inflammatory processes and numerous other complex pathologies play in miscarriage. For example, as new genetic mutations that give rise to disorders are identified, we will be able to go back and literally 'probe' the blocks to identify these molecular abnormalities.

The role of the pathologist with an interest in pregnancy loss is a very important one. Gone are the days when all they could tell us was whether there was a pregnancy present. The new molecular techniques promise to open up another whole dimension in our understanding of the causes of early and late miscarriage.

As we will look at in more detail in Chapter 7, genetic analysis of the products of conception is usually performed only after the third succes-sive miscarriage. Karyotyping or chromosomal analysis of the fetus in this situation will prove to be enormously valuable in establishing the cause of the miscarriage and will have an important influence on the management of the woman's next pregnancy.

Summary

There are many different types of miscarriage, and thanks to the widespread availability of ultrasound, we now have much more knowledge about the development of the young embryo and the stages at which this process most commonly goes wrong. We now understand that the vast majority of miscarriages occur very early and well before eight weeks of gestation. Further, that when the scan identifies a fetal pole measuring more than six weeks' size fetal heart activity must have been present before the pregnancy loss occurred. Not only can the scan identify the stage at which the pregnancy failed, it can also be used to determine the stage that an ongoing miscarriage process has reached. When vaginal bleeding occurs in early pregnancy, the scan can differentiate between a threatened, inevitable, incomplete and a complete miscarriage. In skilled hands the scan can also exclude an ectopic pregnancy. Although ultrasound will never replace the value of a skilled doctor's examination, in early pregnancy it is the fastest and most accurate way to confirm whether the pregnancy is ongoing or has ended. Most importantly, the sight of a beating fetal heart after an episode of bleeding in pregnancy can provide a mother-to-be with more concrete reassurance than hours of verbal reassurance.

Over recent years several important follow-up studies have addressed the important question of whether surgical, medical or expectant management provides the woman who has just miscarried with the best chances of a speedy recovery and the minimum of short- and long-term complications. The advantages of each treatment option invariably depends on the type of miscarriage and the stage in the process that the miscarriage has reached when the woman seeks medical advice. For example, the MIST (Miscarriage Treatment) randomized controlled trial, showed conclusively that there was no difference in the rates of infection between expectant, medical and surgical treatment options. It did however show that expectant management was associated with a higher rate of unplanned surgical curettage at a later interval, which many of us involved in the study had expected to be the case.

I believe that we will need to continue to have all three types of treatment – expectant, medical and surgical – available in the future. However, the finding that both medical and expectant management have a valuable role to play in caring for women experiencing the most common complication of pregnancy is an important step forward and means that we no longer have to expose many young women to invasive surgical procedures. This advance also has significant implications for NHS funding by reducing the need for operating theatres and in-patient beds. The vast majority of women presenting with an early miscarriage are now cared for in an outpatient setting.

PART TWO

UNDERSTANDING THE CAUSES

4

SPORADIC MISCARRIAGE

Why did I miscarry?

In the previous chapter we looked at the different types of miscarriage that can occur. We noted that sporadic miscarriage is the commonest complication of pregnancy and that as many as 25% of all women suffer a single episode of miscarriage. We also noted that recurrent miscarriage is very uncommon and only 1% of couples ever suffer this particularly distressing problem. My reason for emphasising this point again is that the factors which cause sporadic and recurrent miscarriages are different. The aim of this chapter is to look at the reasons why miscarriages occur sporadically. In later chapters of this book we will look in more detail at the reasons why miscarriage may occur repeatedly.

A sporadic pregnancy loss is often described as an isolated episode of bad luck or nature's way of getting rid of a pregnancy that was 'no good'. For many women this seems a poor and possibly unacceptable explanation for the distressing event that they have just suffered. It is important to understand here that often the doctors do not know why the miscarriage occurred, because there are no obvious pointers to its exact cause. Not surprisingly, a woman might assume that her miscarriage was caused by a specific event that occurred in her pregnancy but, in the majority of cases, this is impossible to prove.

Genetic abnormalities in the baby

What we do know is that a genetic abnormality in the embryo or tiny baby is the commonest cause of sporadic miscarriage. Genetic disorders which may result in sporadic miscarriage can be divided into three main headings: chromosomal abnormalities, gene defects and congenital malformations which have a genetic origin, such as spina bifida.

Chromosomes are long strands of genetic material which are housed in the nucleus of our cells. The chromosomes contain the coding for the different genes which make up an individual. There are a total of 46 chromosomes arranged into 23 pairs in each cell of the body. Each pair of chromosomes can be recognised by its size and shape and is numbered. For example, chromosome pair number 1 is the largest and chromosome pair number 22 is the smallest. Chromosomes 45 and 46 (pair 23) are the chromosomes which determine the sex of an individual. The human has over 20,000 genes in total, so each chromosome carries many genes, depending on its size. Each gene is a single unit of 'information' inherited from our parents, and it occupies a specific position on a given chromosome. The genes consist of numerous small segments of DNA (genetic material) which collectively provides a code for a specific characteristic or a particular cell function.

Chromosomal abnormalities

An embryo is created when an egg is successfully fertilised by a sperm. The egg and the sperm each contribute one set of 23 chromosomes from the mother or the father to the embryo. Before, during and after the process of fertilisation these two sets of chromosomes undergo a complex series of divisions and rearrangements. If one of the chromosomes is abnormal, or if during the process of dividing and rearranging, too many or too few chromosomes are left in the fertilised egg, an abnormal embryo or fetus may develop. The vast majority of these embryos miscarry at a very early stage in the pregnancy, because most chromosomal abnormalities are incompatible with life. However, a few continue through pregnancy, resulting in the birth of an abnormal baby or a baby that dies soon after birth. It is not difficult to understand why an abnormal fetus is at risk of being expelled from the uterus. It is much more difficult to explain why some abnormal fetuses fail to be expelled and how the pregnancy can continue developing,

We used to think that some 50% of all early miscarriages are caused by chromosomal abnormalities in the fetus. However, more recent studies undertaken in fertility units that are able to examine the chromosomal make up of all the embryos that a woman produces have suggested that this figure is an underestimate. Chromosome instability is extremely common in human embryos and using new array-based molecular techniques for screening cells it has been suggested that the vast majority (in the region of 80–90%) of early embryos are probably abnormal. However, it would appear that these abnormal embryos find it difficult to implant successfully, since the majority of ongoing pregnancies after 10 weeks result in the delivery of healthy liveborn babies. So it would appear that in humans there must be an important mechanism present in the mother's uterus that helps to limit her investing in the ongoing implantation and growth of embryos that are genetically and developmentally compromised.

It is important for the reader to appreciate that apart from a small proportion of inherited conditions (called parental translocations – discussed later) nearly all the chromosomal defects seen in sporadic miscarriages arise out of the blue (de novo). There are many types of chromosomal abnormality but the most common defects are trisomies, monosomies and polyploidies.

Trisomies

When the cells of the fetus contain three copies of one type of chromosome instead of the usual two, the defect is called a trisomy. Trisomies account for over half of all the chromosomal defects in sporadic miscarriages. The most frequent trisomy involves chromosome number 16 and since it is incompatible with life, no liveborn babies ever have this condition. Some frequently occurring trisomies have been given special names after the doctors who first described the condition.

Down's syndrome is probably the best known and affects chromosome pair number 21. The syndrome is named after Dr John Langdon-Down who was the first person to describe the problem in 1866. All Down's children are affected by a degree of mental impairment but the severity of the handicap is variable. These children share certain physical features, particularly the slanting oriental eyes (that have led to this trisomy being called 'mongolism') and the presence of a single skin crease on the palms of the hands and feet. In addition, the eyes are small, the tongue protrudes and the bridge of the nose is shallow, which often means that the child is snuffly and and very susceptible to colds and chest infections. Babies with Down's are floppy and are more likely to be born with an abnormality of the heart or intestine.

In Patau's syndrome, three copies of chromosome 13 are present. This trisomy is usually fatal within a few days of birth. Tiny eyes, too many fingers and toes and severe heart defects are characteristic. In Edward's syndrome (trisomy 18) the physical malformations include a small receding jaw, low-set ears and the hands are clenched whilst the feet have a curved sole described as 'rocker bottom'. Severe mental retardation is usual and most of these babies die within the first year of life. Other chromosomes often involved in trisomies are numbers 22, 15, and 2.

Most trisomies are due to abnormal division (meiosis) in the egg which occurs before fertilisation. This explains why trisomies are much more common in older women, because they are more likely to ovulate eggs that are abnormal. The best example of this maternal age effect is seen in Down's syndrome (trisomy 21). The chance of having a baby with three copies of chromosome 21 increases with age more sharply after the age of 35 years. Although the majority of trisomy 21 fetuses are miscarried, some do go on to deliver at term and it is estimated that one in 30 babies born to mothers aged over 45 years has the condition. This is one of the commonest chromosomal abnormalities seen in live births.

If you have had the misfortune to miscarry because of a trisomy, you do have a slightly higher risk of suffering another one for the same reasons, even though the chromosome affected may be different. If it is known that your miscarriage occurred because of a trisomy, your doctor will probably advise you to have an amniocentesis or other type of prenatal test in a future pregnancy, to make sure that your next baby is not affected.

Monosomies

When one of the chromosomes is completely missing, the defect is called monosomy. The commonest type of monosomy is only found in girls and involves one of the two X chromosomes, which is why it is called monosomy X or Turner's syndrome. Monosomies are the cause of 15% of all miscarriages but only a tiny number of these pregnancies with one sex chromosome survive to be liveborn. It is estimated that one in 2,500 live births have monosomy X. These girls with Turner's syndrome are short (their growth is seriously affected), have no menstrual periods and are infertile.

Polyploidies

In this condition, the embryo contains one or more extra sets of 23 chromosomes, and accounts for about 20% of all the sporadic miscarriages caused by chromosomal abnormalities. When one extra set appears, the defect is called triploidy and it is not affected by maternal age. It may result from an egg being fertilised by more than one sperm. Many triploidies are miscarried very early, before the embryo has developed. Very occasionally a fetus with triploidy manages to continue to develop into the second trimester and is accompanied by characteristic abnormalities of the placenta (see Chapter 3 – partial hydatidiform moles). These babies never survive to be delivered. Tetraploidies (4 sets of 23 chromosomes) are a much less common type of polyploidy and usually the development of the pregnancy is arrested very early.

Structural rearrangements

These are changes in individual chromosomes, which may arise de novo in the egg or sperm, or may be inherited from one parent who carries a genetic defect in one of their chromosomes. These are a more likely cause of repeated miscarriages and are discussed in Chapter 7.

Other chromosomal abnormalities

Some men have an extra X sex chromosome (bringing the total to 47) . This is known as Klinefelter's syndrome. In other cases, the addition of an extra X or Y chromosome may produce such a mild abnormality that the diagnosis is not made until after puberty or is never made, unless the woman or man happens to have their chromosomes examined for some other reason.

Sometimes an individual may be carrying two different cell lines made up of different chromosome numbers. This is called mosaicism. Mosaic cells occur when a cell divides abnormally some time after fertilisation. Every time this mosaic cell divides, it will produce further mosaic cells. Mosaic cells may also occur as an artefact (an induced artificial abnormality) during the processing and preparation of cells in the laboratory. Unless the mosaicism affects the germ cells (the eggs or the sperms) they frequently go undetected and are not a cause for concern. Certainly, mosaic cells are rarely found in miscarriage tissues.

Overall, the incidence of chromosomal abnormalities found in babies at birth is approximately 0.6% (six abnormalities per 1,000 babies born). If we look at the number of chromosomal defects in babies that are stillborn, the number increases tenfold to 6% (six abnormalities per 100 babies born). This is the tip of the iceberg; the vast majority of chromosomally abnormal pregnancies are miscarried early. It is widely quoted that at least 50–60% of sporadic miscarriages are chromosomally abnormal and, as we discussed earlier in this chapter, the true figure may be significantly higher.

Although chromosomal defects are common, we remain very ignorant about what causes them. We know that many trisomies are increased in older women and that radiation, some chemicals and a variety of environmental factors may underlie some defects. But the cause of most chromosomal abnormalities remains a mystery and is an area which needs further research.

Diagnosing chromosomal abnormalities

This can be difficult to achieve reliably. Although the technology is available to look at miscarried tissues and determine the chromosomes present in them, there are many pitfalls which may prevent you from knowing for certain whether your miscarriage was caused by an abnormality of the chromosomes. The first problem is that in many pregnancies that are miscarried, the fetal tissues are not available to be examined. I hesitate to say that they are lost because this implies that someone has misplaced them. But lost they frequently are, most often in the heavy bleeding that occurs, or down the toilet.

The second problem is that many pregnancies that miscarry are not immediately expelled from the uterus. If the tissues are removed surgically from the uterus by a MVA or ERPC (see Chapter 3) they may be sent to the laboratory for analysis, but if the pregnancy died some weeks ago, it may not be possible to process cells. This may sound rather macabre, so it is important for the reader to understand exactly what the laboratory tries to do to these tissues. They have to separate out the fetal tissues (including the placenta) from all the other tissues (such as maternal blood cells and pieces of the womb lining or decidua) that are present in the pot of products that they receive in the laboratory. Having identified the fetal and placental tissues, these are then processed to determine the number of chromosomes in the miscarriage tissues. This is of obvious value, given that chromosomal abnormalities are the most important cause of miscarriages. In the past, the major problem encountered in trying to get results has been that in order to determine the number of chromosomes in cells from the miscarriage, that these cells were required to grow in tissue cultures in the laboratory. Sometimes they failed to grow because of infection or contamination, which occurred either before expulsion or after collection of the tissues. Sometimes it was not the miscarriage tissue but the mother's uterine lining tissue (decidua) that grew on the tissue culture plates, which explains the excess of female (46, XX) results that we used to receive. Fortunately, there are now more robust techniques available that avoids these complications. A major advantage of these new approaches is that cells do not need to be cultured. Only DNA is needed to make the analysis, which therefore allows us to obtain a successful result in approximately 90% of tests attempted. This is a much higher success rate than we were able to obtain when only tissue culture techniques were available.

This new approach is known as array comparative genome hybridisation (array CGH) and is sometimes referred to as molecular karyotyping or chromosomal microarrays. The underlying principle is that the amount of DNA present for each chromosome in a miscarriage sample can be compared to the known amount of DNA in a normal sample. In practice, this is done by colour coding or labelling the different samples of DNA. For example, the DNA from the sample being tested can be labelled with a red dye and the normal reference (46 chromosome) DNA is labelled in a different colour such as green. If equal amounts of red and green are present (when mixed together this will be viewed as yellow) this means that the number of each of the chromosomes in the miscarriage specimen is the normal 46. However, when the sample DNA for any given chromosome shows an excess of red, then we can conclude that a trisomy must exist for that chromosome. There are multiple variants on this theme, but all of them are essentially based on a known reference standard for each of the chromosomes, whose DNA content can be compared to any miscarriage sample or specimen that is being tested.

As we will see in Chapter 7, knowing the chromosomal makeup of a particular miscarriage is useful not only in diagnosis but in monitoring treatment for the woman with a history of recurrent miscarriages who has been receiving a particular type of treatment. If the next miscarriage analysis shows a normal number of chromosomes, it suggests that the said treatment has been unsuccessful. However, if the chromosomes were shown to be abnormal, this suggests that the miscarriage was due to a random or sporadic genetic abnormality rather than being the result of a treatment failure.

One disadvantage of chromosomal microarrays is that it cannot detect a balanced chromosomal rearrangement, which could be present in either parent who is clinically or phenotypically normal, but whose pregnancy is at risk for a fetus with an unbalanced arrangement due to an excess or deficiency of chromosomal information. In this situation the only way to reach the correct diagnosis is to perform an old fashioned karyotype analysis, which means that a tissue culture is required. Although karyotyping is no longer commonly requested nowadays, it is still useful for the reader to understand how important it is to ensure that the miscarriage samples are processed in the correct way, so that if a formal karyotype is needed that they have the best chance of obtaining a successful result from the tissue culture.

Sadly, there are still some doctors and nurses who do not understand that if the miscarriage tissues are put into formalin (a preservative fluid used to prevent tissues from decomposing before they are examined under the microscope) no chromosomal analysis can be carried out. The formalin 'fixes' the tissues, killing them as it does so. Trying to make the cells grow in culture after they have been exposed to formalin is invariably a hopeless task.

So if you are hoping to have your miscarriage examined genetically, it is worth asking the doctor how the tissues will be stored during their transport to the laboratory. Ideally they should be placed into special cytogenetic fluid (called transport medium). Many laboratories now put some antibiotic into this fluid to reduce the risks of infection. If this is not available, then it is best for the tissues to be sent 'dry' in a sealed container or in some normal saline (salt water of a concentration that does not damage the cells).

I know that many couples I meet feel very upset that cytogenetic analysis of their miscarriage is not usually performed until they have suffered three losses. This does sound very heartless when you have just lost your baby and are desperately trying to understand the reason for the miscarriage. But if we were to do genetic analysis on every miscarriage that occurs, the expense would cripple the NHS which is already hopelessly overstretched! So we have to try and use our resources to the best effect. As discussed earlier in this chapter, the majority of sporadic miscarriages are due to a random numerical chromosomal abnormality in the fetus, which may or may not recur. This is why we are forced to reserve genetic analysis for those women who have suffered repeated miscarriages (see Chapter 7).

I have repeatedly mentioned that chromosomal abnormalities account for more than 60% of all miscarriages in the first trimester and about 10–15% of losses in the second trimester. Of course, there are many other genetic explanations for why a pregnancy may end in miscarriage, but their exact prevalence is unclear. We know that only 20% of all congenital anomalies (meaning that the baby is born with a structural or functional defect or malformation) are due to chromosomal abnormalities. Some 40% are the result of a change in or a mutation of a single gene. But most of the remaining 40% are due to the cumulative effects of multiple different genes.

Of the 20,000 human genes, we currently understand the function of about a third. It is likely that mutations of many of the remainder exert their deleterious effects on the embryo, preventing development and resulting in miscarriage. Finding these genes will probably require DNA sequencing of miscarriages, which is a laborious and expensive process and is only just beginning. That mutant genes cause miscarriages means that sometimes in a given family there are recurrences. In Chapter 7 there is a brief explanation of the various patterns of inheritance for disorders caused by autosomal dominant, autosomal recessive, and X-linked recessive genes.

The other genetic explanation for miscarriage arises when several different genes affect a given organ system. These disorders are considered to be the result of cumulative effects of more than one gene (known as polygenic) or because of an environmental effect which has impacted upon the way a particular gene functions. These interactions between genes and the envrironment are referred to as multifactorial. Collectively these explain most isolated anomalies occurring in a single organ system – congenital heart disease, club foot, pyloric stenosis, congenital hip dislocation, spina bifida. After the birth of one affected child, the recurrence risk for any subsequent pregnancy is usually 2–5%. This is much less than for an autosomal recessive trait (25%) but considerably greater than for the general population (0.1% or 1 per 1000).

Single gene defects

Our genes are arranged in pairs along the length of our chromosomes. For each gene there are two forms, one inherited maternally and one paternally. The alternative forms of a gene are called alleles. Genes may be dominant or recessive. If one or both members of the pair of genes present on the alleles are dominant, they produce a recognisable effect in the body. A single abnormal copy of a dominant allele can override the action of the normal allele. In the case of recessive genes, a noticeable effect is only produced if both alleles of the pair are mutant. Recessive genes are very common, but they will only give rise to a specific disease in the baby if both parents transmit the same recessive mutation gene to their baby. A good example of this is seen in cystic fibrosis. One in every 25 Europeans carries the recessive gene for cystic fibrosis in single dose form. However, the chance of two individuals both passing the recessive allele to the baby is 1 in 625 (1/25 X 1/25). The chance that the two then each contribute their abnormal allele (sperm; egg) is 1 in 4, so the likelihood of cystic fibrosis in any given offspring is 1/2500.

Some gene defects are sex-linked. This means that they are carried on the X chromosome of the mother who, because she has a second normal X chromosome, does not typically suffer from the disorder. She has a 50% chance of passing on her X gene defect to any given child but only her sons will develop the disease. This is because their second sex chromosome is a Y, which cannot provide the balancing benefit of a second X chromosome. Examples of this situation are Duchenne muscular dystrophy and haemophilia.

We are rapidly mapping each of our chromosomes to localise genes that can cause abnormalities. We already know the location of many genetic mutations (abnormalities) and recognise that some of these gene defects give rise to an abnormal baby with a serious disease such as cystic fibrosis, sickle cell anaemia or thalassaemia. It is likely that future research will identify specific miscarriage genes, but at present our knowledge is limited.

Polygenic/Multifactorial defects

When doctors talk about congenital abnormalities, they usually mean that the baby is born with a structural or functional defect or malformation.

Congenital anomalies sometimes, but not always, have heritable tendencies. There is usually increased likelihood of the same defect recurring in relatives (offspring, sibling, parent, or other). A defect restricted to a single organ is usually the result of several genes but no single factor is responsible, giving rise to the terms polygenic or multifactorial. Examples include cleft lip, many forms of congenital heart defects, congenital hip dysplasia and club foot. Couples who have already had a baby with a specific congenital abnormality have an increased risk of another child with the same abnormality. The risk is usually in the region of 2–5%.

An important example of a multifactorial abnormality is spina bifida. Spina bifida is one type of neural tube defect in which the baby's spinal cord is not properly covered by the bony spine. Where the delicate spinal cord is unprotected, it is in great danger of damage and these babies, if they survive, may have very severe neurological problems including paralysis. Spina bifida is a common problem and has a strong genetic link. But it is when the genetic tendency is exaggerated by a factor in the environment, such as poor maternal nutrition (in particular a deficiency in folic acid and other vitamins) that the spinal defect occurs.

As many as 40% of neural tube defects are miscarried and a further 20% are stillborn babies. In total, neural tube defects account for about 5% of all sporadic miscarriages. In the vast majority of cases of neural tube defect, the abnormality cannot be predicted from the woman's or her family's previous history. This is why it is important that all women who are trying to become pregnant are advised to take folic acid tablets, not just those women who have already suffered a neural tube defect. If we could persuade our government to introduce mandatory fortification of foodstuffs such as flour with folic acid we would be able to prevent many other cases of spina bifida too. Fortunately, the sophisticated ultrasound scans that are now available to most pregnant women are capable of detecting 99% of all cases of neural tube defect. I know that this does not remove the pain of being diagnosed as carrying a baby with this problem, but it does allow you and your partner the option of terminating a badly affected pregnancy, if this is your choice.

Drugs, infections, and environmental factors

Damage to the developing embryo before birth may be caused by infections, drugs, irradiation, or chemicals., These can result in congenital anomalies and may sometimes cause miscarriages. A recent example is the Zika virus which leads to microcephaly. About 15–20 drugs taken during pregnancy can cause anomalies (perhaps the most notorious example is thalidomide, which caused limb malformations called phocomelia); exposure to chemicals, irradiation and some metabolic disorders (uncontrolled diabetes) are also culprits. Many environmental factors, such as pollutants, have been associated with structural anomalies and miscarriages (see Chapter 9).

Abnormalities of the uterus and cervix

Abnormalities of the uterus and cervix may also cause miscarriages. The abnormality may be congenital (for example, the mother may have been born with a double uterus or an incompetent cervix) or may appear later on (an acquired abnormality). Examples of an acquired abnormality are uterine fibroids (benign growths in the wall of the uterus) or the development of adhesions within the cavity of the uterus after an infection or surgical procedure.

In early pregnancy, the presence of any of these abnormalities may hinder the embryo from implanting properly in the uterine lining and give rise to a miscarriage. In later pregnancy, the size of a fibroid or the restrictive shape of the uterine cavity may prevent the baby from having enough space to grow to its full size. This situation may result in a late miscarriage or the onset of premature labour.

It is important to understand that anatomical abnormalities of the uterus are extremely common. They are so common that I often find myself wondering whether they should be called 'abnormalities'. Perhaps it would be more sensible to consider them as a variation of the normal shape of the uterus. Certainly, a large number of quite major structural abnormalities of the uterus never cause any trouble at all for a woman during her pregnancies. I can remember many occasions when I have only recognised that a woman has a double uterus (sometimes called a bicornuate uterus) or a uterine septum (sheet of tissue protruding down into the cavity from the top – fundus – of the uterus) after delivering her normal baby at full term! If this same woman had experienced miscarriages, instead of normal pregnancies, she would probably have had tests that would have shown up the abnormality.

If you find this difficult to believe, then I must tell you about a charming 75-year-old lady I performed a hysterectomy upon a few years ago. She was having the operation done because she was suffering from prolapse. The muscles supporting the uterus had weakened and she complained of 'something uncomfortable coming down below' every time she went for a walk. At the operation I discovered that she had two completely separate uterine bodies joined together by one cervix. When I explained this to the lady after she had recovered she asked me what problems this might have caused. I told her that this type of abnormality is associated with infertility, miscarriages, premature labour and babies that are born small in size. She looked at me in utter disbelief. She then went on to tell me (in a gentle manner, suggesting that I was obviously a bit simple) that she had never had a miscarriage. Furthermore, that her six sons had all weighed more than eight pounds and had had to be induced to deliver when they showed no signs of going into natural labour at 42 weeks!

Space does not allow me to continue with more stories like this one. However, I hope the reader has got a feel for the fact that uterine abnormalities do not necessarily give rise to problems in achieving a successful pregnancy. This is why I believe that it is best to only look for these abnormalities in women who have experienced several pregnancy losses, whether they be early or late miscarriages.

There is a growing body of evidence that the presence of a uterine septum can give rise to repeated miscarriages in both the first and second trimester. Furthermore, many recurrent miscarriage clinics believe that correcting this structural abnormality can reduce the risk of miscarriage. The septum is resected through a hysteroscope which is inserted through the cervix. Tiny scissors are then used to cut the septum back to the top of the uterus under direct vision. Copper coils are then inserted into the cavity to keep the raw edges apart while the endometrial lining repairs. (see Chapter 8 for further details)

Infections in the mother and in the baby

One in 20 pregnant women will experience an infective illness during their pregnancy. If this sounds an alarming figure you will be relieved to hear that the majority of these infections are completely harmless. Only a minority of maternal infections during pregnancy are capable of causing damage to the fetus or the newborn baby. When the fetus is infected whilst still in the uterus, the infection is called 'congenital'.

If the baby is infected at the time of delivery, the infection is 'acquired' during the 'intra partum' period. Some infections are only passed to the baby by close contact or breastfeeding after birth and these are 'postnatally acquired' infections.

There are many different possible outcomes to a pregnancy that is complicated by an infection in the mother. The infection may cause an early or a late miscarriage. It may be responsible for the woman going into premature labour or suffering a stillbirth. Some infections will result in congenital abnormalities in the baby, which may be obvious at birth or not be recognised until early childhood. Some infections during pregnancy will be so mild that no specific symptoms are noticed by the mother. Often these mild infections are a source of great anxiety to pregnant women, who fear that their baby is being harmed and, since they have no symptoms, they can do nothing to prevent this risk.

Let me reassure you that the most likely outcome of an infection during pregnancy is an entirely normal baby. Although the word 'infection' may conjure up all sorts of alarming thoughts, particularly if you are pregnant now, it is important for me to stress that most are harmless. Infections during pregnancy are the cause of less than 3% of all congenital abnormalities.

I think it is true to say that almost every viral, bacterial or parasitic infection ever described in medical textbooks has also been claimed as the cause of sporadic miscarriage. Most bacterial and parasitic infections can be successfully treated if they are correctly identified. Some viral infections can be prevented by vaccination. Since treatment may be possible, it is particularly important that we try to identify the infectious organism in the hope that we might be able to prevent some cases of miscarriage.

To do this successfully, we need to know at what point during pregnancy the mother is most likely to catch and pass on the infection and what effect it will have, if any, on her baby. For example, rubella only affects the baby in early pregnancy, whereas cytomegalovirus can infect the baby at all stages in pregnancy. Chicken-pox causes problems early and at the time of delivery, but the middle of pregnancy is not a problem time. The route by which the infection is passed to the baby is also important. During pregnancy, any infectious agent must be capable of passing through the placenta if it is going to infect the baby. During labour the organism may be transmitted by the mother's blood or vaginal fluid secretions.

In this chapter we will look at a variety of bacterial, viral and parasitic infections which may cause sporadic miscarriages. Infective causes of recurrent miscarriage are discussed later in this book (see Chapter 10). I spend a lot of time in the miscarriage clinic answering queries about infections that cause problems in very late pregnancy and in the newborn baby. Strictly speaking these infections should not be included in a book about miscarriage. However, I am going to mention some of them at the specific request of many of my patients!

Viral infections causing sporadic miscarriage

Viral infections during pregnancy are extremely common. The best example is the common cold. During a nine-month pregnancy the chances of a woman developing a cold are very high and usually the baby suffers no ill effects.

Rubella

Many viral infections result in the production of antibodies in the mother, during her first infection, to protect her against future infections with the same virus. A good example of this is rubella (German measles). This infection is important because it has very damaging effects on the fetus if the mother develops the infection in early pregnancy. Many early pregnancies that are infected by rubella miscarry. The virus crosses the placenta and can cause blindness, deafness, heart defects and mental retardation in the fetus. The earlier in pregnancy the woman becomes infected, the more severe the abnormalities in the baby may be. So severe, in fact, that a termination of pregnancy is offered to women who catch rubella in the first 14 weeks of pregnancy. After this date, the fetus may still become infected, but it is unusual for rubella to cause significant damage.

Once a woman has had rubella infection, she is no longer at risk of transmitting the infection to her baby because of the immunity she develops. Rubella antibodies can be measured in her blood and the presence of these antibodies was previously looked for in every pregnant woman in the UK when she first attended the antenatal clinic. However, antenatal screening for rubella susceptibility was discontinued in 2016 since it no longer meets the UK National Screening Committee criteria for a screening programme. Currently the most effective way to protect pregnant women from rubella infection is to ensure they have two measles, mumps and rubella (MMR) vaccinations before they are pregnant. Stopping antenatal rubella susceptibility screening has been made possible by the improved uptake of MMR immunisation during childhood and adolescence – a programme which commenced in 1988. All healthcare professionals should make every contact count and take advantage of existing opportunities to check the status and administration of MMR vaccination. The low numbers of pregnant women who are identified as rubella susceptible need to be advised to avoid contact with the virus (young children are the most common source of the infection) and should be offered vaccination after she has delivered her baby.

If you have suffered the miseries of having rubella as a child or as an adult (when it is usually much more unpleasant) you will almost certainly be immune. I emphasise this point because at least once a month I meet a tearful woman in my antenatal clinic who has been in contact with rubella and is frightened that her baby will be affected. Frequently her distress is because she cannot recall having had rubella in the past. If you find yourself in this situation, please remember that some women have been exposed to rubella but develop such a mild infection (subclinical) that they do not realise they have had it. A simple blood test will tell you whether you are immune. Rubella is not a cause of recurrent miscarriage.

Genital Herpes

There are two main types of herpes virus infection. Type 1 is responsible for cold sores of the lips and mouth. Type 2 is responsible for the ulcers that develop on the vulva, vagina and cervix and are referred to as genital herpes. If a woman develops her first genital herpes infection during pregnancy and it is severe, miscarriage may result. However, the greatest risk for the fetus is when the mother develops a primary genital herpes lesion near the time of delivery. If the virus is being excreted from the lesion (ulcer) it can infect the baby after the membranes have ruptured and during the passage down the birth canal. Although only 10% of babies are infected, the consequences can be very severe, including death of the newborn baby from infection of the tissues surrounding the brain and the spinal cord (encephalitis and meningitis). This is why doctors advise delivery by caesarean section for women who develop a primary genital herpes around the time of delivery. After delivery, the paediatricians will treat the baby with antiviral drugs (such as acyclovir) to ensure that no problems develop.

Infection with the herpes virus produces an antibody response in the mother but this does not protect her from another attack of herpes. However, if you are pregnant it will be comforting to know that the fetus can only be infected during the course of your first herpetic infection and is unaffected by any recurrences that you may experience. I stress this point because I meet many worried mothers who think they should have a caesarean delivery when they develop another attack of herpes near to the time of their delivery. This is not necessary and your baby will not be at risk if the attack is a secondary one. Exciting new research has suggested that it may become possible to vaccinate babies against herpes infection while they are still in the womb, but at the present time this method has only been tried in animals. As with rubella, herpes is not a cause of recurrent miscarriage.

Chicken-pox

The chicken-pox virus is highly contagious, which means that chicken-pox infection is very easily caught. As a result, the vast majority of children (90%) have had chicken-pox before they reach adolescence and infection in pregnancy for the first time is rare. This is another infection which causes great anxiety for pregnant women so I am going to include some details here, even though they are not strictly related to miscarriage problems.

I am puzzled by the fact that I have never been able to find any information about the effects of chicken-pox on the pregnancy when the infection occurs before eight weeks of gestation. I quizzed one of my virology colleagues about this recently, who explained that infection in the very early weeks of pregnancy is not thought to be associated with problems in the baby later on. This is probably because babies infected very early are miscarried, but no one has any proof about this.

If you catch chicken-pox for the first time between eight and 20 weeks of gestation, there is a possibility that the baby will become infected. This congenital infection may give rise to abnormalities affecting the limbs, eyes, skin and brain – the congenital varicella syndrome. The baby may also be growth restricted. It is important to emphasise, however, that the risk is small and that no more than 3–5% of babies will be affected to any degree. If you find yourself in this worrying situation, it is likely that your obstetrician will suggest that you have regular ultrasound scans during the pregnancy to look for problems such as calcification in the baby's head, fluid accumulating in the baby's body cavities (hydrops fetalis) and increasing fluid in the amniotic cavity or pregnancy sac. In the vast majority of cases there will be no problem and the scans will provide you with reassurance.

If you catch chicken-pox after 20 weeks your baby will not be affected by the congenital varicella syndrome. However, towards the end of your pregnancy, the situation is potentially more worrying. The ability of the chicken-pox virus to cross the placenta and infect the baby increases as the pregnancy advances. As many as 50% of babies become infected if the mother catches chicken-pox one to four weeks before delivery. The newborn baby can develop a very severe infection (with pneumonia and encephalitis) because its immune system is not mature enough to deal with the chicken-pox virus. Before this puts you into a panic, let me reassure you strongly that these problems are easily avoided by giving the baby a special injection soon after delivery. The injection is called Zoster Immune Globulin (ZIG) because the proper name for chicken-pox virus is varicella zoster.

If you think you may have caught chicken-pox in pregnancy but you do not develop the typical rash and symptoms, make sure you tell your doctor quickly. A blood test will usually be able to establish whether you are immune or not and, if there is any doubt at the time of your delivery, your baby will be given some ZIG to be on the safe side. Chicken-pox is not a cause of recurrent miscarriage because the mother is immune to future infections.

Parvovirus

This is a virus which appears to be confined to humans. The symptoms of infection with parvovirus B19 are very similar to those of rubella (German measles). Frequently, the infection is so mild that it goes unrecognised. Parvovirus is spread by respiratory droplets (coughing and sneezing) and fomites (any substance which is capable of absorbing and retaining infectious particles – for example, bedding, clothes, carpets and curtains). Although 40% of pregnant women are susceptible to parvovirus infection because they have not previously been infected, it is not a common problem during pregnancy. Parvovirus is capable of causing late miscarriage and intrauterine death, which is usually associated with 'hydrops'

– when the baby accumulates lots of fluid in all the cavities of its body, including the abdomen, chest and ventricles of the brain. However, 80% of pregnancies in which parvovirus infection occurs result in normal live-births. Congenital abnormalities are not associated with this infection, so there has never been any suggestion that termination should be offered to mothers who develop this infection during pregnancy.

Cytomegalovirus

Cytomegalovirus (CMV) infection may affect liveborn infants of term pregnancies, but whether this virus causes early pregnancy loss or recurrent pregnancy loss is not clear. Half or more of adult females have been exposed to CMV. After initial exposure, the virus enters a latent (or quiet) stage and may or may not affect the woman or her offspring. Women with an active CMV infection or reactivation of a previous infection may deliver infants that are in some way affected. CMV infection may be responsible for some early pregnancy losses – this is probably very rare. There is no clear information that CMV infection is responsible for recurrent pregnancy loss. There is no treatment for this viral disease.

Other viruses causing sporadic miscarriages

Influenza infection in early pregnancy may be followed by miscarriage, but it is just as likely that the miscarriage is caused by the very high fevers that the mother develops, rather than the virus itself. Technically speaking, influenza cannot be a cause of recurrent miscarriage since the strains of the virus are constantly changing. This is one of the reasons why flu vaccines do not always prevent further outbreaks of flu.

Infection with the mumps virus is said to occur less frequently in pregnancy, but when it does occur, the risk of miscarriage is high. Similarly, hepatitis A, B and C have all been accused of causing miscarriages. Hepatitis B virus cannot cross the placenta and the baby only becomes infected at or after the time of delivery, so I think that the few reports that have suggested it causes miscarriage are inaccurate and circumstantial. My practical experience from the miscarriage clinic suggests to me that both mumps and hepatitis are very rare in pregnancy. Certainly, the contribution they make to the problem of miscarriage is small.

Rubeola (measles), variola (polio) and vaccinia (smallpox) viruses have all been cited as the cause of sporadic miscarriages in the past. However, vaccination is now eradicating these diseases so successfully that smallpox and polio are virtually extinct. Measles vaccine has not been available for so long, so it will take longer for this disease to be eradicated worldwide. Polio vaccination given during pregnancy has no harmful effect on the fetus and certainly does not cause miscarriage.

Viral infections which may cause recurrent miscarriages.

Some viral infections, such as cytomegalovirus (CMV), can be reactivated. This means that a second episode of CMV infection can be triggered off, under certain very rare circumstances. Some viruses persist in the mother's body and remain infective even after she has developed antibodies to them. The classic example of this is the human immunodeficiency virus (HIV). Since both of these viruses are possible causes of recurrent miscarriage, they are also discussed in Chapter 10.

Bacteria and other organisms causing sporadic miscarriage

Bacterial infections during pregnancy are quite common but usually they do not affect the baby seriously, if at all, until around the time of delivery. Some may cause premature labour, for instance, the beta haemolytic streptococcus and bacterial vaginosis. Since these infections may occur repeatedly, they are also discussed in Chapter 10.

Listeria

Infection with listeria monocytogenes during pregnancy is not common but it may have serious consequences for the baby. Typically, the mother has a short, influenza-like illness in the second or third trimester of pregnancy. The usual symptoms are fever, aching muscles, general malaise, nausea, diarrhoea and abdominal pain. Listeria is a well-recognised, but uncommon, cause of late miscarriage.

The bacteria are present in animals and contaminated soil. They infect humans when they are eaten in contaminated foodstuffs, especially unpasteurised dairy products. In non-pregnant women the infection is often very mild and goes unnoticed, but during pregnancy the infection can be more severe. It seems that listeria find the placenta a particularly comfortable place to multiply. Antibiotics (ampicillin) will cure the infection but the best way to avoid complications to the baby during pregnancy is prevention. If you are pregnant, make sure that you never eat unwashed salad and vegetables and avoid soft cheeses and meat pâtés. If you are in any doubt about whether the product is made from unpasteurised milk, then do not risk eating it.

Brucella

Brucella bacteria are an important cause of infertility and miscarriage in cattle. Different types (species) of brucella affect cattle, goats and hogs. The bacteria invade the animal's placenta, which contains an alcohol called erythritol, and this stimulates the brucella to grow. Brucellosis is now rare in the UK because the disease has been virtually eradicated from our cattle. Brucellosis is sometimes referred to as 'undulant fever' because the symptoms are night fevers which come and go, along with cough, headache, muscle pains and weight loss.

Very occasionally farm workers may become infected because they are exposed to infected cattle. There is also a tiny risk of catching brucella if you eat unpasteurised dairy products. The human placenta does not contain erythritol, which means that the risk of infection is very small, even if you are exposed to infected cattle. If you work on a farm or in a veterinary surgery, simple precautions can reduce the risk of infection. Do not help with lambing or calving. Do not milk cows or sheep that have recently given birth. Nor should you handle miscarried lambs or calves or their afterbirths (placentae). If your partner cannot avoid these contacts, make sure that you do not come into contact with soiled clothing. Careful personal hygiene is all that is needed to prevent person-to-person infection. It is extremely unlikely that you will suffer a miscarriage because of brucella infection.

Chlamydia

Chlamydia are small, infective organisms that are halfway between bacteria and viruses. There are two important types of chlamydia. Chlamydia trachomatis is spread by sexual contact and causes cystitis, a sore vagina and conjunctivitis in the newborn baby. It is a common cause of tubal damage leading to infertility, but it does not cause miscarriage.

Chlamydia psittaci causes miscarriage in sheep and it has been suggested that it may cause miscarriages in farm workers and vets, but this has never been proven conclusively. Infection can cause cough, fever, headache and general flu-like symptoms. If you think there is a risk of being exposed to chlamydia psittaci during your pregnancy, then follow the advice given in the brucella section, on page 49. This is a very rare cause of sporadic miscarriage.

Salmonella

Salmonella is one of the commonest causes of food poisoning, giving rise to sickness and diarrhoea which can be severe. The maternal fever may occasionally cause a miscarriage. Although it may not have any effect on your unborn baby, it is sensible to try and avoid this illness while you are pregnant. Salmonella infection is associated with eating undercooked poultry and eggs. All you need to do to avoid this problem is to follow some simple precautions. Always wash your hands before preparing these foods. Do not let raw meat juices touch or drip on to any other foods in your fridge. Make sure that any poultry or eggs you eat have been thoroughly cooked to ensure that the bacteria are destroyed. Avoid eating mayonnaise and mousses, both of which contain uncooked egg yolks or whites.

Parasites

Toxoplasma

The parasitic organism toxoplasma gondii causes toxoplasmosis. Toxoplasma can sometimes cause miscarriage in early pregnancy and damage to the baby in late pregnancy. It is mainly associated with cats, but sheep can also be infected. Infection with toxoplasma gondii may occur if you eat unwashed vegetables, poorly cooked infested meat or inhale eggs from cat faeces.

The disease itself causes vague flu-like symptoms in the mother, with a low-grade fever and swollen glands, particularly in the neck. Fatigue, headache, a rash, enlargement of the spleen and eye problems are less common. Many women do not recognise that they have had the illness. Toxoplasmosis is more prevalent in communities that have lots of cats or where meat is eaten rare (e.g. France). Recent estimates suggest that two per 1000 pregnancies will be infected with toxoplasmosis in the UK each year.

If the mother acquires her primary (first) infection during pregnancy, she will transmit the infection to her baby in about 40% of cases. I need to emphasise that the fetus can only become infected during the course of the mother's primary infection, which is why toxoplasma infection cannot be a cause of recurrent miscarriage. The baby is most likely to become infected when a non-immune mother is infected near the time of delivery, and may develop congenital toxoplasma or a subclinical infection.

The baby is more severely affected when the infection occurs around the time of conception or during the first trimester of pregnancy. Only 10% of babies will be infected at this early stage in pregnancy but the risk of injury to the baby is high. The injuries include early and late miscarriage, later intrauterine death or liveborn babies with severe neurological problems. Hydrocephaly (water on the brain), cerebral calcification and impaired vision are all possible, but only 10% of infected newborn babies have symptoms and we do not really understand what the later problems may be. However, we do know that congenital toxoplasmosis is a significant cause of mental retardation and blindness worldwide.

The blood tests to diagnose whether you have had toxoplasma in the past or recently are not entirely straightforward. Many false positives and negatives have occurred. However, in the simplest of terms, your blood will be tested for what we call 'IgG toxoplasma antibodies'. IgG is the name given to the class of antibodies which appear in our blood after we have developed immunity to the infection. If it is positive, then you are immune to toxoplasmosis and there is nothing more to worry about.

If the test is negative, this means that you are not immune to toxoplasmosis and may be at risk during pregnancy. The problems come when a woman is retested at a later stage in pregnancy and found to have developed the IgG antibody, which indicates that she has become infected during her pregnancy. Then the laboratory has to go back to the first blood sample and see whether they can find any 'IgM antibody' in it. IgM antibodies are the first antibodies to be made in the immune response and so their presence in the blood sample suggests that the infection is recent. To check that these results are accurate, a 'dye test' then has to be performed which requires live toxoplasma parasites and therefore has to be sent to a special laboratory.

As soon as the maternal infection has been confirmed, the woman will be given the antibiotic spiramycin, because this can reduce the risk of the baby becoming infected by as much as 60%. If the baby is thought to have been infected, the only way to confirm the diagnosis is by taking a sample of the blood from the baby's cord using ultrasound to guide the needle into the uterus (cordocentesis). If the toxoplasma parasite can be found in fetal blood or amniotic fluid, then the mother is at risk of having a baby with serious damage. Some women will want to have a termination at this point, whereas others may want to wait and see whether future ultrasound scans suggest any complications.

About one-third of women build up some immunity to toxoplasma without even realising they have come into contact with it. Nonetheless, if you are pregnant, it is a good idea to try and minimise your chances of being exposed to the risk. Wash your hands carefully after handling cats or kittens and avoid contact with strays. Worm your pet cats regularly. Avoid contact with cat litter. Try to find someone else to remove the soiled litter from the tray every day. If you have to do it yourself, wear rubber gloves and make sure that you wash the gloves and your hands afterwards. Always wear gloves when gardening to protect your hands from contaminated soil. Avoid eating any raw or undercooked meat and make sure that you wash vegetables and salads carefully to remove any soil from them.

The purpose of pre-pregnancy and antenatal screening for women who are susceptible to toxoplasmosis is to reduce the risk of a mother acquiring an acute infection during pregnancy. If she does become infected, it is important to identify her quickly so that the risk of the baby developing congenital infection can be reduced. A recent working party at the Royal College of Obstetricians and Gynaecologists concluded that routine antenatal screening of all pregnant women in this country to detect and warn women who were not immune to toxoplasmosis would not be 'appropriate'. Although this infection causes much anxiety, it is important to remember that the numbers of affected pregnancies are quite small. Furthermore, your antenatal clinic can arrange for you to have your blood checked to see whether you are immune, even though routine screening is not offered to everyone.

Malaria

In countries where malaria is rife, pregnant women are at risk of miscarrying because of the high fevers that usually accompany the infection. Pregnant women are more likely to catch malaria and the infection is often more severe. It is thought that this is because of the altered immune response in pregnancy. Having said this, it is important to remember that the malarial parasite rarely crosses the placenta and gains access to the baby. If it does, the baby is better protected than the mother from becoming infected, because the red blood cells contain fetal haemoglobin (haemoglobin F) which is much more resistant than adult haemoglobin.

It is best to avoid malaria zones when you are pregnant. If this is not possible, then make sure that you take your tablets to prevent becoming infected and continue taking them after you have left that country, for as long as is recommended. New anti-malarial drugs are continually coming on to the market and you should talk to your doctor about which drugs are safe in pregnancy. Chloroquine will not harm your baby, nor will Proguanil if you take folate supplements at the same time. Mefloquin and Maloprim should be avoided in the first 12 weeks of pregnancy. If you have taken these drugs already, do not panic. The most important thing to remember is that a malarial infection is far more likely to cause problems for you or your pregnancy than the drugs you have taken to prevent infection. If you are in doubt about any anti-malarial drug, I suggest you ring up the information centre at the London School of Hygiene and Tropical Medicine. Their experts will advise you.

Hormonal causes of sporadic miscarriage

There is no doubt that the state of a woman's hormones at the time of conception and in early pregnancy may be a cause of pregnancy loss. Getting pregnant and staying pregnant is dependent on the correct balance of reproductive hormones. There are a multitude of different ways in which the balance can go wrong.

In order to understand this, we need to look carefully at the hormonal events which occur during a normal menstrual cycle leading up to a pregnancy. Soon after the menstrual period, the follicle-stimulating hormone (FSH) is secreted by the pituitary gland. This hormone acts upon the ovary. The ovaries contain thousands of eggs which are present at birth. Each egg is surrounded by a group of cells which, as the egg develops, form a small fluid-filled sac, or follicle. FSH stimulates the follicles to start growing. As the follicles develop, the cells which surround the egg start producing oestrogen. This hormone stimulates the growth of the womb lining (endometrium) and the tissues of the breasts.

The rising level of oestrogen in the blood stimulates the brain, telling it that the follicle is mature and ready to ovulate. The brain signals to the pituitary gland to reduce the amount of FSH that it is producing.

The pituitary gland also releases a short sharp burst of the hormone LH (luteinising hormone). This burst of LH (called a pulse) triggers the release of the egg from the follicle, which occurs about 36 hours later.

Ovulation usually occurs when the follicle has grown to about 20mm in diameter (the size of a one pound coin). The egg then passes down one of the fallopian tubes. The space in the follicle which used to be occupied by the egg then becomes filled with blood. The blood forms a clot which is then 'organised' into fibrous tissue. The secretion of LH continues at a lower level and this encourages the remaining cells in the ruptured follicle to form the corpus luteum (Latin for 'yellow body'). The cells produce a bright yellow pigment which stains the whole of the ruptured follicle.

The corpus luteum starts to produce progesterone hormone. Like oestrogen, progesterone has effects on the uterus, breasts and the hypothalamus and pituitary glands in the brain. In the uterus, progesterone makes the cells receptive to a pregnancy by producing the nutrients needed to support a developing embryo.

The corpus luteum is programmed to break down after 14 days if it does not receive the 'message' that a pregnancy has occurred. LH production from the pituitary gland falls after ovulation and without this hormone stimulus to the ovary, the corpus luteum withers and the levels of progesterone fall. The loss of progesterone stimulus to the uterus means that its blood-filled lining starts to disintegrate and menstrual bleeding results. The levels of both oestrogen and progesterone fall, causing a new cycle of follicle growth to start.

If the egg is fertilised by a sperm, this usually occurs in the fallopian tubes and then the fertilised egg (embryo) travels to the uterus, where it implants in the lining of the uterus (endometrium) and grows as a pregnancy. The embryo starts to produce human chorionic gonadotrophin (HCG). The corpus luteum recognises the presence of the HCG as a signal not to break down and to continue producing progesterone. The womb lining does not disintegrate and the menstrual period does not occur. A healthy, active corpus luteum is essential for the pregnancy to continue. If it is damaged and the production of progesterone is poor during the first eight weeks of pregnancy, a miscarriage will result.

The reader will not require more than common sense to recognise that this complex hormonal jigsaw puzzle can go wrong at many different places. If the ovary does not respond well to FSH, the follicles will not grow and the eggs they contain will not mature and be released. If the LH levels in the early part of the cycle are too high and there is no proper LH surge, ovulation may not occur or it may occur too early or too late. These ovulation problems are an important cause of infertility and are frequently seen in women with polycystic ovaries (see Chapter 11). If an egg that is poorly matured is released, the production of progesterone from the corpus luteum may be so poor that the luteal phase (the second half of the cycle after ovulation) is too short and the uterine lining so poorly developed that an embryo cannot implant successfully.

Many cases of miscarriage are claimed to result from a 'deficient luteal phase'. This may be true, but it is important to understand that the success of this phase depends upon a complex sequence of hormonal events that are already in place by the time that the luteal phase starts. If the hormonal events of the first part of the cycle are in any way impaired, the die has been cast. If progesterone levels are low in the luteal phase, this means that the corpus luteum is not functioning properly. If progesterone levels are low in the early weeks of pregnancy, this means that the placental cells surrounding the embryo are not producing sufficient HCG to stimulate the corpus luteum to produce enough progesterone.

I know that many women and their doctors hope that by giving injections of progesterone or HCG, they will be able to prevent a miscarriage. This is a convenient idea but it does not work. This treatment is a good example of 'closing the stable door after the horse has bolted'. Injections of these hormones cannot make a flagging corpus luteum or a flagging placenta come alive again. All they will do is increase the levels of HCG or progesterone in the mother's blood for a short period of time. This may delay the time at which the bleeding and the miscarriage appear to start, but it will not change the overall course of events. The factory producing the necessary hormones to ensure the continuation of pregnancy is not working properly and so miscarriage is inevitable.

In many cases of sporadic miscarriage, the hormonal imbalance which leads to miscarriage is a one-off event and is not likely to be repeated. In those women who have suffered repeated miscarriages, and in particular those women who have polycystic ovaries (see Chapter 11), the hormonal problem will be present in most pregnancies they conceive. These women need careful investigation and to be offered treatment where it is available and appropriate for their problem.

For many years the medical textbooks have stated that other types of hormonal disorders such as diabetes and thyroid problems are a cause of miscarriage. As a result, many doctors have suggested that their miscarriage patients should undergo investigations to see whether they have a previously unrecognised diabetic tendency (glucose tolerance tests) or problems with the way their thyroid gland works (thyroid function tests). I strongly believe that these tests are a waste of both time and money. Women who have these types of hormonal disorders do not go and visit their doctors for the first time with a miscarriage. If you have an overactive or an underactive thyroid, you are much more likely to meet me for the first time in my infertility clinic. A hormone disorder which affects the functioning of every cell in the body (and the thyroid does) will make it very difficult for you to get pregnant in the first place.

However, after you have been diagnosed as having a thyroid problem and been started on the right treatment, you will probably find that you can become pregnant quite quickly and you will not be at any greater risk of suffering a miscarriage than your next-door neighbour who has an entirely normal thyroid gland.

The same is true for diabetes. If you are already a diabetic or suddenly develop this disease, then you will have a variety of medical problems which hopefully will be diagnosed promptly and looked after by a physician. It is true that a woman who has poorly controlled diabetes has a greater risk of miscarriage. She also has a considerably greater risk of producing a baby that has a congenital abnormality. However, when her diabetes is under control she will have no particular problems in becoming pregnant and she will not be at any greater risk of miscarrying. It is very unusual to meet a woman in the miscarriage clinic who has unrecognised diabetes or thyroid disease. Nor is it likely that performing glucose tolerance or thyroid function tests in all miscarriage sufferers will identify women who are 'on the brink' of developing either of these disorders. The perceptive reader will realise, as I say this, that I have used these tests in the past. Yes, I was taught that the tests 'should' be performed. With more experience in looking after women with miscarriage, I have now abandoned them as a routine investigation.

Immunological causes of sporadic miscarriage

Although these mechanisms may be involved in a few cases of sporadic miscarriage, the overall contribution is small. Many women ask me whether asthma, hay fever, eczema and other allergic skin disorders increase the risk of miscarriage but there is no evidence to suggest that this is the case. However, there are some women who have thyroid antibodies (see Chapter 12 for more details) who may be at risk of developing an underactive thyroid gland in the future. In this particular situation it is sensible for the woman to have her thyroid function tests checked on a regular basis to make sure that she does not need to be given thyroxine replacement treatment.

Of course, it is possible that a woman with antiphospholipid syndrome (see Chapter 13) may miscarry her first pregnancy because of this problem, but many studies have shown that this syndrome is more of a problem in women who have miscarried three or more pregnancies. I think it is sensible to reserve the special tests needed to diagnose this problem for recurrent miscarriage sufferers.

Summary

In this chapter we have looked at a wide selection of possible causes for sporadic episodes of miscarriage. Although the broad categories I have used can all make contributions to the problem, it is important for me to emphasise that the most important factors are genetic abnormalities in the baby and infections that occur in the mother. As we will see in later chapters of this book, this is not the case for recurrent miscarriage.

Sensible steps to take to avoid a sporadic miscarriage

- start taking folic acid tablets at least three months before becoming pregnant
- adopt a sensible healthy diet
- stop smoking
- drink alcohol in moderation
- avoid self-medicating and taking over-the-counter drugs – whenever possible
- if you suffer from diabetes, thyroid disease, epilepsy or high blood pressure, consult your doctor, who may suggest that you alter the

type or dose of the drugs you are taking. Make sure that these medical problems are well controlled before you conceive

- keep a record of your menstrual periods so that you do not expose an embryo to X-rays or a drug which may have potential side-effects for a tiny baby
- avoid or minimise contact with farm animals and pets
- avoid travel to malarial zones and countries where the risks of food poisoning or gastroenteritis are high
- ensure that meat is well cooked, vegetables are carefully washed and avoid unpasteurised milk products and pâtés
- ensure that you are immune to rubella infection – and if you are not immune, get vaccinated without delay

Further useful information is included in Part Four – 'Getting ready for the next pregnancy' and 'Coping with the next pregnancy'.

5

WILL I MISCARRY AGAIN? THE RISK OF RECURRENCE

If you have had a miscarriage, this will probably be one of your chief concerns. Let me start by reassuring you that the chances of having another miscarriage are far smaller than your chances of having a successful pregnancy. Hopefully, you will have been looked after by doctors who have explained to you that many cases of early miscarriage are due to bad luck. By bad luck, I mean that the cause of the miscarriage was a random one and is unlikely to occur again.

Many couples I see find it very difficult to believe that their miscarriage was due to bad luck. They want to know what went wrong with the pregnancy. In Chapter 4 we looked at the many different causes of sporadic miscarriage and discussed how it is often impossible for the doctor to know exactly why the miscarriage occurred.

In early miscarriages, this bad luck is often because the fetus has the wrong number of chromosomes, or because the mother had a viral infection in the first few weeks of her pregnancy which affected the baby's development. If you have had a late miscarriage, this may be because the baby had an abnormality but not one that led you to miscarry in the early stages of the pregnancy. It may have been that the baby was normal but you caught an infection (for example, listeria) which was passed on to the baby and caused the miscarriage. Of course, it is just possible that exactly the same thing may happen again in your next pregnancy, but it is highly unlikely. It is much more probable that these problems will not occur again and that your next pregnancy will be trouble-free.

Often women who have experienced a first miscarriage will ask me if there is something wrong with them that will make them miscarry again. This is a very understandable and, I think, a very sensible question. It is very unlikely, however, that there is anything wrong with you which would cause future miscarriages. Although much of this book deals with the causes of repeated miscarriage, it is very important to stress that they are quite rare. However, they cause so much distress that much medical research has been carried out, in order to explain why a small number of couples (no more than 1–2 % of all couples in the population) suffer recurrent miscarriages. Throughout this book I am defining recurrent miscarriage as the loss of three or more consecutive pregnancies. As we noted in Chapter 3, some doctors prefer to include couples with a history of two or more miscarriages in their definition, in which case the scale of the problem increases and as many as 5% of all couples who are trying to have a baby are potentially affected.

Problems with recurrence studies

When I first became interested in the field of miscarriage in the mid-1980s, I looked hard for information that would help me to give couples advice about their risks of miscarrying again. I could find very little data that was useful, because most of what had been written was retrospective. This means that a group of women and their pregnancies are studied and analysed after the outcome of their pregnancies is known.

The problem with this sort of study is that the results may be very misleading. For example, if we study the labour ward register of delivered babies and identify a group of women who have had miscarriages in the past, our study may conclude that the risk of having several miscarriages is very low, because all the women included in this study will have achieved a successful pregnancy. Those women who have miscarried again will not appear on this register. On the other hand, if we study the operating theatre register of women who have undergone ERPCs after a miscarriage, or look at the number of women attending gynaecology emergency clinics for medical or expectant management of their miscarriage, and then look back at their previous pregnancies, our study may conclude that the risk of another miscarriage is very high. This is because there will be some women included in this study who have not yet achieved a successful pregnancy. Nor will this study be able to identify the women who have miscarried in the past, but gone on to have a healthy live baby, because they did not have to undergo an ERPC.

The reason for me describing these issues in such detail is that I think it is enormously important for the reader to understand the shortcomings of retrospective research studies and the value of prospective studies, whatever the subject of the research may be. At the end of reading all the studies that were available in the mid-1980s, the only conclusion I reached was that the risk of a woman miscarrying again after a previous miscarriage was somewhere between 15 and 75%!

The Cambridge miscarriage study

Since this conclusion was of no use to me or the patients I was trying to advise, I set about designing a prospective study that would be able to work out the numerical risk of miscarriage for any woman who was trying to become pregnant. To do this, I had to recruit women to my study before they became pregnant, so that their pregnancy could be followed all the way through. This was no small task, since it can be very difficult to get women to declare that they are thinking about becoming pregnant before they actually fall pregnant. I was helped greatly by my hospital colleagues in Cambridge where I was working at that time (I must mention Peter Braude and Paula Trembath in particular) and also by the local radio and the GPs who helped me to advertise for recruits.

The study proved so informative because the women in this Cambridge population all had their babies and their miscarriages at a single hospital, so that with hard work and dogged determination, it was possible to follow over 400 women during a time period of several years.

The first aim of the study was to find out how many pregnancies ended in miscarriage. We had recruited all the women before pregnancy, in the hope that we would not fall into the pitfalls of previous population miscarriage studies (as described in Chapter 2). We did not miss any of the very early miscarriages, where the women did not need to come into hospital and were dealt with at home. Nor did we end up concluding that miscarriage is more frequent than it really is, because we did not include any woman who came into hospital with bleeding or miscarriage unless we had known about her before she became pregnant. As a result, we were confident about the accuracy of our finding: in a general population of women, 12% of all pregnancies will end in a clinically recognisable miscarriage.

The second aim of the study was to see whether we could find any reasons why these 12% were likely to miscarry. We found no connection between the risk of miscarriage and the previous use of the contraceptive pill or a previous termination of pregnancy (see page 64). Nor were there any general medical disorders in this group of women which put them at greater risk of miscarriage in the pregnancy we followed. We did notice, however, that women who were heavy cigarette smokers appeared to be at greater risk of miscarriage. So too were the women who had had difficulties in becoming pregnant. However, this group seemed to be composed mainly of those women who had experienced a miscarriage and then developed problems in conceiving. The effect of infertility on the risk of miscarriage is discussed in detail in Chapter 13.

The third aim of the Cambridge population study was to assess the risk of miscarriage for a woman who had never been pregnant before, for women who had had a miscarriage and for women who had had a live baby in the past. We were able to show that it is possible to put a figure on the risk of miscarriage in future pregnancy by looking carefully at the outcome of a woman's previous pregnancies. We were able to draw up a table of percentage risks, in the hope that other doctors and their patients would find these numbers helpful when faced with the problem of a recent miscarriage (see Table 1).

Although many previous studies had suggested that miscarriage is more common in first pregnancies (primigravid women), we found that the risk of miscarriage is very low in first pregnancies, about 5%. Among women who had enjoyed a successful pregnancy or pregnancies in the past, the risk of miscarriage was also very low. This low risk of miscarriage was also found in those women whose last pregnancy had been completed successfully, even if she had experienced miscarriages in the past.

TABLE 1: THE CAMBRIDGE MISCARRIAGE STUDY
Effect of past pregnancy history upon the risk of miscarriage (n=407).

Pregnancy history	No of women miscarrying	No of women in category	% Risk of miscarriage in study pregnancy
Last pregnancy miscarried	40	214	19
Only miscarriages in the past	24	98	24
Only pregnancy miscarried	12	59	20
Last pregnancy successful	5	95	5
All pregnancies successful	3	73	4
Only pregnancy successful	3	62	5
Previous termination of pregnancy	2	32	6
Primigravidae	4	87	5

The Cambridge study also showed that a woman's risk of miscarriage increases when she has suffered a miscarriage in the past. After one miscarriage, the risk of a second miscarriage was 20%, which is significantly higher than the miscarriage rate for a woman who has enjoyed a live birth in her first pregnancy or who has never been pregnant before. Before you become distressed by this fact, let me remind you that this figure of 20% miscarriage still means that 80% of the pregnancies in women who have had a single miscarriage in the past will be successful.

It is true that the risk of a further miscarriage does rise as the number of previous miscarriages increases. We found that the risk of miscarriage after two previous losses was 24% and after three consecutive losses, the risk increased to 43%. Once again, it is important to remember that these figures still mean that the majority of future pregnancies will be successful.

Furthermore we were also able to show that if you have had a successful pregnancy in the past, then your risk of miscarriage is lower, even if this live birth was followed by several miscarriages. After two successful pregnancies, the future risk of miscarriage never went above 20%, which is the same level of risk as a woman who has only ever had one miscarriage.

The risk of miscarriage after termination of pregnancy

There was one more group in whom we found a low risk of miscarriage – women who had undergone an uncomplicated termination of pregnancy in the past. I would like to emphasise this point because I know that some miscarriage patients who have had a termination years ago are full of guilt and remorse that the termination may in some way be the cause of the later miscarriages. They may even fear that the miscarriages represent some form of divine retribution for the fact that they voluntarily terminated a pregnancy. I am sure that this is not the case and I hope that you feel heartened by the data in this Cambridge population study, which demonstrated that early, uncomplicated terminations of pregnancy do not increase the risk of miscarriage in the future.

Terminations of pregnancy, however, do have a definite effect on a woman's reproductive health. Approximately one in every 200 women who voluntarily terminates a pregnancy will find that she cannot conceive again. This is usually because of infection at or soon after the termination, which damages the fallopian tubes. Of course, in years gone by when the methods of dilating the cervix and evacuating the uterus were less sophisticated, I think it was true to say that a termination could also have an adverse effect on a woman's risk of miscarriage. The method of termination may have weakened the cervix, leading to incompetence of the cervix in the future. However, this is rarely the case nowadays. A termination of pregnancy is always a sad event and it is quite likely that you will continue to feel emotionally distressed about it for some time. If you are unfortunate enough to then experience a miscarriage, do talk to your doctor about your feelings and try to remember the results of the Cambridge miscarriage study (see Table 1).

Maternal age and the risk of miscarriage

The risk of miscarriage increases as a woman becomes older and, since a woman who has experienced a miscarriage and wants to embark on another pregnancy cannot shed any years, I think it is sensible to consider that maternal age is a significant risk factor for recurrence. We have known for many years that this increase in risk is directly related to the age of the woman's eggs (ova). We are born with all the eggs that we will ever have available to ovulate, whereas men produce new sperm on a regular basis. As the eggs grow older they become more fragile and when they undergo the special cell division called meiosis that occurs before fertilisation, the chance of too many or too few chromosomes ending up in the cell increases. As a result, older women are more likely to ovulate a chromosomally abnormal egg, which when fertilised by the sperm gives rise to a genetic abnormality in the tiny embryo. The clearest example of this maternal age effect is seen in Down's syndrome (trisomy 21). After the age of 35 years the chance of a woman conceiving a baby with Down's syndrome increases sharply – indeed, if you plot a graph of maternal age along the X axis and number of miscarriages along the Y axis, the graph resembles the letter J (which is why many geneticists refer to the J-shaped curve of pregnancy loss) with the upward change in direction occurring at 35 years.

As we saw in Chapter 4, chromosomal abnormalities are the commonest cause of sporadic miscarriage and account for at least half of all early pregnancy losses. So any factor that increases the risk of chromosomal abnormality obviously makes an important contribution to the problem. However, before any reader who is over 35 years of age starts to feel depressed, let me share with you the results of two studies which I think help to make the problem of maternal age a little less daunting. The first is a study carried out in Italy many years ago, in which the doctors followed the outcome of pregnancy in nearly 3000 women in a local community. They showed that the overall risk of miscarriage was 15% (which agrees with the studies of sporadic miscarriage mentioned in Chapter 2). When they went on to calculate the rate of miscarriage by the woman's age, they found that women less than 35 years of age had a much lower miscarriage rate (6%) and in the women over the age of 40 years the figure was 25%. Furthermore, they were able to genetically analyse all of the miscarriages and found that in the 40-year-olds the incidence of chromosomal abnormalities was over 80%.

Where is the comfort in that? I suspect you are asking. Well, try to remember that the vast majority of older women (75% of them in fact) did not miscarry and went on to have a baby. The second study is one that we carried out in the recurrent miscarriage clinic at St Mary's several years ago. We too followed the pregnancy outcome of a large number of recurrent miscarriers and grouped the women by their age. Happily, I can tell you that the risk of miscarriage did not increase significantly when the woman reached 35 years, in fact it only increased when she was in her forties. And even though all of the women attending our clinic have had at least three previous miscarriages, 55% of the 40-plus-year-olds went on to have a live take-home baby. So please don't despair when you hear that miscarriage increases with age. You cannot change your age, but you can take a positive attitude towards your next pregnancy and remember the above points. The outlook is probably not nearly as gloomy as you feared.

Both these studies are complemented by the large population study carried out in Scandinavia that I mentioned at the beginning of Chapter 2. In this the major leap in the miscarriage rate occurred in the women after they reached the age of 40 years when 51% of their pregnancies miscarried and this figure rose to a startling 83% by the time they were aged 45 years or more.

Recurrence data

I think you will also be heartened to hear of the results of a study that we carried out at the recurrent miscarriage clinic at St Mary's Hospital some years ago. We looked at the number of miscarriages experienced by several thousand couples coming to our clinic. We then grouped the women by the numbers of miscarriages that they had had in the past and looked at the outcome of their next pregnancy. We noted that the live birth rate was always higher than 60% until we reached the women who had suffered more than five miscarriages, where the figure started to fall slowly. Indeed, this high likelihood of successful pregnancy, even after miscarrying on three or four occasions, leads some doctors to question whether detailed investigations and treatment are justified for this problem. I have never shared this viewpoint, but I do think the reasoning behind it can be a source of comfort on occasions!

6

RECURRENT MISCARRIAGE

Definitions

The most clinically valuable definition of recurrent miscarriage, in my opinion, is the loss of three or more consecutive pregnancies before the baby has reached viability. Some doctors consider couples who have had two miscarriages to be suffering from recurrent miscarriage. I prefer to use the definition of three losses because, as we have seen in previous chapters of this book, miscarrying twice in a row is much more likely to be due to chance than miscarrying three times in a row.

The other reason I choose this definition is that most of the really robust miscarriage research has been centred upon women with three losses. It is noticeable that when studies have included women with two losses, the 'waters become muddied' and I sometimes suspect that they have been included to boost the numbers of patients in the study. This does not mean that I consider your two miscarriages to be unimportant. On the contrary, I think they are so important that I do not want to risk confusing why they have occurred with the reasons why a woman with three or more miscarriages has lost her pregnancies. The reasons are likely to be different ones.

Incidence of recurrent miscarriage

You may be surprised, and possibly horrified, when I tell you that the incidence of recurrent miscarriage in the population has never been established accurately. There have been lots of studies looking at how many couples are affected by the problem, but they have been bedevilled by all the usual pitfalls of collecting data in a retrospective way. As I mentioned in Chapter 5, if we collect the number of patients who have experienced three miscarriages by looking at the labour ward register, we are likely to underestimate the problem of recurrent miscarriage. On the other hand, if we collect the figures from the operating theatre register for women who have undergone an ERPC to empty their uterus after a miscarriage, or review all the women who attended the gynaecology emergency services who underwent medical or expectant anagement for a miscarriage, then we are likely to overestimate the problem.

I know of no large population study that has examined women with a history of two miscarriages and been able to give a percentage figure for the chances of her having a third or a fourth. The reason for this is that the problem of recurrent miscarriage is quite rare. If we were to set up a national register of miscarriages, it might be possible to come up with a percentage risk, but for any one clinician working in the field, the numbers of women in their local population who experience three or more miscarriages is small. In my miscarriage clinic I see patients from all over the UK, but even this large group does not allow me to work out the overall risk. Couples who have had several miscarriages followed by a successful pregnancy are not usually referred to the clinic. It is the couples who have persistent problems that I see and by definition these are not a representative group. I believe that they are the exceptional cases and not the rule.

What we do know is that compared to sporadic miscarriage, which is very common, recurrent miscarriage is a rare problem. Sporadic miscarriage affects 25% of all women and 15% of all clinically recognised pregnancies miscarry. If we calculate the chances of having three miscarriages in a row from a purely mathematical or statistical point of view, we should be able to work out how many women will miscarry three times in a row because of bad luck. The statistical chances of having two miscarriages is 15% to the power of two and this works out to be 2.3 %. The statistical chance of having three miscarriages in a row is 0.34% – three to four cases per thousand women.

This figure is certainly lower than the most optimistic doctor would probably estimate. If we take an average of all the figures that have been estimated for the incidence of recurrent miscarriage we end up with a figure of about 1% – one per hundred women. This is a significantly larger figure than the one we predicted from the mathematical calculation above (0.34%). It suggests that in addition to random or bad luck cases, a proportion of women miscarry repeatedly because of a specific problem.

Characteristics of women with recurrent miscarriage

If some women with recurrent miscarriages are the victims of bad luck and others have a systematic cause, then the most important aim of a recurrent miscarriage clinic is to try and sort out which women belong to which group. This is not always as easy as it sounds and the next few chapters of this book are dedicated to the ways in which we can try to unravel this problem.

To help us try to distinguish between the two groups, it is useful to look at some general characteristics or pointers about these women and their individual reproductive histories. These pointers cannot identify the cause of the miscarriages on their own, but I often find that they help me determine how to begin my investigations. A good example is the genetic make-up of the miscarried pregnancy. If this was abnormal, it points towards the miscarriage being sporadic. If the chromosomes were normal, we know that this suggests that the woman has an underlying cause for the miscarriages. Recurrent miscarriers have a much greater likelihood of miscarrying a chromosomally normal fetus.

The age or gestation at which the pregnancy miscarried is another useful pointer. Very early miscarriages are often due to genetic abnormalities in the baby or hormonal problems. If the baby has reached a size of eight weeks or more and a beating fetal heart has been seen on the ultrasound scan, a miscarriage after this stage suggests that something has attacked the pregnancy causing it to miscarry. It is still possible that the baby did have a genetic abnormality, but since the majority of chromosomally abnormal pregnancies are lost early the likelihood of a chromosomal abnormality decreases as the weeks of pregnancy increase. Of course there are exceptions to this general rule. Some trisomies (see Chapter 4) may not miscarry until much later in pregnancy and in some cases of trisomy 21 (Down's syndrome) and monosomy X (Turner's syndrome) the baby is born live.

Similarly, a miscarriage that occurs after a fetal heartbeat has been identified is unlikely to be due to an hormonal cause. Although many hormones are needed throughout pregnancy to ensure the well-being of the baby, it is usually only in the early weeks of pregnancy that a hormone deficiency is capable of single-handedly causing the pregnancy to miscarry (see Chapter 11).

In Chapter 3 we defined late miscarriages as pregnancies that are lost after the baby has grown to a size of 13 weeks or more. This is the accepted definition, but the more miscarriage patients I see, the more I think that this definition will change in the future to 10 weeks. Pregnancies lost after fetal heart activity has been visualised may be due to chromosomal abnormality, but there is an increasing chance that it may be due to autoimmune or prothrombotic causes (see Chapters 12 and 13) and sometimes because of an infection (see Chapter 10). Any woman who has visited the recurrent miscarriage clinic at St Mary's will recall how much of the first visit was spent carefully discussing the details of all her previous pregnancies. We will have quizzed you (gently, I hope!) about the findings of any US scans that were performed in the hope that we can work out exactly what size the baby had grown to before the miscarriage occurred. Any baby that measures the equivalent of seven to eight weeks' gestation must have had a fetal heart. This knowledge will point us towards looking at autoimmune, prothrombotic and infective causes as a priority. You will also remember how keen we were to know whether genetic testing or histology was performed successfully on your lost baby.

Another pointer which may suggest that the woman is a recurrent miscarrier is the length of time it took her to get pregnant. Conception delays of more than 12 months are much more common in recurrent rather than sporadic miscarriers. In Chapter 14 we will look at the miscarriage rate in women who have experienced infertility before their miscarriage. It is true to say that difficulties in becoming pregnant affect as many as one in six couples in the general population, but a degree of infertility is present in one in three couples who miscarry repeatedly. In these cases a hormonal factor is a likely cause. In addition, recent research in autoimmune disorders is suggesting that some cases of subfertility and subsequent repeated miscarriages may be due to antiphospholipid antibodies (see Chapter 13).

Recurrent miscarriage sufferers are also more likely to experience a premature delivery or deliver a baby at the right time who is small for dates or has growth restriction. This pregnancy history suggests that there may be problems with the placenta functioning properly or that an infective or autoimmune disorder is the root cause of the problem. In days gone by, a woman with a history of repeated pregnancy losses, premature deliveries and growth-restricted babies was labelled a 'bad breeder'. These old wives' tales were accurate observations, but there were no underlying reasons put forward. The exciting step forward, I believe, is that we are now beginning to understand that all these pregnancy problems are points on a spectrum, or a scale of reproductive disease. Whether you have suffered infertility, early or late pregnancy losses, there is a common thread linking your problems. The factors that make a woman a good or a bad breeder are enormously important and we are starting to understand that the outcome of any woman's pregnancy is largely dictated by events that occur well before the miscarriage or later pregnancy complications occur. Most importantly, the factors which control the implantation of the pregnancy have far-reaching effects on the course of the pregnancy.

The underlying causes of recurrent miscarriage

The term 'recurrent miscarriage' suggests that there is a single underlying cause for the miscarriages. But this need not be so. Some women will suffer recurrent miscarriages because of a single persisting cause. Others will miscarry repeatedly because they have the misfortune to have several different problems. I think this is one of the most difficult things for miscarriage sufferers to understand and to cope with.

If we can identify that you are miscarrying because of problem X and we are able to offer you treatment for problem X, this still does not protect you from miscarrying from problem Y. Worse still, after recognising that you have both problem X and problem Y, this will not protect you from having another miscarriage because of a sporadic cause, such as a chromosomal abnormality of the baby, which can occur 'out of the blue' and by chance. This is why I use every opportunity possible in this book (and with every couple I see in the miscarriage clinic) to stress the importance of ensuring that the tissues from any future miscarriage are analysed genetically.

My reason for emphasising this, is that the results may have important implications for how your next pregnancy should be managed. If your miscarried pregnancy has an abnormal karyotype (chromosomal makeup) the likelihood is that this miscarriage was a sporadic event and unrelated to the previous recurrent miscarriages. In this situation, the treatment you had for this pregnancy should probably be tried again. On the other hand, if the miscarried pregnancy has a normal karyotype, this suggests that the miscarriage is not sporadic and must be considered as a treatment failure. In this situation, it is probably unethical to try the same treatment again and an alternative approach needs to be considered, if it is available.

I think the best way to look at the different causes of recurrent miscarriage is to examine the groups we identified in Chapter 4, which was devoted to the causes of sporadic miscarriages. These same groups apply to recurrent miscarriages, but the proportion of cases in each group is different. For example, the majority of sporadic pregnancy losses are the result of chromosomal (genetic) abnormalities in the baby, which occur out of the blue. In women with recurrent miscarriages, genetic problems in the baby are much less frequent. Inherited genetic problems from one of the two parents are a well-recognised cause, but they are present in no more than 3–5% of couples.

Viral infections are another important cause of sporadic miscarriage, but most viruses do not affect a woman and her pregnancies repeatedly. Instead, other types of infection with bacteria may be important. And whereas structural abnormalities of the uterus and cervix may occasionally cause a sporadic pregnancy loss, they are more usually identified in women who have repeated episodes of miscarriage. Similarly, environmental, hormonal and autoimmune problems seem to cluster in women with recurrent miscarriage, although they may occasionally be responsible for a sporadic miscarriage.

Having said all this, I think it is important to reflect on the fact that whole chromosomes contain many, many genes and that looking at the number and the shape of chromosomes alone, is a crude method of assessing whether a genetic problem is present. In fact, I will go so far as to say that genetic research in the field of miscarriage is still in its infancy. My hope is that when the international collaboration that has developed in order to map the human genome has successfully reached its goal, we will be able to sit down and look at how this fantastic mountain of knowledge can be used to help us understand the causes of miscarriage more effectively. Of one thing I am already quite certain. Our future understanding of miscarriage will not be centred on abnormal chromosomes. It will need to focus on genetic abnormalities and mutations that predispose to abnormalities in the hormonal, infective and immunological mechanisms that control the development of a successful pregnancy. So instead of looking at hormone X, infective agent Y, or antibody Z, we will be examining how a gene mutation leads to the woman being unresponsive to hormone X or more susceptible to an infection with agent Y or the presence of antibody Z.

In Chapters 7 to 13 of this book we will look in detail at the established causes of recurrent miscarriage. A chapter for each of the six categories of miscarriage is needed, so that you, the reader, will be able to recognise how and why the numbers of miscarriages in these groups differ from sporadic miscarriages and also understand why some causes are more important than others. Here again we need to remember that the currently recognised checklist for the causes of miscarriage will undoubtedly have to be rewritten in the very near future. For example, we used to think that the antiphospholipid syndrome (see Chapter 13) should be classified as a maternal disorder. A better understanding of reproductive immunology then prompted us to move this important cause of recurrent miscarriage into the immune section. More recently we have recognised that the phospholipid syndrome is an acquired type of prothrombotic abnormality that makes women more susceptible to miscarrying and that there are many more prothrombotic abnormalities, many of them inherited (genetically determined), which appears to have an adverse impact on pregnancy outcome and may prove to be additional causes of recurrent miscarriage and later pregnancy complications. Where should we put these newly identified defects? In the genetic section, in the immune section, or should we start up a new category on the checklist called prothombotic abnormalities? This is what I finally decided to do for this third edition of my book and created a new Chapter 13.

But the reader needs to understand that this area of medical research is changing so fast that it won't be long before this edition of *Miscarriage* requires further updating to keep abreast of the next set of discoveries that have been made for both genetically determined and acquired prothrombotic disorders. My job will be to perform the appropriate studies which allows us to decide whether they are truly causes of miscarriage (as opposed to casual associations), and if the answer is yes, whether we can develop treatments to combat them.

7

RECURRENT MISCARRIAGE – GENETIC CAUSES

Genetic abnormalities in the baby are one of the most important causes of sporadic miscarriage (Chapter 4). Structural chromosomal abnormalities are also a cause of recurrent miscarriage, but the contribution they make to this problem is smaller.

There are two ways in which a baby might repeatedly end up with abnormal chromosomes. The first is recurrent aneuploidy, which means that in several different pregnancies, the total number of chromosomes is abnormal, either too many or too few. The second is due to abnormalities in one of the parents' chromosomes, which are repeatedly passed on to the baby in each successive pregnancy. These are usually structural abnormalities or rearrangements in one of the parents' chromosomes, called a translocation.

Recurrent aneuploidy

The baby may have abnormal chromosomes because of an event that occurs 'out of the blue', before or after fertilisation of the egg. This is called non-disjunction and results in the wrong number of chromosomes being present in the tiny embryo. Good examples of this are Down's syndrome (called trisomy 21), where the baby ends up with three copies of the number 21 chromosome instead of two, and Turner's syndrome (or monosomy X), where there is only one X chromosome. Many miscarriages are due to polyploidy; too many extra sets of the 23 chromosomes. This is why we use the term 'aneuploid' as an overall description for any pregnancy that does not have the correct (euploid) number of 46 chromosomes.

Although these 'out of the blue' chromosomal abnormalities are most usually associated with sporadic miscarriage, there are some couples who seem to be at risk of repeated sporadic events. They produce chromosomally abnormal eggs or sperm, not as a result of a translocation (see below), but because they have a tendency towards non-disjunction. The tendency may be inherited or induced because of environmental factors. At the present time we do not understand all the mechanisms that cause this problem, although we do know that the risk of trisomies increases with maternal age, while polyploidies are not affected by this factor.

Trisomy is the most common type of recurrent aneuploidy. However, this does not mean that the chromosome involved in the trisomy is always the same. I will always remember the recurrent miscarriage patient I looked after, who had suffered a trisomy 21 miscarriage and then went on to have a trisomy 13 and then a trisomy 7. When she asked me which chromosome would be affected next time, I was completely lost for words and felt nearly as desperate as she did. There was nothing I could do to sort the problem out for her. Happily, I can tell you that she has now had a healthy baby and has recently contacted me to tell me that she is pregnant again. We advised her to have an amniocentesis test to see whether this baby is normal and the report has just come back confirming that she is carrying a normal baby boy.

If you are a recurrent miscarriage sufferer, all this information about recurrent aneuploidy has probably made you feel gloomy. So I must go on to explain that, in fact, the risk of you having another miscarriage after miscarrying a chromosomally abnormal pregnancy is very low. Lower, in fact, than your risk of miscarrying again after you have suffered a chromosomally normal miscarriage. If this sounds confusing, let me put it another way. Chromosomally normal miscarriages are less random than abnormal ones. This is another reason why trying to find out the genetic makeup of the pregnancy that you miscarry is so useful. If the baby was chromosomally normal, this points to the fact that some other cause was responsible for the miscarriage and needs to be looked for.

Of course, the only way to diagnose whether the miscarriage was genetically normal or abnormal is to ensure that the miscarried tissues are analysed. In Chapter 4 we discussed in detail the problems and pitfalls of chromosomal analysis using tissue culture techniques alone and how the introduction of the new CGH array techniques has so greatly improved our chances of a reliable genetic diagnosis for miscarriage sufferers. It might be useful for the reader to recap on some of these points.

Chromosome abnormalities in the parents

In some couples who have experienced recurrent miscarriages, an abnormality in one of the parents' chromosomes may be the cause. Although it is an important cause to identify, this problem is found in no more than 2–3 % of couples with recurrent miscarriage and is extremely rare in couples who have had a single sporadic miscarriage (about 0.3%: three cases per thousand couples). The defect can be in either parent.

The most frequent chromosomal abnormality found in the parents is a balanced translocation. Translocation describes the situation which occurs when a fragment of one chromosome becomes attached to the broken end of another. The cause of this condition is not understood, but it is sometimes associated with exposure to radiation. The translocation is 'balanced' because the abnormality affects only one of the chromosome pairs. This means that the abnormal one is 'balanced' by the normal chromosome, which is why the parent with the translocation appears to be entirely normal. Indeed, the parent with the chromosome abnormality will only be identified if the couple experience repeated miscarriages and the chromosomes are analysed.

The majority of balanced translocations are reciprocal. This means that the translocation involves an exchange of genetic material between one of the two chromosomes making up a pair, with one of the two chromosomes making up a completely different pair. As we saw in Chapter 4, there are 23 pairs of chromosomes and so there are many different types of reciprocal translocation that can occur. Although the individual with the balanced translocation appears normal, when he or she produces eggs or sperm, some will be normal but others will inherit the abnormality. No longer is the abnormality balanced by the second normal chromosome in the pair. If a normal egg is fertilised by a normal sperm, the resulting embryo will be normal. But if one of the abnormal eggs or sperm takes part in a fertilisation, the resulting embryo will inherit the translocation. This may result in the embryo becoming a balanced translocation carrier, like its mother or father, and this is compatible with normal life. On the other hand, it may become unbalanced, and this invariably leads to a baby with such severe abnormalities that it is only very rarely born alive.

Robertsonian translocations are much less frequent and they only affect chromosomes 13, 14, 15, 21 and 22. These five chromosome pairs have a different shape to the others. If you think of a chromosome pair as two strands tied together in the middle (this middle point is called the centromere) you will be able to imagine that there is an upper short arm and a lower long arm to each of the two chromosomes in the pair. Chromosomes 13, 14, 15, 21 and 22 have very short upper arms. In a Robertsonian translocation, the upper short arm of two chromosomes are lost and the long arms fuse together at the midpoint. This means that one of the chromosomes ends up being very small indeed and when it divides at a later date, it is lost completely.

There are some other types of parental chromosomal abnormalities, called inversions and mosaics. Inversions are just like they sound, a piece of chromosome is turned upside down in its position but this only rarely leads to problems. They are usually considered to be a variant of normal. As I mentioned in Chapter 4, some individuals are made up of two different cell lines with different chromosome numbers. This is called mosaicism, but unless the mosaicism affects the eggs or the sperms, they are usually never detected and are not a cause for concern.

If all of these chromosomal variants are counted, the percentage of abnormalities in couples with recurrent miscarriage rises to about 10%. However, it is important to emphasise that it is only the translocations which cause serious problems. Nowadays I always quote the figure of 2–3% when I am talking to recurrent miscarriage couples about the chances of one of them having a chromosomal abnormality. If couples who have had babies with severe congenital disorders are tested for chromosomal abnormalities, the figure may be as high as 20%.

Diagnosing chromosomal abnormalities

Until relatively recently most couples who had suffered recurrent episodes of miscarriages were advised that they should both undergo peripheral blood karyotyping to analyse their own chromosomes. Historically both partners were tested because it is equally likely that the male or the female partner will be the carrier of the translocated genetic material (see Chapter 4 for details). However, we now realise that these very expensive laboratory tests may have diagnosed the exact balanced translocation but that they really did not help to change the management of the couple's next pregnancy. This is because in couples who carry a balanced translocation, the translocation carrier will either create an embryo with their partner that contains the normal chromosome (which is at no greater risk of miscarrying) or alternatively they will create an embryo that contains the unbalanced genetic material. And in the vast majority of cases this unbalanced genetic material will lead to a miscarriage. We realised that it was vanishingly rare for a couple to have an ongoing pregnancy of an unbalanced fetus that was capable of continuing past the second trimester of pregnancy. Furthermore, on the very rare occasions when it did so the baby was stillborn or miscarried at a late stage in the pregnancy, but was never liveborn, which raised the question as to why we were undertaking all these expensive genetic tests but not being able to usefully use the results.

We concluded that it was much more sensible and cost effective to invest the resources on analysing the embryos or other miscarriage tissues from the future pregnancies of the couples that were attending the recurrent miscarriage clinic at St Mary's rather than analysing their peripheral blood karyotypes. Occasionally however, the genetic abnormality identified in the embryo or the fetus will prompt the geneticists to advise that the parents do go on to have their chromosomes analysed and a request for peripheral blood karyotyping to be performed will be made. Hence a few details are useful here as to how the blood samples should be taken and processed to ensure the best chances of obtaining a successful result.

The blood sample needs to be put into a special bottle containing a small quantity of anticoagulant. This is because the test needs to be performed on white blood cells, which can only be separated from the other cells in the blood sample if the blood is prevented from clotting. I emphasise this point because I frequently saw couples who had tried to have this test performed and were told that the blood sample was unsuitable because it had been put into the wrong bottle, which had allowed it to clot. If either you or your doctor are unsure which bottle should be used, it is best to telephone your local hospital or the nearest cytogenetics laboratory and ask them for advice. The test usually takes four to six weeks to be reported, because it has to be sent to a specialised cytogenetics laboratory which has all the techniques required to prepare the white blood cells and make the tissue culture preparations that are required for the genetic analysis. Patients often asked me to 'speed up' the results of the test, but this is simply not possible, because the careful processing of the cells and analysis of the chromosomes takes time and cannot be hurried. The test is very accurate and, of course, because it determines your individual chromosome pattern, it will never change. I mention this point because couples quite often used to ask me to recheck their chromosomes because the original testing had been done some time ago. If the blood sample has been taken the right way, it is only very occasionally that the test fails to give a result and if this does occur, the laboratory will request another sample of blood from you.

If you are advised to undergo karyotyping then it is important that both partners are tested because it is equally likely that the male or the female partner carries the translocation. It is also important to realise that even if you have had a healthy baby in the past, this does not mean that you and your partner's chromosomes are normal. Earlier in this chapter we noted that an individual with a balanced translocation can 'pass on' the normal or the abnormal chromosome in their eggs or sperms. So it is quite possible for you to have a normal baby together and then have several miscarriages. It is also possible that your baby inherits the balanced form of the translocation and you may never know about it, unless you experience problems in the future which result in you, your partner or your baby (now an adult!) being tested.

In summary, although routine karyotyping of couples with recurrent miscarriage can no longer be justified, selective parental karyotyping when an unbalanced chromosomal abnormality or another type of unusual chromosomal abnormality is identified in the products of conception or miscarriage tissues may be.

Genetic counselling

If you are adviseed to undergo katyotyping and you find that you or your partner carries a chromosomal abnormality, it is important that you have the opportunity to talk to a genetic counsellor. They are medical doctors who have specialist training in genetic disorders. They will be able to explain the problem to you in very clear terms, sometimes drawing diagrams or showing you pictures which will help you to understand the abnormality and the problems it could lead to if a baby were to inherit it.

The geneticists I work with always send the couples a letter after the hospital appointment, which summarises all the points they discussed. I think this is particularly useful, since it is often very difficult to take in all of this genetic information at the first sitting! A letter will give you and your partner the opportunity to digest all the information at leisure and go over points that you remain unsure about. Most doctors are quick to refer their patients for genetic advice when they uncover an abnormal karyotype result, but do not hesitate to ask for help if this avenue is not suggested to you immediately.

The genetic counsellor will also be able to give you a figure for your risk of conceiving a baby which will be affected by the problem. This is important because not all chromosome abnormalities carry the same risk of recurrence. Some abnormalities are more likely to result in an early miscarriage, whereas others may lead to later miscarriages or a baby that is born with severe problems. It is also important to remember that the outcome of your next pregnancy may be entirely normal. Often the appointment with the genetic counsellor can result in you feeling much more optimistic than you had thought possible.

Not all translocations have a good prognosis. Some rare types of Robertsonian translocations involve the chromosomes in such a way that any liveborn baby has a severe abnormality and all other conceptions end in a miscarriage. Finding out this information will always be distressing, but it will give you an opportunity to discuss other ways to achieve a pregnancy. Artificial insemination with donor sperm may be acceptable to some couples, and nowadays the option of donor eggs or even surrogacy (see Chapter 14) may also be a possibility.

The genetic counsellor may occasionally suggest that other members of your family have tests to see whether they are carriers of the same translocation. You may have inherited the translocation from your mother or father. Occasionally, the translocation will be a new one, but this will only be established if the rest of your family are screened. It may be that one of your sisters or brothers inherited the same abnormality, or they may have inherited normal chromosomes. All the advice that you need for future pregnancies needs to be offered to them too, so encouraging other members of your family to have these tests will help them greatly.

If you have been found to have a translocation, you will probably be offered the option of having antenatal diagnosis in any future ongoing pregnancy to exclude the baby having inherited an unbalanced form of the translocation. Antenatal diagnosis is the term used to describe a variety of diagnostic tests that are available to establish the chromosomes of your baby during your pregnancy. The aim of these tests is to identify a baby which has inherited an unbalanced translocation, which may lead to severe abnormalities if the pregnancy continues to term. The reality is however, that this rarely proves to be necessary since the vast majority of embryos or fetuses will miscarry before the antenatal tests are undertaken. These tests are discussed in detail below.

Gene defects – new research

We have thousands of genes and of course this means that potentially there are many gene defects (mutations) that could lead to miscarriage. Since our individual genetic code is inherited, it is reasonable to conclude that any genetic mutation which is linked to sporadic pregnancy loss (see Chapter 4) is also a possible cause of repeated miscarriages. This is a fascinating and fast-moving area of research. New genes are being identified on a daily basis and knowledge of the entire code for human genes is nearly finished. Our understanding of single gene defects such as those that give rise to sickle cell disease, Duchenne muscular dystrophy (discussed in Chapter 4) will soon be expanded to include an understanding of the complex interaction of many groups of genes that collectively control our bodily functions. For example, recent reports have identified genetically determined abnormalities in a crucial enzyme that controls the way that our cells deal with free radicals. These free radicals are the toxic chemicals produced every second of our lives as oxygen is metabolised in our bodies. It is ironic to realise that, although we need to breathe oxygen to feed our brain and other body organs, the waste product of this oxygen consumption is actually very toxic to our bodies. If the enzyme (called glucose 6 phosphate dehydrogenase, or G6PD for short) that helps to clear these waste products is not functioning properly, then we start to accumulate free radicals which lead to all sorts of abnormalities, including cancer.

The good news is that the research is also starting to identify that the use of antioxidants may help to reverse this toxic build-up. Further, that there are many natural antioxidants in the form of vitamins and minerals such as vitamin C, vitamin E and zinc and magnesium that may prove to be helpful in combating the damaging effects of free radicals.

However, I need to add a gentle word of warning here. Before any of the readers of this book rush out to buy large doses of vitamins and minerals from the local chemist, they need to reflect on the fact that we do not know whether the use of these compounds in early pregnancy is safe and a good deal of careful research will need to be performed before we can recommend this potential treatment.

Antenatal diagnosis

There are several tests available to identify whether your baby has normal chromosomes. However, it is important to understand that some of the newly introduced and highly sophisticated scans and blood tests we will look at in the following section can only offer you a probability or a risk assessment of whether your baby has an abnormality or not. The only way to accurately diagnose a specific chromosomal abnormality is to perform a tissue culture (karyotype) or use a microarray technique such as CGH – comparative genomic hybridization.

If you need to undertake chromosomal testing to confirm or refute the findings of one of the antenatal probability test that are now so freely available then it will be necessary to take a sample of amniotic fluid, placenta or fetal blood from the baby to analyse. I stress this point because many women I meet believe that the wide variety of blood tests and specialist US scans that have recently become available are sufficient to make an accurate diagnosis and this is not the case. These blood tests are very useful, but they can only offer you a probability that your baby is chromosomally normal or abnormal. They cannot give you a yes or no answer. The only tests that can tell you definitely what chromosomes your baby is carrying are invasive tests, which sample tissue from the baby. These are amniocentesis, chorionic villus sampling, cordocentesis and fetoscopy.

Amniocentesis

If you are advised to have an amniocentesis test, a sample of the amniotic fluid around the baby will be removed from the uterine cavity using a long, thin needle. This test will be done under ultrasound control to allow the doctor performing the test to avoid touching the placenta and the baby. The special needle is introduced through the mother's abdominal wall and the fluid is sucked up into a sterile syringe and then taken to the laboratory for analysis. It is unlikely that the doctor will use a local anaesthetic in your skin if you have this test, for the simple reason that the anaesthetic is usually more uncomfortable to inject into the skin than the thin amniocentesis needle.

After the fluid has been withdrawn, the doctor will scan the pregnancy carefully to ensure that the baby is all right and will probably advise you to take it easy for the rest of the day. There is a small risk of miscarriage following an amniocentesis of about one in 200. In hospitals where many tests are performed regularly by experienced doctors, the miscarriage risk may be only one in 300. The time of greatest risk is within two weeks of having the amniocentesis performed. Having said this, if you experience a complication after this two-week date, I think it will be difficult for me to ever convince you that the amniocentesis test had nothing to do with it. When discussing the risks of amniocentesis, it is also important to remember that only pregnancies which have potential problems are going to undergo this test. Later complications may not be directly related to the needling procedure and may have been going to happen anyway.

The sample of amniotic fluid will be taken to the cytogenetics laboratory. The fluid is spun hard to collect all the cells together in a pellet. These cells come from the baby's skin. They have floated off the surface of the skin into the amniotic fluid, in the same way that our skin cells float off into the bathwater. Many patients wonder why it may take several weeks to get the final chromosome result. The reason is that these fetal skin cells have to be encouraged to grow in tissue culture, or be subjected to specialised tests such as array CGH (see chapter 4 and below for more details). If tissue culture is required, the cells have to be specially prepared and brought to a stage where they are actively dividing (called the metaphase stage) in order to perform the chromosomal analysis. Sometimes the cells cannot be encouraged to grow or are very slow in growing, which can delay your result.

This is why amniocentesis is not usually performed until 14 to 16 weeks of pregnancy. Before this date, the number of fetal skin cells may be insufficient to set up a culture and obtain a chromosome result. Another reason for delaying the test until after 14 weeks is that removing fluid from the amniotic pool before that time may result in problems with the development of the baby's lungs. The downside to amniocentesis is that you will not have the results before about 18 weeks. This means that if the baby has an abnormality and you decide to have a termination of pregnancy, you will have to undergo an induced labour to deliver the baby vaginally (see Chapter 17). The upside is that the risk of miscarriage is low and that amniocentesis is very accurate. It is extremely rare for the results to be wrong.

An exciting new technique which is now available in most specialist centres is called amnio PCR. Using a powerful molecular biology technique – the polymerase chain reaction (PCR) – the DNA (genetic code) present in the fetal skin cells can be multiplied enormously in order to provide sufficient quantities to allow the diagnosis to be made quickly, within a couple of days. Currently trisomies 21, 18 and 13, together with other frequently occurring trisomies and all of the sex chromosome abnormalities, can be reliably identified with this technique. However, the less common chromosomal abnormalities and mosaicism (two different cell lines) may not be identified immediately. To reliably identify these rarer defects, which probably arise in no more than two per 1000 women undergoing antenatal diagnostic testing, the cytogenetic experts will probably want to proceed to the older and more established methods of culturing the cells.

FISH, or fluorescent in situ hybridisation, is another technique which has become widely available in cytogenetics laboratories to quickly test samples for chromosomal abnormalities. This method labels (tags) pieces of DNA from a specific chromosome with fluorescent coloured markers. These are then placed on the amniotic cells or any other cells that are being tested (such as fetal blood cells – see Cordocentesis, below) where they glow (fluoresce) with a specific colour which is easily seen under the laboratory microscope. The beauty of this technique is that the cells being examined do not have to be nurtured to the point where they are actively dividing (the metaphase stage) to see whether the correct number of chromosomes are present. The signal will glow from any cell at any stage of its cell cycle and so this rapidly speeds up the diagnosis of any suspected abnormality. For example, if Down's syndrome is present we would see three signals (one for each of the three copies of chromosome 21) but if the baby is normal we would only see two signals.

Chorion villus sampling

In this technique, a small sample of the placenta is removed through a needle inserted into the uterus via the mother's abdominal wall. For an amniocentesis, the placenta is avoided and the fluid in the amniotic sac is sampled. In chorion villus sampling (CVS for short) the amniotic sac is avoided and, under ultrasound control, the placenta is sampled. Since the baby and the placenta both develop from the same cells, the chromosomes in placental cells are the same as in cells from the baby.

CVS can be performed earlier in pregnancy than amniocentesis, usually between ten and 11 weeks. The tissue obtained is fresh living placenta, which means that culture and chromosomal analysis is much quicker than from the fetal skin cells cultured from an amniocentesis sample. If you have a CVS test, you will probably receive a provisional test result within ten days. Since this test can be performed before 12 weeks, this means that a pregnancy with a severe chromosomal abnormality can be diagnosed in time for a suction termination of pregnancy to be performed. CVS is also used when a specific gene defect is suspected because the tissues can be used for molecular techniques which speed up the results dramatically.

Although the results are available quickly, there are some disadvantages with the CVS test. The first is that the risk of miscarriage seems to be slightly higher. About 1% of all pregnancies that undergo a CVS miscarry. Although this slight increase may be due to the fact that the test is performed earlier in pregnancy and the pregnancy may have been going to miscarry anyway, it is still a concern for both the woman and her doctor. The second problem is that there is some evidence that when the CVS is done very early, the baby may develop an abnormality in the growth of its limbs. The third problem is that sometimes the placental tissues may contain mosaic cells (see earlier) and this can lead to a confusing diagnosis which suggests that the baby has a chromosomal abnormality when, in fact, there is no abnormality. In this situation you will probably be advised to have a later amniocentesis test to check the results. On balance, I think it is reasonable to say that you should be cautious about undergoing a CVS in very early pregnancy.

Cordocentesis

This procedure is very rarely perfomed nowadays but I have included a few sentences about it for the sake of completeness. It involves taking a sample of blood from the baby's umbilical cord which can be directly and rapidly analysed for chromosomal abnormalities. Under US guidance a needle is inserted into the mother's abdominal wall and into the umbilical cord and removes a small sample of blood. This test is only performed after 18 weeks, when the blood vessels in the cord are large enough to be clearly visualised. The risk of miscarriage is the same as the risk for CVS – about 1%.

Fetoscopy

In this investigation a thin, lighted telescope is inserted through the cervix and into the uterus to look at the baby. Some rare liver and skin abnormalities in the baby can be diagnosed with this method and samples of tissues obtained for analysis in the laboratory. It is only performed in very exceptional circumstances and it carries with it a risk of miscarriage of about one in 50.

Ultrasound screening

Ultrasound scans have become enormously valuable in the diagnosis of abnormalities in the baby during pregnancy. The machinery and the quality of the pictures obtained become better each year. However, it is important to emphasise that ultrasound can only pick up structural abnormalities that are present in your baby. Many women I meet are under the false impression that a normal nuchal translucency scan (NTS) at 11–13 weeks or a normal anomaly scan at 20 weeks guarantees her a normal baby. This is not true.

The ultrasound can only see abnormal anatomy. Experienced scanners are able to see tiny pointers that make them suspect that there may be a problem, and they will probably then advise you to have an invasive test to check the baby's chromosomes. But many congenital abnormalities do not have any obvious anatomical or structural markers in the baby. A good example is Down's syndrome. Many babies with Down's syndrome have recognisable heart, kidney and gut abnormalities on the US scan and we are now able to look at the skin creases on the baby's hands and assess the eyelids, which may give us a clue that the baby is affected. Some babies with Down's syndrome have no obvious signs and will not be detected until after the birth.

Cerebral palsy is another good example. There is no antenatal test that can detect cerebral palsy. For decades we have thought that cerebral palsy was the result of a traumatic labour. We now know that many infants with cerebral palsy have developed this problem during the course of the pregnancy but we have not yet been able to identify the trigger(s). We recognise that cerebral palsy is more common in babies born prematurely, but the exact mechanism is not understood.

Over the last few years there have been several 'scare' stories reported in the newspapers suggesting that repeated ultrasound scans during pregnancy may cause damage to the developing baby. Laboratory experiments have suggested that US waves may cause changes in the membranes (covering layers) of cells that potentially could affect the development of the embryo and later growth of the fetus in utero. There are no scientific data to support these assertions and, importantly, a large Swedish study concluded that there is no association between multiple pregnancy US scans and the later occurrence of childhood leukaemia. Several other large studies looking at the follow-up of babies scanned on many occasions during complicated pregnancies have demonstrated that there are no serious developmental abnormalities in these babies. Indeed, the only difference that I am aware of between pregnancies that are scanned regularly and those that are not, appears in another Scandinavian study, which reported an increase in the number of left-handed babies born to the mothers who had received multiple scans and suggested that the sound waves had in some way interfered with the development of the baby.

Many women now opt to have an early scan between 11 to 13 weeks of gestation which measures the size of the fetus and the nuchal translucency (the fluid present behind the neck of the fetus – the nuchal fold). The thickness of the nuchal fold is then fed into a computer program along with the exact age of the pregnancy in weeks and days and the mother's age. The computer then calculates the adjusted risk for this woman having a chromosomally abnormal baby, based on all the information it has been provided with. Once again this is a probability and not a black-and-white answer. The only sure-fire way of establishing that your baby has normal chromosomes is to undergo an invasive procedure such as amniocentesis. The NTS is best at detecting Down's syndrome (trisomy 21) but it is also available to detect other major trisomies.

Although not a guarantee that your baby is normal, I think the NTS scan is particularly helpful for women who have suffered recurrent miscarriages. They are usually, and understandably, fearful that an invasive procedure may result in a further miscarriage or later pregnancy complication. I have looked after many patients in the last few years who have been unsure what to do because they are older than 35 years, and recognise their increased risk of fetal abnormality, but do not want to place themselves at greater risk of miscarriage from amniocentesis. The NTS scan is a good halfway house. In expert hands it is a good predictor of abnormality and normality and many of my patients end up concluding that they would prefer to have an NTS scan and only proceed to have an amniocentesis if the results suggest that they are at significant risk of carrying a baby with a major chromosomal abnormality.

Maternal serum screening

This is the name given to the many special antenatal blood tests which you will probably be offered at the end of the first trimester of pregnancy at your antenatal booking visit or a few weeks later (depending on the screening package that your maternity unit has chosen to adopt). It provides you with a probability (risk assessment) of whether or not there is an increased chance of your baby having a chromosomal abnormality such as Down's syndrome or an open neural tube defect (such as spina bifida). There are a variety of tests on the market measuring two, three, four or more substances in your blood. These are alphafetoprotein (aFP), free beta HCG, oestriol, Inhibin A and pregnancy-associated protein A (PAPP-A). In babies with Down's syndrome the aFP tends to be lower and the HCG higher. Just as with the nuchal translucency scans (see previous page) your age and the exact gestation of your pregnancy are then used to calculate your risk of Down's syndrome.

When the screening test shows a significant chance of having a baby with Down's syndrome it is called screen positive and you will be given the option of having an amniocentesis (see earlier). If the test shows an aFP level indicating an increased risk of an open neural tube defect, a detailed scan will be arranged to look carefully at the baby's head and spine. When you undergo a maternal serum screening test I think it is really important that you remember three things: 1) that a screen positive test does not necessarily mean that the baby has Down's syndrome or a neural tube defect. It only indicates that you are in a higher-risk group and that you need to be offered a further diagnostic test. 2) Although women with screen negative results are unlikely to have a baby with either of these problems, sadly, a few women will. 3) If you decide to have a serum screening test you need to have thought carefully about what you will do if the test is positive. You will be offered an amniocentesis and if you decide to accept and the baby is found to be affected, you will be faced with the choice of whether or not to continue with the pregnancy.

As I mentioned previously, there is no right or wrong answer to these difficult questions. You and your partner will need to make a decision that is right for you. These serum screening tests are very helpful but they can only provide you with a numerical risk. If you need to know for certain that your baby does not have Down's syndrome, or any other chromosomal abnormality, then the amniocentesis or other invasive tests will be required.

Non-invasive prenatal testing (NIPT) and Cell-Free Fetal DNA

The most recent discovery in the fast-moving field of prenatal diagnosis is the discovery of cell-free fetal DNA in maternal blood. This means it is now possible to use entirely non-invasive prenatal testing (NIPT) to detect Down's syndrome in over 99% of cases and three of the other common aneuploidies: Edwards syndrome, Patau syndrome and Turner syndrome are also detectable but slightly less reliably at the current time. Further research and evaluation is necessary before these tests will become available routinely in the NHS, although they are already widely available in the private sector.

NIPT for Down's syndrome works by analysing the DNA fragments present in the maternal plasma during pregnancy. This is known as cell-free DNA. Most of this cell-free DNA comes from the mother (cell-free maternal DNA), but during pregnancy around 10% of the cell-free DNA in her blood originates from the unborn baby (cell-free fetal DNA). Each chromosome has sequences of DNA that are specific to that particular chromosome. It follows that by analysing and counting all the DNA sequences that link or map to each individual chromosome, the total amount of chromosome 21 in the mother's blood can be compared with the amount of the other chromosomes. No attempt is made to separate fetal from maternal DNA. Rather the total amount of DNA is determined (both fetal and maternal) in a given sample. This amount is then compared to the reference amount known to be present in normal pregnancies and the proportion of DNA from any given chromosome to the total amount is also determined. If the total amount and ratios in the sample analysed are similar, the fetus must have the normal chromosome number. If there is more DNA in the sample than expected, that DNA must have originated from the fetus having an abnormal chromosome number. So if the baby has Down's syndrome, there will be slightly more sequences that map to chromosome

21 than expected, indicating that there is more chromosome 21 present than normal. This allows very accurate prediction of pregnancies where the fetus is likely to have Down's syndrome.

Cell-free fetal DNA (cffDNA) comes from the placenta. It is first detectable from about 4–5 weeks' gestation and reaches the required level needed to test for Down's syndrome by 10 weeks' gestation in most pregnancies. The cffDNA is cleared from the maternal circulation within the first hour after birth, and therefore we know that it is specific to the woman's current pregnancy. However, it is important to remember that NIPT for Down's syndrome analyses both the baby's and the mother's cell-free DNA. Inconclusive results happen in up to 4% of cases. This is usually because the proportion of fetal DNA present in the sample is not high enough to give an accurate result. NIPT may then be repeated with the hope that the cffDNA levels will have increased due to the increased gestation.

NIPT detects around 98% of all babies with Down's, Edwards and Patau syndromes. The 99% detection rate for Trisomy 21 is much higher than when using ultrasound and assaying maternal markers (85–90%). Moreover the false positive rate in cell-free DNA of less than 1% is also much lower than the false positive rates of 3–5% which accompany ultrasound and maternal serum markers. Of course an abnormal or positive test result will still need to be confirmed with a CVS or amniocentesis, but far fewer invasive procedures are required with cell-free DNA screening.

False positives with cell-free DNA are most usually found in an unrecognised twin pregnancy in which the deceased twin has a trisomy – thereby explaining the excess DNA present. The viable co-twin by contrast has a normal chromosome number. In this situation an amniocentesis will be required to confirm the diagnosis and reassure the parents that the pregnancy can safely continue and result in a normal, healthy baby. Although there are limitations to cell-free DNA analysis with less information overall being possible to analyse than with CVS or amniocentesis samples, a first trimester screening method that is completely non-invasive and requires only a sample of maternal blood makes cell-free DNA testing an extremely attractive screening tool.

Preimplantation diagnosis

Diagnosing a genetic disorder in a tiny embryo is a very important development which was originally pioneered at the Hammersmith Hospital. It is now possible to determine the sex of a baby and many specific genetic diseases (for example, cystic fibrosis) by removing a single cell from an embryo. Of course, the only way to obtain an embryo is for the woman to undergo an IVF treatment cycle. The embryo created by fertilisation of an egg in the laboratory can then be sampled before the embryo is transferred into the mother's uterus. This cell is then carefully broken up to release the DNA (the genetic code) and, using specialised molecular biology techniques, the genetic code can be identified. If the abnormal genetic code is found, the embryo will not be transferred back to the mother.

I feel compelled to make a further comment before completing this brief overview on preimplantation diagnosis. Numerous patients who I have cared for recently have attended the recurrent miscarriage clinic clutching copies of articles that they have found on the Internet about the use of preimplantation diagnosis, which have alleged that this technique reduces the miscarriage rate in couples who have suffered recurrent pregnancy losses. This is not the case and is sadly very misleading to many desperate couples trying to achieve their ambition of a live, healthy baby. When I read these articles which often misquote the data published in the original scientific papers, I can understand why my patients have come to their conclusions. These data need to be scrutinised much more closely and interpreted a lot more cautiously if we are to prevent false hopes being dashed.

When a couple undergo preimplantation diagnosis they are effectively being screened for chromosomal and other genetic abnormalities in one of the cells taken from an embryo that they have produced as a result of IVF and related specialist treatments. The purpose is to avoid replacing any embryo that is found to be abnormal back into the woman's uterus. It is true that, as a result of this selection procedure, the number of miscarriages that result from those embryos that manage to implant and go on to develop into recognisable pregnancies is low. This is because the commonest cause of miscarriage is a chromosomal abnormality in the fetus. But it is essential that any couple who opt to undergo this complex treatment realise that there is an enormous difference between the number of embryos produced and the number of embryos that progress to become an established pregnancy.

Preimplantation genetic diagnosis is not a cure for miscarriage in couples who can get pregnant spontaneously and without difficulties. It is a highly specialised technique that prevents miscarriages occurring due to chromosomal anomalies in the tiny embryo, because it removes these affected babies from the potential pregnancy pool. However, it does not increase the live take-home baby rate and nor does it shorten the interval to achieving a live take-home baby. This is because for many couples who go through a cycle of treatment there will be no normal embryos to transfer back into the uterus and hence they will have no possibility of becoming pregnant following this treatment cycle. For others, normal embryos may be transferred back to the uterus but there is no guarantee that these will implant – indeed the majority of embryo transfers in even the best IVF units do not result in an ongoing pregnancy. This may sound harsh to the reader but I am confident that it is not as harsh as the reality that some couples find themselves experiencing unwittingly. Namely, that they have undergone an expensive, emotionally and physically exhausting procedure and have not understood that the chances of achieving a healthy baby have not been increased in real terms for the vast majority of couples. There is some evidence that for older women in their middle 40s that IVF with PGD may be beneficial occasionally and certainly if donor eggs are acceptable to the couple this will significantly improve their chances of achieving a successful pregnancy.

I must conclude by stating that I am a great supporter of the advantages that preimplantation genetic diagnosis can provide when the technique is offered to couples with an established risk of conceiving repeated genetically abnormal pregnancies that can be identified accurately. This technique can prevent these couples from ever conceiving pregnancies that are destined to bring further distress and disappointment, but for recurrent miscarriers who do not carry a specific genetic disorder this is not a treatment that will solve your problems.

Summary

Recognised genetic abnormalities in the baby are common in women with sporadic miscarriages and less common in women with repeated miscarriage. A chromosomal abnormality, for example a balanced reciprocal translocation in one of the parents is present in no more than 2–3% of couples who experience recurrent miscarriages. But since the vast majority of their future pregnancies either miscarry early if the embryo has inherited the unbalanced form of the abnormality, or carry on normally if the inherited abnormality is balanced or is not transmitted to the fetus, routine screening for parental chromosome abnormalities is not cost effective and is difficult to justify. By contrast, genetic analysis of miscarriage tissues offers significant benefits in terms of information that can help to plan the management of future pregnancies.

Over recent years the development of new prenatal diagnostic tools to identify pregnancies affected by genetic abnormalities have become more and more sophisticated and informative. Couples are now able to undergo tests of their baby during the first trimester of pregnancy which offer a high degree of accuracy and are completely non invasive and therefore are associated with negligible risks to the pregnancy. These benefits are particularly important to the recurrent miscarriage patients that I see in my clinics since many of them are older women, who recognise that the risks of a genetic abnormality in their baby are higher, but whose greatest fear is to undergo an invasive test during pregnancy that places a normal baby at risk of miscarrying.

It is important to remember that even if your reason for repeated miscarriages has been identified and treated, you are not protected from a sporadic miscarriage caused by an 'out of the blue' chromosomal abnormality in the baby. The most useful way forward is to ensure that any future pregnancy which miscarries is analysed genetically. Knowledge of the chromosomal makeup of the baby will provide you and your doctors with information that will make important contributions to your medical management. It is also likely to be a source of comfort to you and your partner.

8

RECURRENT MISCARRIAGE – ANATOMICAL CAUSES

Much has been written in medical textbooks about the reproductive problems which may result from abnormal development of the ovaries, fallopian tubes, uterus, cervix and vagina. When the structure of these organs is abnormal, they are called 'congenital abnormalities'. The human uterus, cervix and vagina develop from two separate tubes of tissue which normally fuse together in the midline. As a result, most women have two ovaries, two fallopian tubes and a single uterus, cervix and vagina. If this fusion is incomplete, a wide variety of abnormal types of anatomy can result. Abnormalities of these female organs can also be acquired after birth (for example, fibroids) or following an operation on the uterus or cervix (for example, intrauterine adhesions), whereas other abnormalities can be a mixture of congenital and acquired causes (cervical incompetence). Whatever the abnormality is or what has caused it, the methods we use to identify or 'image' these anatomical problems are common to all the different types. At the end of this chapter we will look at these techniques and their practical usage.

Congenital abnormalities of the uterus

No one knows exactly how many women have a congenital abnormality of their uterus. Some studies have suggested that as few as one in a thousand women (0.1%) are affected. Other studies have concluded that as many as one in ten women (10%) have an abnormality. The true incidence is somewhere between these two figures and depends upon the population of women studied. This uncertainty is another good example of how the specialist interest of the doctors investigating women with recurrent miscarriages influences the results. For example, if all women with a history of repeated premature labours or late miscarriages are investigated, it is likely that the number of uterine abnormalities found will be much higher than the figure for women with repeated early miscarriages.

The most frequent uterine abnormality is a bicornuate uterus. This means that the two tubes of uterine tissue (called horns) have not fused together and instead of the rounded dome shape, the uterus has the appearance of two horns joined together at the cervix. Very rarely, the abnormality is so severe that there are two cervices (uterus didel-phys) and two vaginas (bicollis). Occasionally only one uterine horn is present, communicating with a single fallopian tube, and this is called a unicornuate uterus. An arcuate uterus, in which the normal dome of the uterine cavity is flattened, or appears to be slightly heart shaped, is quite common. So too is the presence of a septum in the uterus. If you can imagine a domed ceiling with a curtain hanging down from the centre, then you will understand what a septate uterus is. The curtain can be long or short in length and so we refer to septate and subseptate abnormalities of the uterine cavity.

If you have a bicornuate uterus, it is possible that the baby will not have enough room to grow to its proper size and that you will experience a premature labour or late miscarriage. A bicornuate uterus is also one of the reasons why the baby may be a breech presentation (sitting with his or her bottom above the cervix instead of pointing head downwards). Having mentioned the problems that a bicornuate uterus may cause, I must also tell you that there have been many times when I have only recognised that the woman has a bicornuate uterus after an entirely normal delivery or a routine caesarean section at term. My most memorable case was the pair of healthy twins I delivered at 36 weeks, each twin delivering out of their own uterine horn.

In the past, open surgery to correct a bicornuate uterus was recommended. This entailed a major pelvic operation during which the two horns of the bicornuate uterus were opened and stitched back together to form a single uterine cavity. Although supporters of this treatment claimed that the women they operated upon had a high live birth rate in future pregnancies, it was later realised that about one-third of these women never became pregnant again. The scar tissue and pelvic adhesions caused by their surgery resulted in them becoming infertile. I feel strongly that this is much too high a price to pay for a treatment which has never been demonstrated to offer benefit in a proper controlled trial. Fortunately, open surgery has fallen out of favour and I know of no clinicians who now offer this treatment to women with a bicornuate uterus and a history of recurrent miscarriage.

Some doctors believe that a septum in the uterine cavity is a major cause of infertility and repeated miscarriages. The septum is usually thin and has no proper endometrial covering, so it is argued that the embryo cannot implant properly on this surface, which may result in the woman experiencing difficulties in becoming pregnant. Alternatively, the embryo may start to implant on the septum, but because of the poor blood supply and thin endometrium, the pregnancy cannot continue and an early miscarriage is likely. I am sure that this is a valid explanation for a few cases of miscarriage, but it has always struck me that it goes against the laws of probability to assume that every embryo makes a beeline for the septum rather than choosing another more promising site to implant in the uterus.

Certainly there have been numerous papers published on the incidence of uterine septae in women with a history of infertility and of recurrent miscarriage. The figures quoted have varied greatly, because once again they reflect the specialist interests of the doctors involved. However, one very important Spanish study has helped to put the problem into perspective. These doctors found that the incidence of septae in women who were undergoing laparoscopic sterilisation after completing their families was in the region of 3%. This is not significantly different from the incidence of septae found in women being investigated for infertility. Furthermore, in a study performed at the recurrent miscarriage clinic at St Mary's several years ago, we also found that 3% of our patients had an intrauterine septum. These results emphasise the importance of always including appropriate control groups when trying to establish the incidence of a particular disorder in women presenting with a history of repeated pregnancy loss.

If you have a septate uterus, the doctors may suggest that they cut out (or 'resect') the septum with the help of an operating hysteroscope. This is a fine telescope which is inserted through the cervix into the uterine cavity. At the tip of the telescope is a pair of fine scissors which are used to carefully resect the septum. In fact no single piece of tissue is removed or cut away. Instead, as the scissors cut into the fibrous septum they effectively "untether" the bunching up of the cavity (or hanging curtain) that the septum created. This swiftly opens up the fundus (top of the womb cavity) making it more dome shaped. I confess to the reader that it was only very recently, when looking up some old research papers, that I discovered how ancient this technique of septal resection is! The first septal resection was carried out blindly by a Dr Ruge in 1884 long before fibre-optic telescopes or proper anaesthetics were available. Nearly a hundred years later, in 1974, Dr Edstrom performed the first septal resection under direct vision using one of the newly designed operating hysteroscopes.

The current-day procedure is usually performed quickly under a light general anaesthetic and does not require an overnight stay in hospital. I tend to leave two coils in the cavity at the end of the procedure to help keep the raw edges of the uterine wall apart for the next 4 weeks. During this time I usually suggest that the woman takes some oestrogen and progesterone hormone treatment in order to speed up the healing over of the endometrial lining at the resection site. After the hormonal course has been completed, the two coils are easily removed in the outpatient clinic with minimal discomfort and the woman can then embark on another pregnancy without any further delays. I have certainly used this technique for many of my miscarriage patients, who appear to have been cured by this simple operation and gone on to have successful pregnancies.

Indeed, we have been so impressed by the outcome data that we now routinely offer a hysterosocopy to any woman who is referred to us with a history of five or more unexplained consecutive miscarriages, in order to exclude a septum or other structural abnormality within the cavity. We also go on and resect the septum during the same procedure if we find one and leave coils in the cavity and give the woman a four-week course of HRT to promote swift healing of the cavity. In addition, if the 3D scan suggests that the recurrent miscarrier with three or more losses has an abnormally shaped cavity, or has experienced delays in conceiving, when she is first referred to our clinic, then we will schedule her to have a hysteroscopy sooner rather than later and resect any septum that we find.

However, I think it is important to point out to the reader that this is one of the few treatments that I perform for women attending the recurrent miscarriage clinic at St Mary's that has not been formally validated by a well-designed, multi-centred, randomised controlled trial. Such a trial would of course be extremely difficult to undertake and to persuade patients to join since it would involve comparing the future pregnancy outcome of recurrent miscarriers with a septum who undergo resection treatment and those who have no surgical intervention. Several units have tried to start such a trial (mine included) and then been forced to give it up because all the women who are eligible to become trial participants want to be in the treatment group, despite the fact that there is no robust evidence to suggest that it is going to resolve their problems. A recent Cochrane review article confirmed the lack of evidence to support this surgical procedure and agreed that good trials are urgently needed. I hope that we can undertake such a trial but continue to have doubts as to whether we will ever be able to randomise sufficint numbers of women to the no treatment arm. However, we are all agreed that an open pelvic operation (see earlier) to correct a structural abnormality of the uterine cavity is likely to cause more harm than good, cannot be justified and should definitely be avoided.

Diethylstilboestrol

A variety of congenital uterine abnormalities, particularly a T-shaped uterine cavity, are found in some of the daughters of women who were treated with diethylstilboestrol (DES) in pregnancy. DES is a synthetic oestrogen and ironically it was first prescribed in the late 1940s for women who were threatening to miscarry! It did not stop the miscarriages, a fact that was known as early as 1953, but it was only when it was realised in the 1970s that this drug caused problems in the daughters of the women who had been treated that it was withdrawn from the market. The problems ranged from an increased risk of developing autoimmune diseases such as lupus and rheumatoid arthritis to the development of vaginal tissue abnormalities, called vaginal adenosis. The most serious problem was the occurrence of a rare type of vaginal and cervical 'clear cell' cancer. DES-related abnormalities are very rare these days because only a few daughters exposed to the drug are still of childbearing age. Thankfully the problem is virtually extinct now.

Fibroids

Uterine fibroids are very common, and may cause both infertility and miscarriage. In fact, fibroids are the most common benign (non-cancerous) growth in women and as many as 50% of women will eventually develop one or more fibroids. Fibroids can vary in size from a small pea to a large melon and vary in number from one to a hundred. The amazing thing about fibroids is that no one really understands how they develop. Since they are the cause of many obstetric and gynaecological problems, I always think it is strange that we still do not know how to prevent them from growing in the uterus.

They are rare before the age of 20 years, and do not develop after the menopause, which points to the fact that their growth is influenced by our reproductive hormones. There is obviously a genetic tendency to develop fibroids, since they are often found in several women in the same family and are much more frequent in Afro-Caribbean women. Fibroids can grow in any part of the uterus. If they are in the wall, they are called intramural fibroids. If they are on the outside of the uterus, they are called subserous, or pedunculated if the fibroid is attached to the outside surface of the uterus by a stalk. When the fibroids protrude into the uterine cavity, they are known as submucous fibroids and occasionally these may form a polyp attached to the endometrial lining by a stalk.

Many women with fibroids become pregnant without any delays and experience no complications during their pregnancies. However, some fibroids can enlarge the uterus and distort the uterine cavity to such an extent that they cause serious reproductive problems. Submucous fibroids are the worst offenders and if they grow near the opening of the tubes into the uterine cavity, or occupy a large surface of the uterine cavity, the woman may present with infertility. The endometrial lining over the surface of submucous fibroids has a poorer blood supply and this is probably what makes it difficult for an embryo to implant (infertility) or to continue to develop successfully (miscarriage).

In later pregnancy, fibroids in any position may cause problems. They grow along with the rest of the uterus under the influence of the hormones of pregnancy. Many of the problems they cause are beyond the scope of this chapter, but a few points need to be mentioned here. Sometimes their growth outstrips their blood supply and the fibroid starts to degenerate – this is most commonly experienced between 20 and 28 weeks of pregnancy. Fibroid degeneration in pregnancy can be very painful and the inflammation that it causes may make the pregnancy go into labour prematurely. When they are very large, the fibroids may limit the growth of the baby. If the fibroids are positioned low in the uterus, near the cervix, they can cause difficulties with the delivery. The risk of these complications is one of the reasons we try to remove large fibroids before pregnancy.

If you are found to have a fibroid polyp, the doctors will advise you to have it removed from the uterine cavity. Fibroid polyps can usually be dealt with simply by performing a hysteroscopy (looking inside the cavity with a telescope) which allows a targeted or directed polypectomy to be performed. The decision to remove a submucous fibroid will very much depend upon the results of the imaging which will demonstrate the position and size of the fibroid and what percentage is protruding into the cavity and what percentage is sitting within the womb wall.

It may be possible to perform a transcervical resection of the fibroid with the help of a specialised operating hysteroscope (see earlier), which is undoubtedly the best approach. Once again, it should be emphasised that an open pelvic operation is always more complicated and carries with it many more problems in the post-operative period, the most serious of which is not being able to conceive due to scar tissue and adhesions. Nevertheless, open surgery is sometimes required particularly for very large fibroids in recurrent miscarriage women who also need to have future assisted fertility treatments such as IVF. In this situation, the presence of a large uterine fibroid may make it very difficult for a future embryo transfer to be successfully performed.

The most appropriate method of dealing with intramural fibroids and subserous fibroids will also depend on their size and position. If you are advised to have it removed, the operation is called a myomectomy (a 'myoma' is a fibroid). It involves an open operation, cutting through the muscular wall of the uterus in order to shell out the fibroid, which is surrounded by a tough fibrous capsule. The operation can be very bloody and much care is taken to try and reduce the bleeding during and after the operation by very carefully stitching the muscle walls together. Open surgery for fibroids is best done by experienced fertility doctors, in order to reduce future complications.

Laparoscopic (or keyhole) surgery can also be used to remove fibroids in certain patients. The suitability of this type of procedure will depend on the position and size of the fibroids. If the fibroids are too large, it will make it very difficult to impossible to manoeuvre the telescopic instruments that need to be inserted via entry points or ports through the abdominal wall. In addition, if there are any adhesions or endometriosis in the abdominal or pelvic cavities resulting from previous surgery or an episode of pelvic inflammatory disease, their presence can distort the pelvic anatomy and make a laparoscopic approach dangerous.

Having said all that, it is clear that when careful selection of suitable patients is undertaken, that laparoscopic myomectomy may be a better option for women, particularly in terms of overall blood loss, length of time spent in hospital and greatly reduced post-operative recovery and convalescence times.

Minimally invasive treatments for fibroids

In the future it may be possible to avoid open or laparoscopic surgery altogether for fibroids in women who want to preserve their fertility.

Uterine artery embolization

This effectively means blocking off the main blood vessels to the uterus and hence the vessels feeding the fibroids. It is now a well-accepted method of treatment for symptomatic uterine fibroids. In brief, a radiologist inserts a catheter into an artery in the woman's groin and feeds it up and along until the uterine artery is reached. Then particles of polyvinyl are inserted into the vessel and the procedure repeated on the other side of the uterus. UAE compares favourably to open and laparoscopic myomectomy surgery in reducing heavy menstrual bleeding and reducing pressure symptoms for women with large or multiple uterine fibroids. Around 80% of patients will be asymptomatic or have significantly improved symptoms when reviewed after one year from the UAE procedure and this improvement is accompanied by a reduction in the size and volume of the fibroids that varies from 40–70%.

On the face of it, UAE may appear to be an appealing option for women with large or multiple fibroids who are having difficulty conceiving or suffering recurrent miscarriages because it avoids all the complications associated with surgical operations. Since this treatment reduces the fibroid volume it should theoretically improve the chance of a successful pregnancy. However, UAE may lead to adverse effects on any future pregnancy. Follow-up studies suggest that the procedure may reduce the quality and depth of implantation, resulting in the placental blood supply being compromised and poorer growth of the baby. It may also increase the risk of uterine rupture in late pregnancy or during labour. Perhaps the most worrying side-effect for women in their forties who are still trying to achieve a successful pregnancy, is that UAE carries with it a 1–2% risk of premature ovarian failure. As such, patients who want to become pregnant need be fully informed about the potential side-effects of UAE on fertility and on future pregnancies. Another complication of UAE is that it is invariably associated with severe pain for at least 48 hours after the procedure. This frequently necessitates an inpatient stay for one to two nights so that the woman has the option of intravenous pain relief. It is thought that the severe pain results from the fact that the UAE procedure causes the cells in the fibroid and uterine muscle to die because their blood supply is cut off. When this happens in our body organs it is referred to as ischaemic cell death and the pain stems from the fact that these ischaemic cells release chemicals called cytokines that are extremely irritant and painful.

Magnetic Resonance Imaging

Magnetic resonance guided focused ultrasound (MRgFUS) is another treatment option for women of reproductive age with symptomatic uterine fibroids. The procedure is carried out with the patient lying prone (face down) on a bed that is wheeled inside the MRI scanner. The high-energy US is generated from below the woman's abdomen in contact with the MRI bed. Using a real-time MRI scan to visualise the uterus and the fibroids it is then possible to ensure that the US beam is positioned so that after it passes through the abdominal skin and muscular wall that it is focused on a small area of the fibroid within the uterus. When turned on, this very high-powered US energy heats up the tissue at the tip of the focal point until the cells die. The cells then become liquefied and the watery part of the cells starts to be absorbed which results in the tissues starting to shrivel up and shrink in overall size. Colour-coding software allows the operator to see when the tissues have reached the correct temperature and have undergone cell death. This small area of treated tissue is called a sonication and when the first is completed the operator can then move the focus of the beam to an adjacent small area and another sonication is performed. Gradually the whole of the fibroid being treated becomes a confluent (continuous) area of these sonications and the operator can then move on to the next fibroid. The overall size of the fibroid or fibroids scheduled for the MR treatment will therefore determine how long the whole procedure will take. But in women with a large volume of fibroids, it is not uncommon for the treatment to take several hours to complete.

At the end of the procedure a final MR image is taken after some contrast has been injected into the IV drip that has been placed in the woman's forearm. This allows us to see exactly how much of the fibroid has been successfully treated, since the dead cells can no longer take up the contrast material and they therefore appear as a dark area on the MR scan. However, the live cells do take up the contrast material via their active blood vessels and can be clearly seen on the MR images. The greatest advantage of this procedure is that it can be carried out as an outpatient treatment and the patients require very little analgesia or pain relief. The woman is able to get up and walk out of the radiology department after the procedure and go home and carry on her life normally that evening.

We now have many years of experience of using this treatment at St Mary's and it is fortunately very rarely associated with any serious complications. Occasionally it may cause pain if the US beam hits a nerve root particularly those near the spinal column. The other problem is that previous scar tissue on the skin may absorb the high intensity US rather than transmitting the beam to the uterine fibroids. This can give rise to skin burns which is why women with large or thick scars are usually considered unsuitable for this type of treatment. It appears that MRGFUS has no adverse effect on future fertility and that the pregnancies which have occurred following the treatment have not been affected by any of the serious complications associated with UAE. Nevertheless, it is probably best reserved for women with moderate-sized fibroids giving rise to symptoms of pain and bleeding. It is unlikely to be particularly helpful for those women with very large volumes of fibroid tissue giving rise to pressure symptoms on the bladder or bowel. This is because the shrinkage of the fibroid size is rarely more than 20 to 30% and in some very large fibroids this will not materially change the pressure symptoms. In addition it may not be possible to access MRI facilities for the very long periods of time that are likely to be necessary if treating very large fibroid volumes.

The newest development in minimally invasive treatments is the SONATA system. This involves the use of transcervical radiofrequency probes placed in the uterine cavity which are able to ablate the uterine fibroids and the procedure is monitored and guided by an integrated sonographic system. The benefits are that no incision is required and the treatment does not require general anaesthesia or hospitalisation. The early results are promising but will need further careful evaluation before it can be adopted more widely as an accepted treatment option.

Intrauterine adhesions

These are also referred to as synechiae or scar tissue and are fine bridges of fibrous tissue which cause the walls of the uterus to stick together. These adhesions stop the endometrium from thickening at the appropriate time in the woman's menstrual cycle. In mild cases, this may prevent an embryo from implanting successfully. In more severe cases, the woman may stop having periods altogether although she will often experience pain and discomfort at the time when the period should have come. Intrauterine adhesions almost always follow a surgical procedure in the uterine cavity, such as a D&C or an ERPC after a miscarriage, termination of pregnancy or following a manual removal of the placenta. As such, they are another type of acquired uterine abnormality.

Adhesions in the uterus are really very common. In fact, the more you suspect that they may be present, the more you find them. I frequently meet women who have no periods but experience cyclical abdominal pain for several months after a miscarriage which has required a surgical evacuation (ERPC). Experience has taught me to do nothing in the short term and wait for a few months – the problem usually resolves spontaneously. The traumatised uterine lining starts to regenerate and the periods come back with no adverse consequences. When the problem continues, it is advisable for the woman to have the adhesions divided under a light anaesthetic using a hysteroscope (see earlier). If there are a lot of adhesions in the cavity, your doctor will probably insert a plastic coil into the uterus after dividing the adhesions with the hysteroscope. The coil (intrauterine device, or IUD) ensures that the walls of the uterine cavity stay apart, giving the endometrial lining time and space in which to regenerate. Some doctors also advise a short course of hormone replacement therapy, to help the uterine lining to heal more quickly (see septal resection section).

Fortunately, uterine adhesions are almost always responsive to treatment and do not usually cause long-term problems. I mention this because many women I meet in the miscarriage clinic worry about the effect of repeated ERPCs on their womb. Let me reassure you that it is much better to have a carefully performed ERPC if you have failed to empty the womb after a period of conservative management (even if you do have the bad luck to develop some adhesions) rather than risk infection of the remaining tissues in the uterus. Infection can cause much more severe problems and is a very real cause of future infertility.

Cervical incompetence

The cervix needs to remain closed during pregnancy to allow the fetus and placenta to develop to a size that will allow a viable baby to be delivered. However, if the muscles of the cervix are weak, the cervical canal may start to open during the second trimester of pregnancy, most usually at or around 20 weeks. This situation is called cervical incompetence and may occasionally be due to a congenital abnormality of the muscles of the cervix. In days past, cervical incompetence was not infrequently caused by forceful wide dilatation of the cervix at the time of a D&C or a termination of pregnancy. Nowadays, doctors are very conscious of this potential problem and routinely use drugs to prime or soften the cervix to make it more pliant before starting the uterine evacuation. They are also careful not to dilate the cervix more than 10–12mm when they are operating on the uterus. Occasionally, damage to the cervix may result from a difficult vaginal delivery where the cervix is torn by the forcep blades, ventouse cup or a particularly large baby.

The cervix also needs to remain closed so that the membranes surrounding the baby are not exposed to the vaginal environment. The vagina contains many bacteria which normally do not cause any harm to the pregnancy because the cervix is closed. However, if the muscles of the cervix start to open, the bacteria present in the vagina may then cause inflammation of the membranes which are protruding into the vagina. The woman may experience an increase in her normal vaginal discharge and a feeling of heaviness in the vagina as the cervix shortens and starts to dilate. The inflammation causes the membranes to weaken and sometimes to burst, releasing liquor from the pool around the baby. When the waters break, it is usually only a matter of time before the uterus starts to contract. The reason for this is twofold. Firstly, the membranes release a variety of chemicals when they rupture, which encourage the uterine muscles to contract. Secondly, the bacteria present in the vagina now have easy access to the uterine cavity and within a very short period of time the fetus and placenta become inflamed and infected, which further encourages the uterus to expel its contents. Once infection has set in, it is not possible to save the pregnancy, even with the use of antibiotics. An infection in the uterus is a very serious problem for the pregnant woman, and she needs to be delivered promptly to ensure that she does not develop a life-threatening systemic (generalised) infection.

For some women, there may be no symptoms or signs such as vaginal discharge, broken waters and uterine contractions. Instead, with very little or no warning, the cervix may suddenly open and expel the pregnancy from the uterus. Most commonly, the woman suddenly feels that she wants to open her bowels and on reaching the toilet realises that what she is feeling is the baby miscarrying through the open cervix. The placenta may deliver spontaneously, but more often it is retained in the uterus and has to be removed manually with the help of an epidural or general anaesthetic. I have always thought that nature is particularly unkind in this situation – the woman fails to keep the baby in the uterus, but then has to go through manual traction to get rid of the placenta.

Classical cervical incompetence is described in the textbooks as a 'painless' and sudden opening of the cervix. It has been considered an important cause of late miscarriage for decades. My practical experience is that a painless opening of the cervix during the second trimester of pregnancy is a relatively rare event. If I take a careful history from a woman who has suffered a late miscarriage there are almost always pointers that the opening of the cervix was accompanied by painful uterine contractions or broken waters. Furthermore, I regularly see patients in my recurrent miscarriage clinic referred to me as cases of 'cervical incompetence', but further questioning reveals that the baby had died in the uterus during the second trimester of pregnancy and it was necessary to use drugs to induce the uterus to contract and expel the dead baby – a very different set of affairs to the spontaneous opening of an incompetent cervix.

I am not suggesting that cervical incompetence does not exist, but I do want to state that it is quite rare. More importantly, you need to realise that if causes other than this weakness of the cervical canal are not looked for, it is unlikely that we will find the root cause of your problem. In the past, I think that cervical incompetence has been used as a dustbin diagnosis into which all previously unexplained late miscarriages have been thrown. An infection in the vagina which ascends (travels up) into the uterine cavity is undoubtedly a cause in some cases, and in Chapter 10 we will look at this problem in more detail. However, I firmly believe that many cases of late miscarriage, previously considered to be another example of cervical incompetence, are due to the antiphospholipid syndrome of pregnancy (see Chapter 13). This is an autoimmune disorder, which can be difficult to identify in some women, but undoubtedly is the cause of a wide variety of pregnancy losses. In the miscarriage clinic at St Mary's, we spend a lot of time looking for these antiphospholipid antibodies together with other prothrombotic or pro-clotting disorders in the patients referred to us with late miscarriages. Many of these women have been told that they have an incompetent cervix, but after careful questioning and a study of their medical records, we frequently find that there is more to the story than a weak cervix. I think every woman who suffers a late miscarriage or a premature delivery should be screened not once, but repeatedly, for evidence of the antiphospholipid syndrome. My reasoning is quite simple. Treatment for this problem is extremely effective and can transform a high risk of miscarriage into a high chance of a live birth.

Surgical treatment of cervical incompetence

True cervical incompetence is uncommon in my opinion, but this chapter would be incomplete without describing the treatment method of 'cerclage' – where a stitch is inserted into the cervix to stop the cervix from dilating. Several operations have been tried to achieve this aim, the most famous of which have been named after their inventors, Mr Shirodkar and Mr McDonald. Essentially, the technique is the same. Under a general anaesthetic, the cervix is examined with a speculum inserted into the vagina. A strong mersilene tape or thick nylon stitch (which cannot dissolve like other types of suture material) is inserted into the cervix with a special needle at the 12 o'clock position and brought out at the 3 o'clock position. Further stitches around the circumference of the cervix bring the needle back to the 12 o'clock position, where a strong knot is tied. Personally, I prefer the nylon sutures, which I find easier to insert without having to pull too hard on the cervix. The nylon sutures also appear to cause less tissue reaction and scar tissue to form in the cervix.

The success of the suture depends upon how high up the cervix the operator can insert the stitch. Indeed, the original Shirodkar method involved careful dissection of the bladder off the front of the cervix in order that the stitch could be placed even higher in the cervix at the level of the internal cervical os. This is the junction at the top of the cervical canal where the canal opens into the uterine cavity. Whereas the McDonald suture was inserted at a lower level in that portion of the cervix which is easily visible in the vagina. These McDonald sutures are not nearly as successful as the Shirodkha sutures for several reasons – firstly because the suture is lower meaning that the membranes around the baby are nearer to the naturally occurring bacteria in the vagina. Secondly, because the presence of the stitch material acts like a foreign body that provokes an inflammatory response in the vagina and this chronic focus of inflammation results in a copious watery vaginal discharge for the remainder of the pregnancy which eventually weakens the fetal membranes encouraging them to be break. After the waters have broken around the baby an ascending infection invariably occurs sooner or later and then the process of labour leading to cervical dilataion, uterine contractions and delivery are inevitably going to follow. This is why my personal preference is to perform a Shirodkha suture insertion high in the cervix and then bury the suture material beneath the vaginal mucosa so that there is no foreigh body or uncovered stitch material to generate a vaginal discharge. I am sure this makes a very mjor contribution to the very high success rate we have achieved at St Mary's for women with a late miscarriage or very early preterm birth in their past history.

If you undergo cervical cerclage, you may be given some medication to quieten the uterus if it becomes irritable as a result of manipulating the cervix. You will probably be advised to rest in hospital overnight before going home again.

Of course, not all stitches are successful and sometimes the trauma of inserting it may cause the cervix to start bleeding, the uterus to start contracting, or the waters to break. In this situation, the stitch must be taken out without delay to avoid the risk of strong contractions ripping the stitch out of the cervix and causing even more damage to the torn cervix as it dilates. Similarly, if an infection develops or is suspected, the stitch should also be removed quickly, because it will encourage further infection, which can ascend into the uterus with serious consequences for the mother (see earlier). If the procedure is uncomplicated, then the stitch will remain in place until about 37 weeks, then it usually needs to be removed to allow a normal labour to progress. Removing the stitch is much less of a problem than putting it in, and is usually managed with a local injection of anaesthetic into the cervix.

The decision to insert a cervical cerclage may be based on the obstetric history of painless cervical dilatation, the findings of an US scan or as an emergency procedure, which is referred to as a rescue cerclage. Most doctors plan to electively insert the suture between 12 and 14 weeks of gestation. Only a small minority of doctors advise that the cervical suture should be inserted before pregnancy. I have never thought this approach to be very sensible, since it means that any pregnancy that dies in the first trimester cannot miscarry without removing the stitch. As you will remember from previous chapters in this book, early miscarriage is much more common than late miscarriage and so the risk of this complication is quite high.

During the late 1980s the Medical Research Council (MRC) of England mounted a large multicentre trial of cerclage treatment. Sadly, the results were disappointing. The MRC study demonstrated that women who did have a suture inserted delivered their babies a few weeks later than the women who did not have a cervical suture. As a direct result of the longer gestation time, the weight of the babies in the suture group was higher. It was concluded that for every 13 sutures inserted, one baby would be prevented from delivering prematurely. However, the number of live take-home babies did not increase. Furthermore, the suture group spent considerably more time during their pregnancies in hospital and required more medication for infection and other complications than the control group of women who had no suture. I think it is important for the reader to have these details about the MRC trial results because I frequently hear them being misquoted. I can see no value in a treatment method that requires 13 procedures to be performed to increase the gestational age of one baby, if that one baby does not leave hospital alive and well.

A subsequent randomized controlled trial published in the *Lancet* showed that the insertion of a Shirodkar suture in women with a short cervix did not substantially reduce the risk of early preterm delivery. It did confirm however that routine sonographic measurement of cervical length at 22–24 weeks identified a group at higher risk of early preterm birth.

Nonetheless, as I mentioned above, I have been using high cervical sutures for many years in carefully selected cases, and the results have been extremely encouraging. I suspect that this improved success (when compared to the MRC results) is due to the fact that the length of the cervix is markedly increased when the sutures are inserted higher. A recent retrospective study showed that the higher a cerclage was placed within a shortened cervix, the lower the subsequent odds of preterm birth. The study went on to suggest that it was worthwhile continuing to monitor the length of the cervix using ultrasound after the procedure, as those in whom the cervix failed to elongate remained at higher risk of preterm delivery. You will note that I mention length rather than how tightly closed the cervix becomes after the stitch is in place. I suspect that a longer cervix not only prevents the membranes around the baby from being exposed to infective organisms in the vagina, but also makes the successful ascent of these organisms into the uterine cavity less likely for purely mechanical reasons.

A recent Cochrane review concluded that cervical cerclage reduces the risk of preterm birth in women at high risk of preterm birth and probably reduces the risk of perinatal deaths. Risk was quantified by the history and the length of the cervix. The question of whether cerclage is more or less effective than other preventative treatments, particularly vaginal progesterone, remains unanswered. As such, current NICE guidance offers the patient a choice between prophylactic vaginal progesterone and cervical cerclage when an ultrasound suggests that the cervix has shortened to less than 25mm. It is suggested that if the patient has a history of a previous second trimester loss or a history of cervical trauma, one should recommend cerclage. In the absence of this history, vaginal progesterone should be recommended.

There have also been reports of the use of a cervical stitch inserted by the abdominal route either before or during pregnancy. This method involves a major operation to open the abdomen and identify the top of the cervix from above. Not surprisingly, the advocates of this technique claim an excellent success rate, although it is important for the reader to note that this method has never been assessed in a controlled trial. In women where a transvaginal cerclage has failed, there may be an indication to offer them a transabdominal cervical cerclage prior to their next conception.

Cervical cerclage has always been a very controversial issue in the management of recurrent miscarriage and it continues to be so since a randomised treatment trial of sufficient numbers is unlikely to be completed for women with repeated late miscarriages. Armed with the facts, you, the reader, will now be in a position to make up your own mind about this treatment if it is ever offered to you.

Methods of diagnosing anatomical abnormalities

There have been many techniques used to identify anatomical abnormalities. Each has merits and disavantages and it is important for the reader to recognise that different doctors will use different methods, usually dictated by the facilities and expertise that are available to them.

Laparoscopy and hysteroscopy

Telescopic techniques such as laparoscopy and hysteroscopy are almost always available and in experienced hands can successfully diagnose most of the abnormalities discussed in this chapter. Laparoscopy is a good way of assessing the shape, size and position of the uterus, tubes and ovaries. Many suspected congenital abnormalities will be visualised in this way and, when attached to a video camera, the laparoscope will also provide a pictorial record of the problem. A blue dye is flushed through the cervix and into the uterus. This then fills the tubes and spills out through the fimbrial end into the abdominal cavity. During laparoscopy, this allows direct visualisation that the tubes are open. Hysteroscopy is a particularly useful tool, because in addition to diagnosing abnormalities, it can also be used to treat problems such as submucous fibroids, polyps and adhesions, without the need for an additional procedure. Small scissors or a looped cutting wire can be inserted into the uterus alongside the hysteroscope to remove tissues under the telescopic control. However, these techniques usually require a general anaesthetic and a short stay in hospital of less than 24 hours. They are relatively safe but of course all operative procedures carry with them a small risk of complications. This is one of the reasons why so many alternative methods have been tried, in an attempt to identify non-invasive techniques which are just as accurate.

Hysterosalpingogram

A hysterosalpingogram (HSG) is a X-ray examination of the uterine cavity (hystero-) and the fallopian tubes (salpingo-). The procedure is performed as an outpatient and you will be asked to lie down on a couch in the X-ray department. The doctor will insert a speculum into your vagina and very gently hold the upper lip of the cervix to steady it whilst inserting a tube into the cervical canal. A special radiopaque dye is then injected into the cervical canal and passes up into the uterine cavity and along the fallopian tubes. The HSG needs to be performed in the X-ray department because your abdomen will be screened with a special low-dose X-ray machine whilst the dye is being injected. A television screen will monitor the passage of the dye as it outlines the cavity and the tubes and then several hard copy X-ray films will be taken.

The HSG is usually performed by an experienced radiologist because, in addition to the permanent films taken, useful information can be gathered from watching the passage of the dye during the screening procedure. The HSG is a good method of diagnosing a cervix that is wide (and possibly incompetent), the shape of the uterine cavity and whether adhesions or fibroids are present and distorting its outline. Most congenital abnormalities will be clearly visible using this technique. Since the inside surface of the fallopian tubes is also visualised, HSGs are also used to investigate women who have experienced infertility, to see whether their tubes are open or distorted in some way. The HSG can cause some discomfort but this is not usually more severe than period pain. Some women tell me that they found the HSG very painful but painkillers can be given if you need them. After all the films have been taken, the instruments will be removed from your vagina and you will be able to go straight home.

A few last points need to be mentioned about HSGs. Since the test involves X-rays, it is performed in the first ten days of the menstrual cycle and before ovulation to avoid the risk of irradiating a fertilised ovum or young embryo. Of course, it is possible to perform the test during the second half of the cycle as long as you have used a barrier method of contraception to avoid pregnancy in that cycle. The HSG will be postponed until another date if you are having your period. This is because the pressure of the injected dye is thought to increase the possibilities of pieces of endometrial lining being dislodged backwards into the abdomen and pelvis, where it may cause endometriosis. If you have ever had a uterine or pelvic infection it is very important to tell the doctors this before the HSG is performed. They will probably suggest that you take a dose of antibiotics before the procedure and one immediately afterwards. This is because pelvic infections have a nasty tendency of recurring and the organisms that cause them are often lying quietly in the cervix. This is particularly true for infection caused by chlamydia. If the chlamydia are washed up the cervix and uterus along with the injected dye, a pelvic infection may result and this may have a serious effect on the tubes, possibly causing future infertility. I think there is a lot to be said for giving every woman who has an HSG some prophylactic antibiotics to cover the procedure. Another modality for assessing the uterine cavity and tubal patency is Hysterosalpingo-contrast sonography, or HyCoSy. It is similar to an HSG, but uses ultrasound and a contrast medium instead of X-rays, limiting the patient's exposure to ionising radiation.

Magnetic resonance imaging and computerised tomography

MRI and CT scans are sophisticated imaging methods which can provide very detailed information about the pelvic organs. They are 'gold standard' for diagnosing anatomical abnormalities but may not be routinely available because the equipment used is very expensive. This means that there may be long waiting lists for these procedures. Furthermore, since the radiological expertise required to interpret the images is specialised, very few gynaecologists have much personal practical experience in interpreting the test results. This is an important point because the only way to forward research in this area is by comparing results obtained from a large number of different units and this is just not feasible at the present time.

Ultrasound

Ultrasound has the enormous advantage of being widely available and in experienced hands it can be very informative. I consider myself very lucky to have an excellent ultrasound service, headed by a radiologist who oversees all the gynaecology scanning. As a result, the ultrasound reports for all the patients seen at my recurrent miscarriage clinic are extremely accurate and I am confident that we diagnose the presence, size and location of any uterine fibroids, the presence of adhesions and pick up congenital abnormalities in the majority of cases. Not everyone working in this field has access to such a good service, but it is worth striving for since ultrasound is non-invasive, non-painful, cheaper than all other alternatives and has no complications.

Some units prefer to rely on an HSG but it is useful to remember that these can only help to identify submucous fibroids or large intra-mural fibroids big enough to indent the uterine cavity outline by their pressure. They also take up much more time to perform and require access to radiology screening facilities. Furthermore, the introduction of three-dimensional and now four-dimensional US scanning has truly lived up to its name. It really adds a different dimension to imaging the shape of the uterine cavity. As one of my patients said to me after her 4-D scan – 'I felt as though I could reach out and touch my uterus, the picture was so clear.' The big difference with 3 and 4-D ultrasound is that it is possible to get an impression not just of the outlines of the uterus but also of the volume of the uterus, which is enormously valuable when assessing the potential contribution that a congenital abnormality or a fibroid is making to a woman's recurrent miscarriages.

For women whose anatomical problem requires further investiga-tion, and in particular those women with subfertility, a HSG, HyCoSy, laparoscopy and hysteroscopy may be required to finalise the diagnosis.

Summary

Having described the various anatomical abnormalities that may be a cause of repeated miscarriages, examined the ways in which we can iden-tify these problems and discussed the methods available to treat them, I think it is important for me to mention again that no one knows the true number of these abnormalities in the general population. All the available evidence points to the fact that a surprisingly large number of women are born with anatomical abnormalities of the uterus and in many cases they cause no problems at all. It is only if the woman experiences problems in getting pregnant (infertility) or staying pregnant (miscarriage) that these structural abnormalities are noticed.

I want to emphasise this point because it is difficult to know whether these structural abnormalities are really an important cause of recurrent miscarriage. The question that is still not answered is whether these congenital abnormalities cause recurrent miscarriages or whether they are casual associations, only identified when the woman experiences problems. If this is the case, then we run the risk of exposing many miscarriage sufferers to needless anxiety and operative procedures to 'correct' a supposed abnormality which, in truth, is just a variant of normal. Hopefully, the introduction of 3-D and 4-D scans may help to resolve this problem. Doctors in this field need to ask themselves whether they are treating themselves or the patient because they are, understandably, under pressure to do something. Although the newly developed surgical techniques are likely to make a valuable contribution to the management of a few specific cases of uterine abnormality, the message for the future is really 'hands off' and instead of operating, doctors must spend the time examining the other causes of early and late miscarriage, in particular the antiphospholipid syndrome. Finally, I must state again that I believe that true cervical incompetence is a relatively rare problem.

9

RECURRENT MISCARRIAGE – MATERNAL DISORDERS AND ENVIRONMENTAL FACTORS

Maternal disorders

Certain maternal diseases may be the cause of recurrent miscarriages. Women who suffer from connective tissue and rheumatological disorders or have chronic kidney (renal) or liver (hepatic) failure are at greater risk of miscarrying repeatedly. This is because the disease may cause such severe metabolic and hormonal disturbances that a pregnancy cannot be supported. In the case of women being treated with dialysis, miscarriage is very common, and it is unusual for such women to have successful pregnancies. However, it should also be mentioned that fertility itself is very low in women with untreated kidney or liver failure, and it is unusual for them to fall pregnant in the first place. As a result, the overall number of pregnancies miscarried for this reason is small.

It is interesting to note that if the woman receives a successful organ transplant, her fertility improves dramatically and she is much more likely to fall pregnant. Despite all the drugs that the transplanted woman has to take for the rest of her life, they do not increase her risk of miscarriage.

We now know that these drugs do not increase the risks of a fetal abnormality significantly, although for many years it was generally presumed that the steroids, and other immunosuppressive drugs used in these women, would cause developmental problems in their babies. I mention this point because, over the last 25 years, progress in the field of transplantation has been enormous. As a result, there are many young women who have undergone a successful kidney transplant and not surprisingly want to have a baby. Thanks to the significant improvements in the drug regimens now available to prevent organ rejection, this has now become possible and with specialist care many of them will be able to achieve their dream. Furthermore, we are now in a position to reassure them that their risk of fetal abnormality and miscarriage is not high, although frequently their pregnancies have to be delivered early to prevent blood pressure problems in the mother and growth problems in the baby.

It is also true that women with congenital heart problems, infection with tuberculosis and a variety of blood disorders have an increased risk of miscarriage. However, serious maternal disorders are more usually associated with problems in becoming pregnant, rather than staying pregnant. They do not make a significant contribution to the overall numbers of miscarriages. Certainly, relatively rare maternal medical disorders are correspondingly rarely causes of miscarriage.

Historically, several maternal disorders used to be listed under this section, but our improved understanding of the mechanisms involved in these disorders has demonstrated that they should now be classified differently. For example, diabetes mellitus and thyroid disfunction are now more sensibly considered as potential hormonal causes of miscarriage (see Chapters 4 and 11). Diseases such as lupus and phospholipid antibody problems might once have been considered 'maternal diseases'. They are, of course, but they themselves are caused by more generalised autoimmune disorders in the mothers. Our knowledge of these autoimmune disorders – and the problems they can cause during pregnancy – has mushroomed over the last twenty years. We now recognise that although we used to classify them in the autoimmune section (see Chapter 12) that the problems that they cause in pregnancy are usually due to the prothrombotic tendencies which develop in both the mother and the placenta. This is why I decided that in this third edition of my book, that they warrant a separate chapter (see Chapter 13).

Since the first edition of this book was published in 1997 we have come to realise that there are a lot of other factors (both inherited and acquired) in addition to the antiphospholipid syndrome which put the woman at risk of becoming more susceptible to developing blood clots in any of the blood vessels in her body, and particularly in her placental vessels, when she is pregnant. As a result, the search for prothrombotic risk factors has become a fast-growing and very exciting area of research.

I am often asked whether miscarriages are more common in women with gastrointestinal disorders such as Coeliac disease, Inflammatory Bowel Disease, and Irritable Bowel Syndrome. Coeliac disease is a common disorder in which foods containing gluten (wheat, barley and rye, but not oats) trigger local inflammation of the small intestine, which improves when gluten is excluded from the diet. Untreated or poorly controlled Coeliac disease is associated with higher rates of miscarriage, fetal growth restriction, preterm birth and maternal anaemia. However, I am happy to report that women who are able to manage their gluten sensitivity successfully do not appear to have any increase in their risk of miscarriages or any other pregnancy complications. Similarly, with Irritable Bowel Syndrome, those women who manage to keep their symptoms under control by carefully avoiding trigger foods and situations that they find stressful, do not have a higher incidence of miscarriage. For all these women, careful dietary control together with folate and vitamin B supplements should be started preconceptually.

The situation for women with Inflammatory Bowel Disease (IBD) – both Crohn's Disease and Ulcerative Colitis – is different, since these women are suffering from a generalised (or systemic) inflammatory disorder which affects many organ systems in their bodies. When their disease flares they become generally very unwell and frequently require high dose steroids to bring the inflammation under control. In this situation they are less likely to try to conceive or to be able to, and their doctors will be advising them to defer a pregnancy until their symptoms are under control – firstly to ensure that their baby is exposed to only the smallest possible steroid dosage and secondly, because flares are more likely during pregnancy in women whose disease is active at the time they conceive. When women with IBD are in remission and have good symptom control, they may well become pregnant and although they are likely to have more complications in later pregnancy, such as preterm birth and fetal growth restriction, there are no data to show that an increased risk of early miscarriage is one of them. High-dose folic acid, Vitamin D and Vitamin B12 supplements are all recommended during the preconception period and throughout the first trimester of pregnancy to reduce the risk of miscarriage and birth defects.

Asthma, hay fever and allergies

Approximately 3% of all pregnant women will have asthma but their symptoms may be missed because most pregnant women develop a degree of breathlessness. Asthma is often triggered by exposure to foods, chemicals, dust, pollen and smoke or follows a viral chest infection. Roughly speaking, one-third of women with asthma find that their symptoms improve during pregnancy, for one-third there is no change and for the remaining third the symptoms worsen. Inhaled steroids and bronchodilator drugs have no effect on the fetus and can be used without any concerns. However, those women who require oral steroids for an asthma attack during pregnancy are at risk of developing pre-eclampsia and having a baby with growth restriction or IUGR. Mothers who are able to breast feed should be encouraged to do so since breast feeding reduces the risk of the baby developing future allergies or atopy. It is important to note here that there is no reason for women to be denied anti-histamine medication during pregnancy if they have bad hay fever or other allergies.

Histamine intolerance

Over the last few years I have met an increasing number of women with a history of miscarriage, who have been told that they have histamine intolerance. This means that they have problems dealing with the histamine content of some foods they eat because they have developed a deficiency in the enzyme diamine oxidase (DAO) that breaks down or degrades the histamine that is present in certain foods. Alternatively, they may have an acquired imbalance between their histamine levels and DAO levels. Foods that are known culprits include red wine, ready meals, preserved foods and additives, cured meats, matured cheeses, tomatoes, aubergines, cocoa and chocolate, nuts and some pulses. Histamine is also found in mast cells in our blood and tissues and when these cells become activated, either by foods or numerous additional triggers such as pollen and other allergens, they release histamine which causes a local inflammatory response. This may lead to gastrointestinal upsets or blotchy, itchy skin and if your symptoms are severe it may be worth considering adapting your diet to exclude certain foods to see whether your symptoms improve. Of course, being able to identify women who have histamine intolerance does not necessarily mean that the histamine intolerance has caused the miscarriages. But nevertheless, there has been much interest in whether this is a possible new avenue of research and understanding into why some miscarriages occur.

Obesity

I think it is very important for me to emphasise to everyone reading this book the very damaging effect that obesity is having on our reproductive health. Throughout the world, the problem of obesity is quite literally growing and has now reached epidemic proportions. Indeed, the World Health Organisation was forced to change the criteria for defining obesity some years ago and raised the threshold values because the problem was becoming so common and sadly, the tide shows no sign of turning. Essentially, we measure weight by calculating an individual's Body Mass Index or BMI. This is a simple calculation of their weight in kilos divided by their height in metres squared (Wt/Ht2). A normal value is when your BMI falls within the range of 18.5 to 25. If your BMI is less than 18.5 you are underweight. If your BMI is over 25 you are overweight, but because so many people nowadays have a BMI in excess of 25, the range for overweight is now 25 to 29.9 and then when you reach a BMI of 30 you are classified as obese. Between 30 and 34.9 you are Class I obese or moderately obese. When the BMI exceeds 35 the individual is classified as seriously obese and when the BMI reaches 40 or over you are now referred to as morbidly obese. Sadly, there is an increasing number of people who have become extremely obese and have a BMI in excess of 50, which places them at very significant risk of many health problems, not least of which is their reproductive health.

We have known for many years that women who are overweight or obese find it more difficult to become pregnant. They also develop many more complications during their pregnancy and during the postpartum period. Indeed, it is now recognised that obesity increases the risk of just about every complication of pregnancy including miscarriage (both early and late), gestational diabetes, raised blood pressure and pre-eclampsia, preterm birth, rates of caesarean section, urinary tract infections, wound infections and, of course, obesity in pregnancy significantly increases the woman's risk of a blood clot or venous thrombotic event (VTE). She is also more likely to have anaesthetic complications including failed epidural or spinal regional blocks leading to the need for general anaesthesia which is far riskier for the pregnant than the non-pregnant woman due to the potential problem of gastric reflux and poor access to her veins. The other thing to mention here is that in the last confidential enquiry into maternal deaths in the UK, 50% of all the mothers that died were overweight or obese.

Being obese also has very serious consequences for the unborn baby who is at greater risk of having a congenital anomaly or birth defect, being stillborn or suffering a neonatal death. In addition, these babies are at a great risk of being born overweight (macrosomic) with all the accompanying delivery complications of high birth weight and of becoming an obese infant with a greatly increased risk of diabetes and heart disease in later life. The transmission of the problems that accompany obesity therefore, start in utero (in the womb) and become a legacy that your baby has to live with for the rest of his or her life.

We have known for over a decade that there is a specific link between miscarriage and obesity, and several studies have shown that women with a BMI of over 25 are more likely to have a sporadic or single miscarriage. More recent studies performed in recurrent miscarriage populations have further shown that a high BMI is directly linked to recurrent episodes of miscarriage. For example, one study from our unit at St Mary's identified that nearly one third of our patients were overweight and that 20% of them were obese. When we followed them up during their next pregnancies, there was a significantly increased risk of a poorer outcome when the woman's BMI was over 30.

However, many women that I see in the recurrent miscarriage clinic who are very overweight or obese, find it very difficult to accept that this is a problem that they really need to tackle before they become pregnant again, if they are to give themselves the best chance of a successful pregnancy outcome. Many of them respond to my initial suggestion that their high BMI is contributing to their miscarriages by saying that they have several friends or neighbours who are far larger than themselves and who have had several children and experienced no such trouble. Others become very angry and upset with me and tell me that I am insensitive and do not understand how difficult it is to lose weight or are frankly disbelieving that there can be a causal connection. So, over the years I have tried to find the best way to explain the link between obesity, conception delays and recurrent miscarriage.

Currently, my preferred way of triggering the best response from my patients is to explain that their body fat is not just a layer of padding, but an organ in its own right, in the same way that our skin – which covers the whole surface of our bodies – is an organ. Furthermore, I stress that this fat organ is producing all sorts of inflammatory chemicals or cytokines. I then go on to explain that there is a growing body of evidence to show that obese women produce more harmful cytokines in their fat cells and these appear to have a damaging effect on the metabolism of their ovaries and their endometrium or womb lining. In the ovary, this translates into them not ovulating so efficiently and for some women, particularly those with polycystic ovaries (see Chapter 11), their cycle may lengthen or become very infrequent because of their poorer ovulatory function. Certainly, there is very good evidence to show that women with a high BMI who manage to successfully lose weight, find that their cycles become more normal and that their ovulatory function improves.

In the womb lining the situation appears to be slightly different. Recent studies suggest that obese women have altered levels of certain endometrial proteins that play an important role in the body's response to inflammatory conditions. When there is an increase in the central fat compartment, this leads to the release of various inflammatory proteins which increase in proportion to the severity of the obesity. One hypothesis is that these proteins are markers of an ongoing inflammatory reaction in the endometrial lining of obese women with recurrent miscarriage, which may explain why they are experiencing poorer chances of implantation and lower ongoing pregnancy rates. Alternatively, it may be that increased levels of other endometrial proteins in the endometrium leads to the lining of their blood vessels behaving abnormally. This is called vascular or endothelial (the name for the cells lining the blood vessels) dysfunction and is well recognised to be a characteristic of chronic inflammatory conditions such as obesity.

Most importantly, we also know from recent research studies that losing weight and reducing a woman's BMI has an immediate and beneficial effect on both her ovulatory function and her ability to implant an embryo successfully. So, it is really important for all of the readers of this book to understand this point and if they are overweight or obese to tackle their problem straight away. I emphasise this point again and again in my clinic because losing weight is something that you will have to do yourself and my advice would be to adopt a vigorous exercise regime in addition to calorie counting your food intake. I have noticed that women who burn off their weight with exercise rather than calorie restriction to the point of near starvation, are much more likely to succeed in their weight loss goal. So, if this applies to you please start your new weight-loss diet and exercise programme today – not tomorrow, next week or next month – today please.

Environmental factors

Adverse reproductive outcomes have increased over the last 50 years and this trend cannot be explained by better methods of diagnosing problems and genetic tendencies alone. We know that childhood cancers, autism, birth defects such as hypospadias and gastroschisis, premature delivery and reduced fertility have increased by 10–40 %. Testicular cancer and hypothyroidism (underactive thyroid) have seen a dramatic increase in the western world. There is a growing body of evidence to show that environmental exposures may be contributing to these poorer health outcomes. Chemicals in pregnant women can cross the placenta and accumulate in the fetus, with long-lasting consequences. Worldwide, there has been a dramatic increase in chemical manufacturing over the last 70 years and this growth is predicted to continue for many years to come. Perhaps most worrying is the fact that current regulation of the manufacturing industry means that research must be able to prove that the substance causes harm before any steps are taken to limit exposure. Whereas in the pharmaceutical industry, research must be able to prove safety before the public can be exposed to that drug.

Environmental exposures are synthetic chemicals and metals found in our air, water, soil, food and consumer products. These chemicals include pesticides and herbicides which have been implicated as endocrine (hormonal) disruptors, causing cancers and neurodevelopmental disorders. Metals include lead, mercury and arsenic, all of which appear to lead to impaired cognitive ability (brain function) and abnormal development of the nervous system. Air pollution has been linked to reduced fertility, birth defects and poorer pregnancy and child health outcomes. The phtahlates found in many personal consumer products have been implicated in birth defects and poor neurodevelopment.

Although many environmental factors have been accused of causing miscarriages and fetal abnormalities, performing studies that can accurately identify a single agent as the cause may be impossible. Numerous drugs and environmental chemicals have been shown to cause damage in laboratory animals but there are very few data available on the effects of these agents on humans. Much of our human knowledge is based on 'clusters' of miscarriages that occur in a certain geographical area or in a particular workplace. Having noted the miscarriages, a search is then started for a potential cause. In this situation, control groups are often lacking and are even more difficult to recruit. As a result, allegations that a specific factor is to blame may become accepted in the minds of all the individuals involved.

It is impossible, in a single chapter, to cover all the environmental factors that have been implicated as a cause of miscarriage. I think it would be most useful for the reader if I focus on those potential causes that have been the source of the most concern and anxiety to the miscarriage patients attending my clinic. Effectively, this means a brief summary of the questions I am asked most frequently.

Alcohol

Any woman who has a heavy and regular alcohol intake will increase her risks of experiencing both early and late miscarriages. All the research data point towards the fact that the alcohol has both teratogenic (early) and toxic (later) effects on the fetus, and that this is related to the doses of alcohol taken by the mother. During the first few months of pregnancy, large quantities of alcohol can cause severe abnormalities in the development of the baby.

In alcoholic mothers, there is a distinctive pattern to these abnormalities which is broadly known as the 'fetal alcohol spectrum disorder' (FASD). This includes fetal alcohol syndrome which can be difficult to recognise in newborns and the diagnosis is made most accurately around four years of age. The main characteristics are intrauterine growth restriction followed by immediate failure to thrive after delivery and persistently poor postnatal growth below the expected milestones. There is a characterisic facial appearance which includes microcephaly (small head) and thin upper lip, short upturned nose, flattened nasal bridge and general underdevelopment of the middle of the face. There are also severe central nervous system signs seen in the newborn baby, such as irritability, hyperactivity, poor muscle tone, and poor sucking ability. At a later date the neurodevelopmental problems become evident, including attention deficit disorder, language delays and mild to moderate mental retardation.

It is important to realise here that it is the abuse of alcohol rather than any alcohol that is the culprit. In the 1990s it was thought that the fetal alcohol abuse syndrome affected 1 in 1000 live births. However, this figure was based on studies from the United States where the incidence is very much higher than in Western Europe. Since alcohol consumption in the United States is generally much lower than in Europe, this inverse relationship between background drinking levels and the incidence of FAS in the US has been called the 'American Paradox'. The incidence reported more recently is 6 to 9 cases per 1000 live births. There are two additional risk factors associated with FAAS. In virtually every instance in which a child has been born with FAAS, his or her mother was noted to be a smoker and of low socio-economic status, which suggests that poor nutritional status in these women influences the way in which the alcohol intake adversely affects the developing baby.

Some reports have also suggested that moderate regular drinking also increases the risk of miscarriage, milder fetal abnormalities and the possibility of a baby who is growth restricted when delivered, but these data are much weaker.

It is obviously sensible to reduce your alcohol intake to a minimum during pregnancy, especially during the first three months. However, there is little data to suggest that the occasional drink is harmful in later pregnancy. Studies looking at the effects of alcohol in pregnancy are often difficult to interpret because there are many factors to confuse the result. For example, alcoholics are usually smokers as well and tend to have a much poorer diet – so how do we establish which factor(s) caused the miscarriage?

Smoking

Women who smoke cigarettes regularly during pregnancy run a greater risk of miscarriage than non-smokers. In a detailed review of the effects of nicotine on the function of the ovary, uterus and placenta, cigarette smoking was shown to have a direct effect on the ability of the placenta to invade and proliferate (grow), particularly in the first three months of pregnancy. As I mentioned above, the effects of smoking are often difficult to separate from the effects of alcohol. It is also likely that the increased risk of miscarriage in smokers is in part due to the fact that women who smoke heavily during pregnancy tend to have a poorer diet. Certainly there are many reports that demonstrate that smoking in pregnancy can lead to a reduction in the supply of oxygen and nutrients delivered to the baby. Not only are these babies smaller (or lighter) than average, some of them are actually growth restricted and suffer from developmental problems. Interestingly, the placenta in smoking mothers is significantly larger compared to non-smokers. This increase in the size and weight of the placenta is an adaptive response to the reduced oxygen available for the baby in smokers. The tree-like projections or villi, which make up the placental lobes, produce many more capillaries (tiny blood vessels) in order to increase the surface area over which oxygen can be extracted and delivered to the baby. For similar reasons, the placentae of pregnant women who live at high altitudes are also larger.

It is important for pregnant women to understand that the significant increase in the risk of stillbirth that smoking exposes them to comes from both passive and active smoking. This is why you should avoid spending any length time in a smokey atmosphere during your pregnancy. If your partner smokes, encourage him to quit immediately or at least insist that your home is a smoke-free zone. Many antenatal clinics now offer carbon monoxide testing so that you can see whether you are surrounded by and inhaling other people's smoke on a regular basis.

Smoking also has an adverse effect on a woman's ability to become pregnant. Valuable new information has been gained from studies of in vitro fertilisation and other assisted reproduction techniques. Smoking appears to reduce the optimal functioning of the ovary in a dose-dependent manner. It may also affect fertility via effects on the function of the fallopian tubes and uterus. Although the mechanisms are not fully understood, we have known for some time that smoking is associated with a reduced incidence of uterine fibroids, endometriosis and even uterine cancers. This suggests that smoking inhibits the ability of the uterine cells to proliferate (multiply and divide). There is no doubt that men who smoke heavily are at greater risk of having both low sperm counts and producing abnormal sperm. Quitting smoking usually improves the sperm count and motility within about three months. All in all, smoking has a very adverse effect on reproductive outcome.

Coffee

Coffee and other caffeine-containing drinks (such as tea and cola) have also been implicated as a cause of miscarriage. An Italian study reported that more than six cups of coffee per day was accompanied by a higher rate of miscarriage. Larger reviews have given inconclusive results, but all suggest a possible association. In reality, most pregnant women seem to find coffee unpalatable, particularly in the first few months when the risk of miscarriage is greatest, so I think it is unlikely that they will be consuming large quantities. However, if you have suffered unexplained miscarriages, reducing your coffee intake may be a sensible precaution to take in your next pregnancy.

Cocaine

The use of cocaine and other illegal drugs of addiction is an established risk for early miscarriage and late pregnancy complications, such as preterm labour and placental abruption. There are also studies to suggest that marijuana and some of its derivatives (cannabinoid compounds) cause miscarriage and a slowing of embryo development. One study looked at the enzyme which breaks down the naturally occurring (endogenous) cannabis-like substances that we all have in our bodies. The researchers showed that when the levels of this enzyme are low in our bodies the build up of endogenous cannabinoids is associated with an increased miscarriage rate. The potential power of these observations is that the development of a routine test for this enzyme may become a useful test with which we will be able to predict the risk of miscarriage. It also raises the possibility that more research into targeting this endocannabinoid system could help to develop novel treatments for infertility.

X-rays

There is no doubt that ionising radiation can harm the fetus if the doses are high. There have been many sad examples of the damaging effects of radiation. The lessons that we have learnt from the nuclear disasters at Hiroshima, Sellafield and Chernobyl have alerted us to the fact that exposure to radiation has immediate and long-term effects. As a result, every newly qualified doctor is concerned about the potential problems that may result from a pregnant woman undergoing X-ray investigations. I entirely approve of this concern, but it is also important to mention that if you need an X-ray while you are pregnant, it is very unlikely that it will cause any damage to your baby. The doctors looking after you will only advise you to have an X-ray if they feel it is absolutely necessary. I am often asked whether a termination of pregnancy should be offered to a woman who has had an X-ray without knowing that she was pregnant. Let me assure you that the only risk of abnormality to the baby would occur if you had had a large series of X-rays before the eighth week of pregnancy and, even then, this risk is only 0.1% (one in 1,000 cases). A single X-ray will cause no harm.

The long-term effects are a result of the damaging effects that irradiation has upon human gametes – the eggs and sperm cells. We know that men and women exposed to radiation accidents have an increased risk of producing children who develop childhood cancers. Until very recently, we also thought that this risk increased with the dose of radiation that the parent had been exposed to preconceptually (before pregnancy). This was known as the Gardner hypothesis after the scientist who first described the observation. However, several later studies cast doubts on the association between the dose of radiation exposure preconceptually and the child's susceptibility to cancer. The highest rates of childhood leukaemia and non-Hodgkins lymphoma were found in the children of men working in the radiation industry who had never been exposed to radiation before their partners became pregnant. It is still not clear what the mechanism is to account for the increase in childhood cancers in the children of these workers and trying to find the answer to this important question is an ongoing problem.

Video Display Units (VDUs)

I used to receive a lot of anxious enquiries from patients fearful that VDUs may be the cause of miscarriages. Let me reassure you that using a VDU will not cause you to miscarry. Nor is there any association between VDU usage and birth defects in babies. Several large research studies have been carried and have reassuringly concluded that VDUs do not increase the risk of miscarriage. These studies have also demonstrated that even if your job demands that you work in front of a VDU screen for long periods of time each day, you are not at risk.

Air pollution

Exposure to common air pollutants such as ozone, carbon monoxide and particulate matter have been associated with reduced fertility and a variety of adverse pregnancy outcomes. It may increase the risk of early pregnancy loss according to some recent studies from the USA. Ozone is a highly reactive form of oxygen and is found in urban smog. The mechanism is not clearly understood but may be due to an increase in inflammation of the placenta and oxidative stress which can in turn interfere with fetal development. Exactly when in pregnancy it has the greatest effect requires more research. However, both acute and chronic air pollution in the few days prior to delivery has been linked to stillbirth.

Toxic metals – lead, mercury and arsenic

Lead is a naturally occurring heavy metal that has significant harmful effects on fertility, pregnancy outcome and child development. Lead crosses the placenta and is associated with miscarriages, poor fetal growth, preterm birth, reduced birth weight and various mental health problems. Children exposed to high levels of lead can suffer serious neurological and behavioural defects and stunted growth. Lead levels are very carefully regulated in the UK and nowadays most countries have now banned lead paints and reduced the lead content of gasoline, but there may still be risks of lead leaching into domestic drinking water from lead-lined pipes in very old plumbing systems. There have been several famous clusters of lead poisoning in the US that deserve a brief mention. When the city of Flint in Michigan diverted their water supply from Detroit to the Flint river to cut costs, corrosive substances in the new water supply allowed lead to leach out of the plumbing. Fertility rates plummeted by 12% and fetal deaths increased and were undoubtedly underestimated since pregnancy outcome data were only available after 20 weeks' gestation and the true miscarriage rate following this environmental disaster will never be known accurately. A similar story in the Washington DC area in the late 2000s similarly led to a drop in fertility.

Arsenic is a metal found in soil, water and some foodstuffs. Rice based foods are the most common source since rice naturally absorbs arsenic from the environment. The health risks assoociated with arsenic include a variety of cancers and learning disorders in children. Easy ways to lower the risk of exposure are to avoid giving rice-based cereals to children and cooking rice in extra water and pouring off the excess before serving and eating it. You may not realise that rice flour is frequently used in gluten-free recipes. I am told that the basmati rice grown in

California, India and Pakistan contains the lowest levels of arsenic, but the alternative if you are really worried about this risk is to switch to other grains such as quinoa and faro.

Mercury is a very toxic metal and can pollute air, water and high levels can accumulate in fish, particularly oily fish such as salmon and tuna. During pregnancy the mother absorbs the mercury through her gut, which then accumulates in the placenta and can enter the fetal blood circulation, causing growth restriction and brain damage. The mercury is later excreted in breast milk and, since it then accumulates in the newborn's brain, leads to behavioural disorders and mental retardation.

Some types of mercury (inorganic mercury) have been used in dental amalgam (fillings) for 150 years. Concerns have been raised that the mercury vapour, which is released in small quantities during the placement or removal of amalgam, could be harmful to dental workers and their assistants. It is obviously sensible to reduce exposure to any vapour or compound but the reports that dentistry workers are at greater risk of subfertility and menstrual problems have never been confirmed. Theoretically, the removal or placement of fillings in a pregnant woman could allow mercury vapour to cross the placenta and affect the baby's brain, as noted above. However, a previous directive from the Department of Health on the safety of dental amalgam concluded that there was no evidence of any harm being caused to the fetus. Nonetheless, the advice offered was that women should avoid having amalgam fillings during pregnancy. I must add here that they were also advised that there was absolutely no need to have fillings removed before pregnancy. I mention this point because several of my miscarriage and subfertility patients have told me that they have rushed off to have all their amalgam fillings extracted and replaced with ceramic alternatives. This can be a costly procedure so before you consider it do remember that there is no data to implicate amalgam as a real cause of pregnancy loss.

Microwaves, electromagnetic fields and radios

Most homes and many workplaces now have microwave ovens and I am often asked whether they may cause problems during pregnancy. There is absolutely no scientific data to support the 'scare reports' that they do and you need to treat these stories with a large pinch of salt. Similarly, there have been occasional reports suggesting that miscarriage and other problems in pregnancy are more common in women who live in the vicinity of electrical substations, electromagnetic fields and radio stations. There is nothing to support these allegations, but they have certainly been the source of considerable anxiety. Please ignore them!

Ultrasound

I am frequently asked whether ultrasound can cause damage to a pregnancy. Several large studies have looked at this issue carefully (see Chapter 7) so I feel confident in stating firmly that US causes no problems for either mother or baby. Low-frequency ultrasound is used in manufacturing watches and fine tools. There are a few reports suggesting that female employees in this field experience more headaches and episodes of vertigo (dizziness). There has never been any suggestion that low frequency ultrasound can cause miscarriage. The ultrasound used to perform obstetric scans is of high frequency.

Over the last few years there have been several 'scare' stories reported in the newspapers suggesting that repeated ultrasound scans during pregnancy may cause damage to the developing baby. Laboratory experiments have suggested that US waves may cause changes in the membranes (covering layers) of cells that potentially could affect the development of the embryo and later growth of the fetus in utero. There are no scientific data to support these assertions and, importantly, a large Swedish study has been published which has concluded that there is no association between multiple pregnancy US scans and the later occurrence of childhood leukaemia. Several other large studies looking at the follow-up of babies scanned on many occasions during complicated pregnancies have demonstrated that there are no serious developmental abnormalities in these babies. Indeed, the only difference that I am aware of between pregnancies that are scanned regularly and those that are not, is that a recent Scandinavian study reported an increase in the number of left-handed babies born to the mothers who had received multiple scans. The fear here was that the sound waves had in some way interfered with the development of the baby.

Many women are anxious that vaginal ultrasound probes may cause them to bleed, or aggravate a pregnancy that is threatening to miscarry. This is not true, and avoiding a vaginal scan may obstruct the vital monitoring of your pregnancy.

Hazards in the workplace for women during pregnancy

Over the last few years, I have been asked to give several lectures to industrial employers about the potential hazards that pregnant women may encounter at work and, in particular, whether the workplace can contribute to a woman's risk of miscarrage. Nowadays, employers are much more conscious that they must protect women in the workplace from being exposed to physical stresses and toxins that could have an effect on their ability to conceive and the outcome of their pregnancy. I have already mentioned VDUs and X-rays. All radiographers have to wear protective lead jackets when they are in contact with X-rays, whether they are male or female. It is common for female radiographers to be moved to other duties in their department when they are pregnant, although the risks to their baby are negligible because of the strict rules that apply at all times for these workers to protect them from radiation exposure. Other potential hazards for pregnant women at work can be summarised into three broad groups – physical, chemical and biological stresses.

Physical stresses

We know that severe fatigue (tiredness) can be associated with an increase in the risk of miscarriage, premature delivery and low birth weight babies. It can also increase anxiety, stress and the risks of high blood pressure. By fatigue, I mean the physical tiredness of lifting heavy loads, excessively long working hours and long periods of standing. More recently, it has been suggested that women who work regular night shifts may have a higher risk of various pregnancy problems.

The reader might be interested, at this point, to learn about the origins of maternity leave. At the end of the last century, a French obstetrician called Adolphe Pinard (the metal ear trumpet used to listen to the baby's heartbeat was named after him) noticed that women who worked in the laundry in his district in Paris had a high risk of premature delivery. He reasoned that this was related to the hard work involved in beating the laundry on the banks of the River Seine.

Dr Pinard persuaded the laundry owners to excuse pregnant woman from the most tiring duties after they reached 32 weeks (I presume that they had to do the ironing rather than the beating and the mangling). As a result, these laundry workers delivered their babies at term. In his treatise, which was published in 1895, he commented that if the laundry workers were excused hard physical work towards the end of their pregnancies the outcome of their pregnancy was as good as the wealthier folk whom he also looked after and who did no work at all. Dr Pinard's observations were the first steps towards the introduction of maternity leave for all pregnant women in the Western world.

Interestingly, one century later, European studies have revisited the association of hard physical work and the risk of preterm delivery and miscarriage in pregnant women. The conclusions are rather different and they suggest that it is not just hard physical effort but the lower socio-economic status of the pregnant woman that determines her being at greater risk of premature birth and pregnancy loss. Presumably this is because of poorer nutrition, the greater likelihood that she smokes, lower take-up of the antenatal services that are offered in our hospitals and other factors that we do not yet fully understand. These studies have fuelled the effort in the UK to encourage employers to provide comprehensive information to their female pregnant workforce about the importance of diet and avoiding smoking. The Tommy's campaign has actually set up a Pregnancy Accreditation Scheme for UK employers which lays out the optimal requirements for pregnant women in the workplace.

Chemical hazards

There are many toxic chemicals that can affect a woman's reproductive performance. Our knowledge that occupational exposure to lead can cause miscarriages, stillbirth and infertility has led to lead levels being carefully regulated in the UK. Mercury is a very toxic organic metal which is widely used in the process of gold extraction. Heavy mercury pollution is found in the air, rivers and fish in the goldfields of Brazil, where many of the pregnancy and childhood studies have been carried out (see earlier in this chapter).

Carbon monoxide gas, produced by coal and gas fires and smoking cigarettes, crosses the placenta and may lead to the baby receiving less oxygen. Ethylene oxide, which is used to ripen fruit, has been shown to increase the risk of miscarriage, so wash your fruit carefully before eating it.

A wide variety of solvents used in manufacturing industries can be the cause of miscarriages if pregnant women are overly exposed to them during their work. Fat-soluble organic solvents can cross the placental barrier and inhaling these compounds may lead to pregnancy problems. Healthcare professionals and workers in the clothing and textile industries are the most likely to experience exposure. A Canadian study looked at a very large cross-section of women working in factories, laboratories, pharmacies, dry cleaners, garages, funeral parlours, carpentry workshops and artists' studios to name but a few! They found that hydrocarbons, phenols, trichloroethylene, xylene, vinyl chloride, acetone and related compounds were the most common solvent exposures. The study showed that the incidence of congenital abnormalities was increased among the pregnant women exposed to organic solvents during pregnancy but only in those women who described symptoms of exposure. This suggests that the potentially damaging effects of these solvents may be avoided if employers provide well-ventilated working premises and if pregnant women are vigilant about wearing protective clothing and avoiding areas at work where they can smell chemicals. Miscarriages were also more frequent in the women exposed to organic solvents, together with an increase in babies with low birth weight, premature delivery, fetal distress in labour and neonatal complications.

Methylchloride is a solvent used in the furniture refurbishing industry for paint and varnish stripping. It used to be widely available in hardware and retail shops. It has been banned in the European Union since 2012 following case reports of serious toxicity and health impacts including liver and kidney failure and an increased incidence of cancers including brain, liver and lymphomas.

Vinyl chloride can also increase the risk of miscarriage in the wives or partners of male workers (plasterers, for example), if they are exposed to contaminated clothing. The same is true for pesticides used by agricultural workers.

Surgery and anaesthesia

As many as 2% of all pregnant women undergo surgery and anaesthesia during pregnancy and so it is not surprising that many patients ask about the potential risks both of the operation and of the anaesthetic drugs that are used. The safety of surgery in pregnancy is difficult to estimate because there are so many factors that need to be taken into consideration. What is certain is that no doctor is going to suggest that you have an operation whilst you are pregnant unless it is absolutely necessary. However, if you do have the misfortune to need an operation in early pregnancy the chances of you miscarrying will be determined by the type of operation you have to have, your underlying problem, your stress levels, whether you have a fever and possibly by the anaesthetic agent. Abdominal surgery after the pregnancy has reached the second trimester is generally considered to be safer than surgery carried out earlier in pregnancy. However, I suspect this just reflects the fact that the vast majority of miscarriages occur before the end of the first trimester of pregnancy. It is impossible to establish whether a miscarriage occurring to a woman who has to have an operation early in pregnancy was caused by the surgery or whether it would have happened anyway. Abdominal surgery in the third trimester of pregnancy increases the risk of making the uterus irritable, which may lead to threatened preterm labour. If you do have to have an abdominal operation in late pregnancy it is likely that the doctors will give you some tocolytic (uterus quietening) drugs to reduce the chance of this complication occurring.

Doctors and nurses working with anti-cancer drugs have an increased risk of miscarriage if they do not use protective gloves when they are administering the drugs. Anaesthetic gases have also been implicated as a cause of miscarriage and of low birth weight babies amongst anaesthetists and operating department staff. However, these data are not very strong or convincing and, perhaps most importantly, date back to a time when ventilation and scavenger systems in hospitals and dental operating rooms were not nearly as efficient as they are today.

Biological hazards

Many biological agents can affect a baby if the mother is infected during pregnancy. Many of these infectious organisms are mentioned in Chapters 4 and 10. In most cases, the risk of infection for a woman at work is no greater than the general risk of contracting the infection in the community. However, there are some women at greater risk of infections during pregnancy, such as laboratory, healthcare and nursery workers. I have already discussed the importance of women who are exposed to animals and animal products when they are pregnant (Chapter 4).

Male environmental hazards and factors contributing to miscarriage

It is important to remember that it is not just women who are exposed to environmental hazards that can affect reproduction. Men who work with lead, certain chemicals such as hydrocarbons and steel welders may develop sperm problems leading to subfertility. The declining sperm counts that have been noted in European countries over the last few decades are not fully understood. However, it is thought that a variety of toxins and pollutants, including a steady increase in the quantities of oestrogen hormone in our water supplies, may be the culprits. It has also been suggested that there is an increased risk of premature labour in the female partners of men who work in the glass, clay, stone, textile and mining industries. Further studies are needed to confirm these observations. What is certain is that the children of men who are heavy smokers and or have been exposed to radiation leaks are at risk of developing leukaemia.

More recently attention has turned to analysing the levels of DNA fragmentation in the sperm of men whose partners are experiencing both fertility and recurrent miscarriage. The sperm DNA fragmentation rate is – as it sounds – a measure or index of how damaged or fragmented the genetic code or DNA contained in the sperm has become. Most cell types in our bodies are able to repair damaged DNA, but sperm lose this capacity during their development and have to rely on repair mechanisms within the egg. If the sperm has acquired a lot of damage during its production and storage in the male reproductive tract there may be too much damage for the egg to repair. Another consideration is that as the damage increases it becomes more likely that any repair process will give rise to genetic mutations that could lead to serious abnormalities in the embryo.

It is clear that high sperm fragmentation rates are associated with longer time intervals for couples to become pregnant, poorer embryo development and an increased risk of miscarriage. Indeed some studies have suggested that high sperm DNA fragmentation rates may double the rate of miscarriages. We also know that DNA fragmentation is increased by smoking, alcohol, cannabis, sexually transmitted infections, obesity, steroid drugs, and a wide variety of other environmental factors. Importantly, fragmentation rates are often higher in older men which may well explain the higher rates of miscarriage and developmental abnormalities that have been reported in pregnancies conceived with men over the age of 45–50 years.

What is not understood is whether the use of antioxidant medications (including a variety of vitamin supplements) is able to reduce sperm DNA fragmentation rates in couples that are suffering recurrent miscarriages. This is an important question to address because men are able to make a completely new set of sperm every 3 months, in contrast to women who are born with all the eggs that they will ever have. So any intervention that reduces DNA fragmentation should only take a few months to take effect and result in improved sperm parameters for that man. So in addition to the various laboratory techniques that can now be used to measure DNA fragmentation rates, some units are exploring ways in which the total oxidant status and antioxidant capacity of sperm samples can be studied. If successful this would identify a group of men who may be eligible to enter a well-conducted trial to see whether anti-oxidant therapies for men with high sperm DNA fragmentation rates can reduce the miscarriage rate.

Summary

Many maternal disorders and environmental factors have been blamed for causing miscarriages and later problems in pregnancy. The reader will have noticed that many of these factors are difficult to research properly. The mother's age, body mass index (BMI), social habits, socio-economic status and previous pregnancy history all have a contribution to make and if she is exposed before or during pregnancy to a potential toxin, the dose and the timing of exposure appear to be critically important in determining whether problems result.

Historically, investigations for couples suffering from recurrent miscarriages were almost exclusively reserved for the female partner. Occasionally the possibility of a genetic problem may have prompted the request for a male partners to undergo chromosomal or peripheral blood karyotyping (see chapter 7). But in the majority of cases no interest in the contribution that the male makes to the problem was even considered. The realisation that high sperm DNA fragmentation rates are associated with an increased risk of miscarriage opens new doors to the investigation of these couples. It also offers the potential to explore whether giving these males antioxidant treatments improves the DNA fragmentation rate and whether this in turn helps to reduce the miscarriage rate. Well-designed, randomized trials to answer these questions are urgently needed.

In the meanwhile, the most useful advice I can offer to miscarriage sufferers is to resist the temptation of interpreting scary newspaper and magazine articles as medical fact. The stories that sell newspapers are not necessarily representative of the scientific truth. Take comfort from the fact that pregnant woman are treated as very special people in our society. No employer wants to risk exposing them to agents that could cause them harm. Many of the industrial regulations that are in practice today are over-protective, but it is as well that they remain in force.

10

RECURRENT MISCARRIAGE – INFECTIOUS CAUSES

For many years, doctors have suspected that infections are a major cause of premature labour and miscarriages. I am certain that they are, and some of the latest research into miscarriages suggests that a genetic predisposition to infection (only detectable with the use of sophisticated molecular biological techniques) has a significant part to play in determining whether a baby in utero develops an infection or is capable of fighting it off. Until these molecular techniques have been fully explored, we can only try to identify specific infective organisms that could realistically be the cause of recurrent miscarriages.

It is important to remember that a germ, bug or infective organism capable of causing repeated miscarriages is an unusual beast. It needs to be able to persist for long periods of time, and to produce minimal symptoms in order to escape diagnosis. After being diagnosed, it then has to be resistant to treatment with twenty-first-century drugs or, alternatively, be able to reinfect the woman after the treatment has been stopped. I know of very few germs capable of all these feats.

Some medical textbooks still advise doctors to perform a TORCH screen for women who have suffered repeated miscarriages. The problem with TORCH screens is that they provide us with very little useful information with which to help and advise the miscarriage sufferer. When one of the tests in the screen is positive, much distress and anxiety results, although the positive result is usually caused by high levels of antibodies in the woman's blood. This occurs because she has been exposed to an infection in the past and, in most cases, is therefore immune (protected) from future infections. Nevertheless, one of the main aims of this book is to provide you, the reader, with accurate information so that you can make up your own mind as to whether test A, B or C may help you. I therefore feel that a brief discussion about TORCH screening needs to be included.

T stands for toxoplasma – and in Chapter 4 we looked at how this organism can only infect a fetus during the course of the mother's first infection. So, by definition, toxoplasmosis cannot be a cause of recurrent miscarriage. There is one exception to this rule and that is when toxoplasma complicates a pregnancy in a woman whose immune system is suppressed, for example after a kidney or liver transplant.

O does not stand for any bug but conveniently makes up the TORCH acronym. In my reckoning, O ought to stand for 'other', because I hope that in the future we will be able to identify other organisms and other inherited immune problems in both the mother and the father.

R stands for rubella, and as the reader will have realised after reading Chapter 4, a mother infected with rubella (German measles) produces an antibody response during her first infection which protects her against future infections with the rubella virus.

C stands for cytomegalovirus (CMV) and since CMV can be reactivated in certain situations, it is possible that CMV infection is the cause of some recurrent episodes of miscarriage. (CMV infection is discussed in detail below.)

H stands for herpes and, once again, Chapter 4 showed that maternal herpes virus infections only affect the fetus during the first herpes infection, although the mother may experience repeated episodes herself.

Viral infections which may cause recurrent miscarriages

Some viral infections, such as cytomegalovirus (CMV) can be reactivated. This means that a second episode of CMV infection can be triggered off, under certain circumstances. However, this is very rare and probably only ever occurs in women whose immune system is compromised. For example, those women who are taking immunosuppressive or cytotoxic drugs, such as steroids and anti-cancer drugs. Some viruses persist in the mother's body and remain infective. The classic example of this is the human immunodeficiency virus (HIV). Since both of these viruses are possible causes of recurrent miscarriage, they are discussed here.

Cytomegalovirus infection in pregnancy

CMV is one of the herpes group of viruses and is usually acquired by close physical contact or by infected blood, urine or secretions of saliva and breast milk. In industrialised countries such as the UK, as many as 50% of women have never had an infection with CMV. The maternal infection is usually mild, with fever, sickness, enlarged lymph nodes and an abnormal white blood cell count – it is frequently unrecognised. During pregnancy, 1% of these susceptible women (one in 200) will acquire their first (primary) CMV infection. Among these 200 women, the CMV virus will probably be transmitted to the fetus in 40% of cases, which potentially involves one in 80 of the babies born to affected mothers. Babies born with congenital CMV infection are at risk of mental retardation, but the number of affected babies is very small.

At-risk groups, such as hospital, laboratory staff and nursery workers, need to take simple aseptic precautions such as careful handwashing. At the present time there is no specific treatment available for confirmed cases but this is likely to change in the future with the development of more sophisticated antiviral agents. If you suffer a CMV infection during your pregnancy, the chance of it causing a severe problem for your baby is very small. In the UK, a proven CMV infection is not considered a valid reason for suggesting a termination of pregnancy.

Human Immunodeficiency Virus (HIV)

We know that HIV can be passed on (transmitted) to the baby in utero. Most of the available data concerns the risk of vertical transmission (the direct passage of the virus from mother to baby during pregnancy and immediately after delivery). The current gold standard treatment for HIV positive women is to treat them with antiretroviral (ARVs) drugs throughout their pregnancy and this has dramatically reduced the 30% background rate of vertical transmission from mother to baby. These ARV drugs may be given as single agents or as combinations or cocktails of drugs.

With optimal care delivered by a multidisciplinary team, in which the woman receives regular ARVs, is monitored throughout pregnancy for her viral load and CD4 count to assess her disease response and is also given advice specific about delivery and breastfeeding, the vertical transmission figure falls to under 1%.

If the woman is on regular ARVs and careful monitoring reveals that the viral load remains low (<50 HIV RNA copies/ml), HIV positive mothers can be safely delivered vaginally and be treated similarly to non-HIV infected mothers. For those mothers who have a persistently high viral load, delivery by elective caesarean section is protective for the baby and results in a lower vertical transmission rate. This suggests that the passage of infected blood from mother to baby at the time of delivery must be an important risk factor. Perhaps just as important is the exposure of the baby to vaginal secretions during delivery. Certainly, the risk of HIV transmission to the firstborn twin delivered vaginally is greater than the risk to the second twin.

Recent studies have concluded that when the viral load is higher (>400 HIV RNA copies/ml), delivery by urgent caesarean section is recommended and that these mothers should be advised to avoid breast feeding and feed their babies exclusively with formula feed from the time of birth to reduce the postpartum vertical transmission rate from mother to baby.

Sadly, these measures are not practical or affordable for pregnant women in developing countries where the prevalence of HIV is much higher. For example, in sub-Saharan Africa, babies who are bottle fed have a much higher risk of dying from gastroenteritis, and since the diarrhoea, vomiting and consequent dehydration claim an enormous number of infant lives, breast milk offers them the best chance of surviving the first few months of their lives.

In the western world, the new drug therapies available for HIV positive women have significantly improved the lifespan of these women who can now expect to have a relatively normal lifestyle and life expectancy. The unanswered question remains, however – namely, since the HIV infection is persistent does this mean that this virus is a potential cause of recurrent miscarriages?

Bacteria and other micro-organisms

Syphilis
Syphilis is a proven infectious cause of recurrent miscarriage. Fortunately, it is now a relatively rare cause in developed countries because all pregnant women are screened for the infection at their first antenatal clinic

visit. Nevertheless, during the last decade there has been an increase in the number of cases of syphilis reported in pregnant women. Which is why I think it is important to continue to look for this infective organism routinely among the pregnant women I look after today. I have always argued that it is very important to do so because this is an infection that is easily diagnosed and successfully treated with penicillin antibiotics. If it is missed, two patients – the mother and the baby – will suffer unnecessary problems. Although relatively few cases are found, I think syphilis deserves a special mention here since the incidence has increased as a result of HIV infection and other sexually transmitted diseases.

In the days when syphilis was common and untreated, this infection caused a lot of miscarriages. Syphilis is referred to in the French literature of the last century as 'la plus grande avorteuse' (the greatest abortionist). The organism is called a spirochaete and its proper name is treponema pallidum. Syphilis is spread by sexual contact. It crosses the placenta and the risk of miscarriage and congenital infection is greatest soon after the mother becomes infected. When the mother is infected shortly before conception, the baby is invariably affected and the likeliest outcome is miscarriage. If she becomes infected during the first trimester of pregnancy, the risk of miscarriage is lower, but congenital infection and abnormalities in the baby are still a big problem. Typical features in the newborn baby are an enlarged liver and spleen, pneumonia, anaemia, jaundice, retarded growth, snuffles, skin ulcers and bone problems.

Many textbooks still state that the syphilis organism cannot cross the placenta until 16 weeks of gestation. This is not true, but the reason for this misunderstanding is interesting. Many years ago it was noted that mothers who were treated for syphilis before 16 weeks delivered babies who appeared not to have the obvious pointers of congenital syphilis. We now realise that a baby's immmune system is not capable of mounting the special inflammatory response – the characteristic skin lesions of syphilis – until about 16 weeks of gestation. However, the organisms can be found in the body of the fetus long before this date.

Streptococcus B
This bug is present in the vagina of one in ten women during pregnancy. Unlike the streptococcus A, the B strain is quite resistant to the acid environment of the vagina and grows well in amniotic fluid. In many

women, the streptococcus B bacteria cause no harm, but if the woman experiences a premature rupture of the membranes, this streptococcus can infect the amniotic fluid and the premature baby, causing a severe infection. Respiratory difficulties are the biggest problem in premature babies and male babies are more susceptible to the infection than female babies. The infection of the baby can occur during the vaginal delivery and may result in pneumonia and sometimes meningitis.

The reason why I have included a brief paragraph about this infection in a book concerned with miscarriages is that some women with a history of late miscarriages appear to be chronic carriers of the streptococcus B. I have met several women in my miscarriage clinic who have had repeated problems with streptococcus B and it leads me to wonder whether this organism is actually capable of causing the premature rupture of membranes, as well as infecting the amniotic fluid after the membranes have ruptured. If an infection is suspected at any stage during pregnancy, because of a past history of the problem, or because the pregnant woman has developed a vaginal discharge, it is important that vaginal swabs and a urine sample are taken promptly to look for the streptococci.

If the vaginal swab is positive, this confirms that the woman is a carrier for the Group B streptococcus. However, there is no point treating the infection during pregnancy, since the organisms will return or recolonize soon after the treatment is completed, and it is important to avoid repeated courses of treatment which will lead to antibiotic drug resistance. However, the finding that she is a streptococcus B carrier should be recorded in her maternity notes so that everyone is alerted to the importance of starting a course of penicillin antibiotics as soon as she goes into labour. This is to protect the baby from being affected by the infection during the delivery and in order to ensure that high maternal blood levels of the antibiotic are achieved swiftly, the first doses are usually given intravenously.

However, if the organism is detected in a urine sample, this requires immediate treatment with penicillin to eradicate the organism from the urinary tract. If the infection goes untreated, the inflammation and irritability of both the urinary and reproductive tracts that may follow often leads to the onset of a preterm delivery.

As well as culturing vaginal swabs, streptococcus B can also be identified using a rapid molecular technique called the polymerase chain reaction or PCR which takes just a few hours to perform and report the results.

This test offers very reliable results in pregnant women during labour both before and after the membranes have ruptured.

Mycoplasma and ureaplasma

If you have already done some reading about the infective causes of recurrent miscarriage you will have noticed that, so far, I have made no mention of mycoplasma or ureaplasma infections. These organisms are very common and are found in the vagina or cervix of as many as 70% of all women who are sexually active. During the first trimester of pregnancy, they can be identified by vaginal and cervical swabs in many women. They are of low virulence and do not usually cause an obvious discharge or infection, although they are an occasional cause of post-partum (post-delivery) fevers. Because these organisms are so common and can often be cultured in miscarriage tissues, it has been suggested that they may be a cause of sporadic miscarriage. However, prospective studies have compared the miscarriage rate in women with and without mycoplasma and ureaplasma organisms before conception and during the first few months of pregnancy, and they have not detected any increase in the number of sporadic miscarriages.

Since these organisms are so often found in the vagina and cervix, it has also been suggested that they may be the cause of some recurrent miscarriages, possibly because their constant presence sets up a low-grade inflammatory process in the endometrial lining of the uterus or womb, which is called chronic endometritis. Certainly, chronic endometritis is an important cause of repeated miscarriages in animals. Based on this theory, one study many years ago looked at the effect of treating women sufferers with tetracycline antibiotics before they became pregnant. Although the live birth rate was said to increase with the antibiotic treatment, no control groups were included and later studies did not confirm any advantage. It is important for me to remind the reader that tetracycline must never be given to pregnant women because this particular antibiotic is deposited in and discolours the babies' bones and teeth which causes them to turn green.

Fortunately, this type of uncontrolled treatment was never generally adopted because it did not take long for doctors to realise that using a 'broad spectrum' antibiotic like tetracycline (meaning that it can be used against a wide variety of infections) meant that other organisms present in the vagina would be prevented from growing too. Many of these organisms are necessary to keep the vaginal environment healthy and if broad spectrum antibiotics are used routinely, they can cause more infective problems than they solve. I am sure that most women reading this book can remember an occasion when they have developed a vaginal thrush infection after taking penicillin antibiotics for an infection somewhere else in their body, such as a dental abscess or a chest infection. The thrush infection is an overgrowth of yeast organisms in the vagina, which are normally kept under control by the normal housekeeping bacterial organisms. The antibiotics disturb this equilibrium allowing one organism to become predominant and the result is the thick curd-like itchy vaginal discharge that characterise vaginal thrush infections. Fortunately, they are usually self-limiting, and it is just a matter of time before the vaginal environment gets back to normal.

Bacterial vaginosis

We have known for some time that another vaginal infection called bacterial vaginosis is an important risk factor for premature rupture of the membranes and preterm labour. It may be of interest to the readers of this book, since we have noted in previous chapters that the difference between a preterm labour and a late miscarriage is often a grey area. If bacterial vaginosis can be the cause of some premature labours at 26 weeks of gestation, it is logical to consider that the same problem may be the cause of some late miscarriages, say at 20 weeks of gestation.

Bacterial vaginosis (BV) is a condition in which the normal vaginal organisms (which are predominantly lactobacilli) are replaced by anaerobic bacteria, the most common of which are gardnerella vaginalis and mycoplasma hominis. The vaginal secretions become more alkaline or less acidic, as the numbers of lactobacilli decrease and the numbers of anaerobic bacteria increase. The resultant vaginal discharge has a characteristic fishy smell. Bacterial vaginosis is best diagnosed not by culturing swabs but by looking at a smear taken from the top of the vagina at either side of the cervix (in the fornices). The smear of discharge is placed on to a microscope slide and fixed in methyl alcohol. The slides are then stained with Grams stain and examined under the microscope. The smears are graded – I (normal), II (intermediate) and III (bacterial vaginosis) – based on the presence or the absence of the lactobacilli and the numbers of anaerobic bacteria in the smear. The finding of a grade III smear is an indication for offering treatment with antibiotics.

We still need to do a lot more research about the triggers that cause bacterial vaginosis. We know that Afro-Caribbean women, smokers and women who use antiseptics when bathing or vaginal douches have a greater chance of developing the infection, but this does not explain why bacterial vaginosis develops. Many studies have reported that bacterial vaginosis increases the risk of late miscarriage, premature rupture of the membranes and premature delivery. Since prematurity is the most important cause of neonatal mortality and bacterial vaginosis can be successfully treated with antibiotics such as clindamycin or metranidazole, it was obviously important to find out whether antibiotic treatment for bacterial vaginosis can prevent premature delivery.

One randomized controlled trial in a low risk population of pregnant women showed that the risk of late miscarriage and preterm birth is reduced by screening women for BV in early pregnancy and treating them with oral clindamycin tablets. However, researchers in no less than eight randomized controlled trials have found that there is no benefit in screening and treating all pregnant women for BV to prevent preterm birth. On the other hand, a Cochrane review of numerous studies concluded that detection and treatment of BV in early pregnancy might prevent preterm delivery in a subgroup of women with a previous history of preterm birth. This finding raises the possibility that there must be other factors acting together with the infection which leads to the woman with bacterial vaginosis going into premature labour. So we are still in the dark about how we should manage bacterial vaginosis infections in pregnancy. What we do know now is that the predictive value of a positive test in early pregnancy is poor and it is important that we do not give pregnant women unnecessary antibiotic drug treatments during pregnancy. This is particularly important now that we know that it is not going to affect their pregnancy outcome – at least in terms of the risk of premature delivery.

The possibility that bacterial vaginosis is a cause of infertility and early pregnancy loss has also been studied. In infertility patients undergoing IVF treatment it has been shown that bacterial vaginosis present at the time of the treatment cycle does not affect the chances of conception. However, one small study did suggest that after achieving a positive pregnancy test, the risk of a very early miscarriage was increased twofold. In this study, early pregnancies included bio-chemical pregnancies as well as pregnancies visible on early US scans. The authors suggested that this could be because the bacterial vaginosis causes endometritis (inflammation of the womb lining) which could adversely affect implantation and early embryo development. Of course, an alternative explanation for these findings could be that they are due to the abnormally high oestrogen levels that develop in women who are undergoing ovarian stimulation, IVF and embryo transfer. Whichever, since the outcome of IVF treatment is unaffected by the presence of BV it is important to understand that screening and treating women before IVF treatment is not just unnecessary but may also be disadvantageous, since the use of antibiotics will encourage the growth of antibiotic-resistant organisms which may then become introduced into the embryo culture system as a result of the vaginal egg collection procedure. Whether the same observations about BV can be made in naturally occurring pregnancies is unclear.

Many years ago we undertook a study at the recurrent miscarriage clinic at St Mary's which showed that about 20% of women with a history of late miscarriages have BV infection, compared to only 9% of women with a history of early miscarriages only – a similar figure to the incidence of BV in the general population. What we wanted to find out was whether treating the infection at an early stage in pregnancy was useful, or whether BV can recolonise (redevelop) at a later stage and would therefore require repeated courses of antibiotic treatment. We followed these women through their next pregnancies and concluded that recurrent late miscarriage patients, found to be positive for bacterial vaginosis in early pregnancy, were unlikely to have the infection present later in pregnancy or at the time of delivery. Faced with all of this evidence it is difficult to justify telling a pregnant woman with a history of late recurrent miscarriage that screening for BV and treating any BV infection found will be the answer to her problems. The search for infective organisms that are a real cause of late miscarriage continues.

Future developments and the new microbiome research

The most recent developments in our knowledge of how infection may lead to miscarriage and other pregnancy outcomes and complications, comes from our understanding that so much of what goes on in our bodies is determined by microbes – the collective term for bacteria, yeasts and viruses often referred to as bugs, germs, or infective organisms. In addition to the important part they play in causing pathology or diseases, these microbes also play a key role in maintaining human health and in particular reproductive health.

The fact is that we humans provide a wonderful environment to grow and cultivate microbes and, over time, these bugs have become so accustomed to the different conditions found on and within our bodies that we have become outnumbered. For every human cell in our bodies, there are at least two bacterial cells or microbes to match it. This means that depending on our age and health status, we are carrying around anywhere between 10 and 100 trillion microbial cells. I was fascinated by a review article on the importance of our human microbiome entitled 'Microbes Maketh Man' (and Woman of course!) and to read that although we humans have approximately 20 thousand genes, there are more than nine million bacterial genes in our gut alone.

However, the relationship that we share with our bugs is a very special one because it is mutually beneficial, by which I mean that both we humans and the bugs benefit from the fact that we are living side by side. We give them a home, and they return the favour in the most extraordinarily helpful ways. For example, our gut can host up to 2kg (nearly 5lbs) of microbes that actively help us by digesting food and producing essential vitamins and energy products, breaking down medicines into useful compounds that our bodies can use, as well as helping stop other harmful organisms from causing infection. During the first few years of life, microbes even help to develop and train our immune system.

The reproductive tract is no different and it is thought that a disturbance in the finely tuned balance of bacteria in the reproductive tract or the overgrowth of harmful organisms, can influence the ability of a woman to conceive, increase the risk of miscarriage and cause preterm birth. We know that 'healthy' microbes like the Lactobacillus species (the same microbes that are used to make yoghurt) are abundant in the female reproductive tract and can help prevent infection, which is particularly important during pregnancy. Recent research from my colleagues at Imperial College, London has shown that in healthy pregnancies there is a shift towards the vagina being colonised with a few specific types of lactobacillus. They have clearly shown that poor pregnancy outcomes such as preterm birth are associated with an abnormal vaginal microbiome where a wide range of different microbes become dominant and replace the healthy lactobacilli. Interestingly it appears that the abnormal microbiome may be made worse by the use of prophylactic antibiotics which further encourage the growth of diverse organisms.

It seems likely that the vaginal microbiome also influences the chances of implantation success or failure, so we will now need to see whether there is a relationship between the development of an abnormal vaginal microbiome where the lactobacilli are replaced by various hostile bugs and miscarriage. Alternatively, since the uterus has its own microbiome and the placenta also develops a distinctive microbiome, it may be that these factors influence whether a pregnancy is miscarried or continues successfully. During childbirth, the newborn baby is exposed to the mother's microbes as it passes through the birth canal and this exposure appears to have long-term health consequences such as an increased risk of asthma or obesity in those who come into contact with 'bad' bacteria.

Perhaps the most exciting aspect of this new avenue of research is trying to understand the interactions between all of these different microbiomes, including the gut microbiome, and the maternal host and the impact they all have upon the mother's immune response in pregnancy. This is where setting up a laboratory pipeline that is able to perform individual metabolic profiling for women with pregnancy complications is so important. Each one of the microbiomes mentioned above is a product of an individual's genes and their interaction with environmental factors. This gives rise to a specific phenotype or characteristic appearance of that individual, which in turn produces metabolites or downstream products which can be measured in simple bodily fluids that are routinely collected, readily available and do not require invasive procedures to obtain them, such as blood, urine, saliva and faeces. Many pregnancy research groups are setting up storage banks of multiple samples from individual women that can be used to answer critical questions both now and in the future. I am confident that it will not be long before we are able to assess a woman's risk of miscarriage, the underlying causes of her pregnancy losses and predict her response to new treatments, using this kind of metabolic profile technology.

11

RECURRENT MISCARRIAGE – HORMONAL CAUSES

An abnormality of the hormones is often the underlying cause of many cases of recurrent miscarriage. In Chapter 4 we discussed the fact that getting pregnant and staying pregnant is dependent upon a complex hormonal jigsaw puzzle and we looked in some detail at the hormonal events which occur during a normal menstrual cycle leading up to a pregnancy. A quick look back to this section of Chapter 4 may be useful for some readers at this point.

We noted that ovulation, implantation and the early stages of pregnancy require an intricate hormonal (endocrine) environment, which is very finely tuned and has the potential to go wrong at many different stages. Of course, in many cases of sporadic miscarriage, the hormonal imbalance resulting in a miscarriage is a one-off event and is unlikely to be repeated. In this chapter we need to look at those hormonal problems which are likely to be a recurrent cause of pregnancy loss. Strange as it may seem, I think it is fair to say that of all the proposed causes of miscarriage, hormonal factors have been the most studied and yet they remain the most controversial.

Diabetes

Some of this controversy is historical. Not unreasonably, any long-standing (chronic) hormonal problem was considered to be a potential cause of miscarriage. Since women who are diabetic continue to be diabetic, they were thought to be at risk of repeated miscarriages because the problem was present in each of their pregnancies. We now know that well-controlled diabetes is not an important cause of miscarriage. But if you are diabetic and your diabetes is poorly controlled, then you do have a higher risk of miscarriage. You will also be at risk of developing a serious fetal abnormality, which is why it is very important that your sugar levels are well controlled at the time you become pregnant and during the pregnancy. Fortunately there is a very good blood test called glycosylated haemoglobin A1c that assesses how well the glucose levels in your body have been controlled over the last few months. When the HbA1c levels are high they reflect the fact that your sugars have been out of control many weeks before and this test therefore gives us some idea as to whether the tiny embryo has been exposed to a potential danger. On the other hand, if the HbA1c levels are normal this is reassuring and also helps to give the diabetic mother confidence that she is controlling her sugar levels well despite the added complication of being pregnant.

Women with poorly controlled diabetes may also experience problems in becoming pregnant and this is probably because the high glucose levels cause a break-up (fragmentation) and hence a reduction in the cells that make up the tiny embryo, which occurs before the embryo has even had a chance to try to implant in the uterine lining. The newest molecular biology techniques have also allowed us to see that high glucose levels encourage the normal process of programmed cell death to become unbalanced. Instead of there being a careful balance between cells that are being protected and cells that are being allowed to die, the cell-death-promoting pathways go into overdrive in the tiny embryo. I am conscious of the fact that all this scientific detail may sound a bit frightening, but I have included it in this edition because so many of my patients have asked me about the mechanisms involved and really want to understand the situation. Once again I want to emphasise that if your diabetes is well controlled, you are no more likely to miscarry than a non-diabetic, and it is very unlikely that you will need any help in becoming pregnant.

Many years ago we undertook an audit of all the patients attending our recurrent miscarriage clinic over a five year period, looking specifically at whether they had any history of diabetes or gestational diabetes. Gestational diabetes is a type of diabetes which is induced by pregnancy, but which usually disappears when the baby is delivered. We found that the incidence of diabetes in this large group of several thousand recurrent miscarriage sufferers is significantly less than the incidence in the general population. This study confirmed my belief – based on practical experience – that diabetes is never first diagnosed when a woman presents herself at a recurrent miscarriage clinic. In my view, screening for previously undiagnosed (occult) diabetes in women with recurrent miscarriage, by performing glucose tolerance tests, is invariably unhelpful, is a waste of resources and cannot be justified financially.

Thyroid problems

For similar reasons, screening recurrent miscarriage sufferers for previously undiagnosed thyroid disease is not a very helpful exercise. Although abnormalities of the thyroid gland may be a cause of infertility (both overactive and underactive thyroids may result in difficulties for a woman who is trying to become pregnant), I have rarely met a recurrent miscarrier in whom I have diagnosed overt thyroid disease which was unrecognised before then. The clinic audit that I mentioned in the previous paragraph also included a search for thyroid abnormalities. The results showed that thyroid abnormalities were no more common among recurrent miscarriers than in the normal female population, of whom about 3% have established thyroid disorders.

Recurrent miscarriage patients do seem to have a greater tendency for the presence of thyroid autoantibodies in their blood. For some time now, it has been suggested that the finding of these antibodies may be a way to identify women who have undiagnosed thyroid disease, or may be at risk of developing a future problem with their thyroid gland, or alternatively may be at greater risk of miscarriage.

All of these suggestions have been the subject of numerous research studies both at St Mary's and other units, and the results have been inconsistent. At St Mary's we screened several thousand women visiting our miscarriage clinic for the presence or absence of thyroid antibodies, and we were forced to conclude that their risk of future miscarriage was not dependent on their thyroid antibodies. It is true that they do have an increased incidence of thyroid antibodies (both the thyroid peroxidase and thyroglobulin types) but we did not find this correlated with abnormal thyroid function testing. We did identify some women with very high levels of antibodies who are undoubtedly at risk of developing an underactive thyroid at some point in the future.

We always advise these women to have their thyroid function checked every 3 to 6 months in the future and to watch out for any symptoms of an underactive thyroid.

The TABLET study is a randomized, controlled trial in which the main question being addressed is to see whether prescribing low doses of Levothyroxine, which is a drug or supplement used to treat an underactive thyroid, reduces the risk of miscarriage in women who have thyroid antibodies even though their thyroid hormones are in the normal range. The results are eagerly awaited.

Hyperparathyroidism

Primary hyperparathyroidism (pHPT) is the third most common endocrine or hormonal disorder after diabetes and thyroid disease. It affects between 1 in 400 to 1000 people in the general population and women are twice as likely to be affected than men. Although most cases are diagnosed in late middle age, it is recognised that approximately 1% of cases come to light during pregnancy. Interestingly, pHPT in pregnancy has been associated with an increased risk of miscarriage, pre-eclampsia, IUG restriction, premature delivery and neonatal tetany due to low calcium levels. We recently undertook a prospective study in our clinic at St Mary's, to establish the incidence of undiagnosed pHPT in women with a history of recurrent miscarriage. We measured their serum calcium, phosphate, parathormone and vitamin D levels and after treating any vitamin D deficiencies with supplements we re-checked their calcium levels. If still elevated, they were followed up by the specialist endocrine team and pHPT was confirmed in 0.34% of the women studied. They underwent surgery to remove abnormal parathyroid tissue from where it was found on the edge of their thyroid gland in their neck, and the calcium and HPT levels returned to normal almost immediately.

This prevalence figure of 0.34% in women with a history of recurrent miscarriage is very much higher than the 0.05% (1 in 2000) figure found in non-pregnant women between 20 and 40 years of age. This supports the earlier observational reports that pHPT gives rise to a threefold increase in miscarriage. Of course, we now need to follow these women and study the outcome of their future pregnancies since we still do not know whether the pHPT was a causal factor or merely associated with their previous miscarriages, but this study offers the potential of another curative treatment if studies of larger numbers of recurrent miscarriage women confirm these findings.

Progesterone deficiency

We have known for nearly 60 years that progesterone hormone is essential for the maintenance of early pregnancy. Progesterone is produced by the ovary in the corpus luteum – this is the follicle which still contains cells and is left behind in the ovary after the egg has been released (see Chapter 4 for details). In the 1970s a scientist called Csapo performed some very delicate animal experiments and showed that if the corpus luteum was removed surgically from the ovary before seven weeks of pregnancy, then miscarriage inevitably resulted. After this date, removing the corpus luteum does not cause a miscarriage, because the placenta has implanted successfully and taken over the production of progesterone which is necessary to support the pregnancy. Further evidence that progesterone deficiency can determine the outcome of an early pregnancy comes from our recent discovery that anti-progesterone hormones can be used to terminate a pregnancy before nine weeks of gestation. After this date, this method of termination is not very effective.

It is important for the reader to understand how this works. The ovary produces progesterone until the placenta has implanted properly and can manufacture its own supply for the baby. If the corpus luteum is not functioning properly, for example, because the ovulation was poor (suboptimal), the production of progesterone will be low and the pregnancy may not implant successfully. After the placenta has taken over the production of progesterone and the corpus luteum has withered away, low progesterone levels demonstrate that the placenta is not functioning properly, so effectively the pregnancy has already failed.

An inadequate corpus luteum is quite common in women with a history of recurrent miscarriage. It is sometimes referred to as luteal phase defect, or corpus luteum deficiency. There have been many studies looking at the incidence of this problem among miscarriage sufferers and the figures quoted have varied from 20 to 60%. However, low progesterone levels in the luteal phase of the cycle and an endometrial lining which is retarded (behind) in its development are the characteristic findings. Much research has been carried out as to which are the most useful investigations and tests to make the diagnosis of corpus luteum or luteal phase defect. The problem with many of these investigations is that they can only be carried out in cycles where it is known that a pregnancy has not occurred. For example, taking a biopsy of the endometrial lining can only be done in a non-conception cycle, since the biopsy may interfere with the implantation of a tiny embryo. Some of the more recent research suggests that luteal phase defects may be due to the endometrial lining failing to respond adequately to normal circulating progesterone levels. This may well be one of the reasons why attempts at treating corpus luteum and luteal phase defects with progesterone have been so disappointing.

Progesterone and HCG treatment in early pregnancy

As I have mentioned in Chapter 4, many women and their doctors hope that injections of progesterone hormone will salvage their pregnancy and prevent a miscarriage. Armed with the facts above I think that most readers will realise that no amount of injected progesterone can make the placenta implant more successfully at this stage of pregnancy and come alive again. Furthermore, the amount of hormone contained in an injection is very small – a drop in the ocean compared to the quantities that a healthy corpus luteum and a healthy placenta are producing in a successful pregnancy. Injections of hormone in the early weeks of a pregnancy at risk may prolong the miscarriage but they cannot reverse it. My view is that this is why all those clinical trials of treatment with progesterone in early pregnancy have repeatedly failed to show any benefit. In summary, low progesterone levels in early pregnancy are the result rather than the cause of miscarriage.

Nevertheless, since so many doctors and their patients continued to hope that progesterone suppositories in early pregnancy might improve outcome, the UK Medical Research Council agreed to fund a large multicentred randomized controlled trial to answer the question once and for all. The PROMISE trial recruited nearly 1000 women with a history of 3 or more early miscarriages and gave them daily progesterone supplements (or dummy/placebo suppositories) during the first trimester of pregnancy. The trial concluded unequivocally that progesterone supplements do not improve outcomes in women with a history of unexplained early recurrent miscarriages. This was true whatever their age, ethnicity, medical history and pregnancy history. Nearly two-thirds of the women in the trial had a successful pregnancy outcome, whether they were randomized to the progesterone or the placebo. A secondary outcome of the trial is that no harmful effects of progesterone treatment for women or for their babies were identified and progesterone treatment does not delay the process of miscarriage significantly. Amongst those who miscarried, there was no difference between the treated and untreated women in the stage at which they miscarried.

I should mention here that if you have been undergoing assisted fertility treatment, such as in vitro fertilisation (IVF), you will probably have been treated with regular progesterone or HCG injections from soon after the embryos were replaced in your uterus. Many IVF units believe that this is an important aid to the successful implantation of the embryos, particularly when drugs have been used to desensitise or down regulate the pituitary gland before inducing the ovaries to produce multiple eggs (see Chapter 14). Although there are no research data to specifically confirm this hypothesis, the concept is a sensible one, in my opinion. If progesterone treatment is to be of any benefit, it should probably be started before implantation takes place. There are a few recent studies which suggest that giving patients progesterone in the luteal phase of their menstrual cycle (after ovulation and at the time of implantation) may be helpful in improving the implantation rate, but there is certainly no benefit in giving this hormone in early pregnancy.

In theory, treatment with HCG in the luteal phase (second half of the menstrual cycle) should stimulate the corpus luteum to produce progesterone. However, since abnormal HCG production is often a reflection of the fact that the embryo is abnormal it is hardly surprising that none of the many studies that have been undertaken have shown that HCG supplements in pregnancy improves outcome.

A small study of women with unexplained recurrent miscarriages has suggested that HCG is only useful in a subgroup of miscarriage sufferers who also have irregular menstrual cycles (oligomenorrhoea). This has prompted a proposal to perform a multicentre trial of HCG supplements in early pregnancy for women with recurrent miscarriages and irregular cycles. However, this study was inconclusive and I think it is important for us to remember that pregnancies recruited to a study between six and eight weeks of gestation are likely to be successful anyway. As we have seen earlier in this book, the majority of early miscarriages will already have been determined by this date.

Hormonal events before ovulation

In recent years we have shifted our focus away from looking at abnormal hormone levels in early pregnancy as the most likely cause of early miscarriages, because we recognise that the hormonal events that occur before ovulation dictate the quality of the luteal phase of the cycle and, as a result, determine whether a fertilised egg will implant successfully in the womb lining. It is interesting to remember at this point that as many as one-third of all recurrent miscarriage sufferers have also had problems in becoming pregnant. When this subfertility is looked at more closely, it becomes evident that recurrent miscarriers usually suffer from ovulatory problems, rather than sperm problems or tubal disease.

These findings all point to the likelihood that subfertility and early miscarriage are two different types of the same reproductive disorder, both of which start with an abnormality in the follicular phase (first half) of the menstrual cycle, before ovulation has occurred. The consequent luteal phase is then unable to support implantation of the embryo (subfertility) or the implantation process is faulty and continuation of an early pregnancy is impossible (miscarriage).

We now need to turn to the problems that can develop in the follicular phase, before ovulation has occurred. Undoubtedly there are many, but during the last 25 years it has become increasingly clear that high levels of luteinising hormone have an unfavourable effect on a woman's ability to get pregnant. You may remember from Chapter 4 that luteinising hormone (LH) is one of two gonadotrophin hormones secreted by the pituitary gland in response to another hormonal signal from the hypothalamus in the brain – gonadotrophin hormone releasing hormone (GnRH).

Early in a normal menstrual cycle, follicle-stimulating hormone (FSH) is secreted and makes the ovarian follicles start to grow. As the follicles enlarge in size, they produce oestrogen. The rising levels of oestrogen 'feed back' to the brain, telling the hypothalamus that the egg is nearly ready to be released from the follicle and the production of FSH is slowed. The levels of LH are quite low during the early phase, but around the middle of the cycle, in response to the message from the hypothalamus triggered by the higher oestrogen levels, the pituitary gland releases a short sharp burst of LH, known as the LH surge. This LH surge releases the egg from its follicle (see Chapter 4).

High LH levels

Several problems may occur if the levels of LH are too high during the follicular phase of the cycle. Perhaps the most important is that ovulation may not occur at all (known as 'anovulation'), despite the high levels of LH which have been present during the follicular phase, because the LH surge needed to release the egg does not occur. This is a common and important cause of infertility. In fact, it was the dramatic effect that high LH levels have upon a woman's ability to become pregnant which first brought doctors' attention to this problem.

In 1985, the first publication from an assisted fertility unit suggested that when LH levels were high at the time that the eggs were harvested in women undergoing IVF treatment, the fertilisation of these eggs was poor. During the next few years, numerous studies were conducted, all showing that high LH had a very detrimental effect upon fertility. Not only was fertilisation compromised, but those eggs that did fertilise were less likely to divide into embryos, the embryos were less likely to implant in the womb lining and, of most interest to the readers of this book, the embryos were more likely to miscarry. Of course, it was possible that these high LH problems were a complication of IVF treatment, but when women undergoing fertility treatment that did not include IVF were also studied, the same correlation of poor implantation and high miscarriage rates was noted if they had high LH levels before ovulation.

The reader who remembers me talking about the Cambridge pregnancy loss study in Chapter 5 will recall that we were fortunate enough to have a captive population of women with no infertility history, who had volunteered to join the research programme before they became pregnant. They provided us with an opportunity to see whether the LH and miscarriage story held up for women who were not undergoing infertility treatment. We took blood samples from them on day 8 of their menstrual cycle and then watched what happened in their next pregnancy. The results were quite dramatic. We found that high LH levels in the follicular phase of the cycle did appear to be a risk factor for a future miscarriage. Whatever the past obstetric history, the finding of elevated LH levels before pregnancy resulted in a higher miscarriage rate. These women also took longer to fall pregnant. Women with a history of successful pregnancies and women with a history of miscarriages ran a higher risk of miscarrying if they had high LH levels before conception, when compared to women with the same past obstetric histories who had normal LH levels before conception.

Of course, this study can be criticised because we did not measure the LH levels in the cycle in which the woman became pregnant and we know that LH secretion can vary from cycle to cycle. Nonetheless, at the time it was performed in the late 1980s, the results of this research project offered us the potential of a simple test with which we might be able to predict those women who were at risk of miscarriage in future pregnancies. Although LH testing became a part of the routine investigations carried out in the recurrent miscarriage clinic at St Mary's for many years, our most recent hormonal studies have led us to realise that this test is not nearly as useful as we had originally hoped it would be.

Numerous theories as to why high LH levels may lead to miscarriage have been suggested, some more plausible than others. There are three potential places that may be adversely affected by high LH levels – the ovary, the egg and the endometrial lining. The ovary may respond to high circulating LH levels by producing inappropriate amounts of hormones at the wrong time, leading to an imbalance that does not favour successful implantation and the development of the early pregnancy.

Another theory is that high LH levels cause the egg to mature too early in the follicle and that when the egg is released, it is old, less fertilisable and less capable of implanting sucessfully or, if it implants, it is not able to progress into a viable pregnancy. Certainly there are data from animal studies to support this hypothesis, but in humans it is virtually impossible to perform the experiments necessary to address this question directly. Nevertheless, the LH surge is meant to occur in the middle of the cycle, which ensures that the egg is of optimal maturity and quality when it comes into contact with the sperm and the endometrium is at its most receptive.

However, I think the most plausible explanation is that the high LH levels cause problems in the endometrial lining, making it less receptive for a tiny embryo to implant. Certainly, if implantation is adversely affected, this might explain why miscarriages are sometimes the consequence for women with abnormally high LH levels. However, at the present time it is too early to say whether abnormally high levels of LH hormone contribute directly to an unreceptive endometrium, or whether they are just a downstream marker of some other hormonal problem that we have yet to discover.

Polycystic ovaries

Most women have high levels of LH during the surge that occurs normally just before ovulation, but it is only women with polycystic ovaries who produce high levels of LH at other times in their menstrual cycle.

The term polycystic literally means 'many cysts'. This description is a bit misleading and, for many women, it is worrying, because the use of the word 'cyst' may conjure up the vision of diseased ovaries and can even raise the suspicion that the cyst on the ovary is cancerous. So it is important for me to emphasise strongly here that polycystic ovaries are not cancerous or even pre-cancerous. Furthermore, all normally functioning ovaries contain cysts, which should be referred to as follicles. As we have seen earlier in this chapter and in Chapter 4, an ovary without follicles would mean an ovary without eggs and in that situation there would be no chance of a successful pregnancy.

When doctors talk about polycystic ovaries (in contrast to polycystic ovary syndrome – see later) what they are referring to is the appearance of the ovary on an ultrasound scan. Compared to normal ovaries, polycystic ovaries are usually slightly larger in size and contain more follicles. The characteristic scan picture shows that the follicles are positioned around the outside of the ovary and that the central tissue of the ovary (the stroma) is increased. Perhaps the best way to picture a polycystic ovary is to imagine a string of pearls. The pearls are the follicles arranged around the ovary in the same way that a necklace sits around the wearer's neck.

Polycystic ovaries are very common. About one in five women in the general population have them and they do not cause any problems. Indeed, most women with polycystic ovaries do not realise this unless they have an ultrasound scan. These women have regular periods, normal fertility and no hormonal problems. We also know that polycystic ovaries run in families, so it is likely that they are inherited.

Polycystic ovary syndrome

Some women with polycystic ovaries (PCO) also have polycystic ovary syndrome, which means that they develop certain symptoms because the polycystic ovaries are the cause of an hormonal imbalance. Their periods are irregular, light and may disappear altogether. This is because the follicles in their ovaries do not develop to the right size and so ovulation does not occur. Since the hormones produced after ovulation are missing, the endometrial lining is not shed regularly. These women usually present to their doctor because of difficulties in becoming pregnant. Others are troubled because they develop unwanted facial and body hair, which is called hirsutism.

When the syndrome is present, the woman usually has raised LH levels and may also have abnormally high testosterone levels. Testosterone is the male hormone which all women produce in small amounts from the ovaries. However, it should be mentioned here that some unfortunate women are extremely sensitive to the effects of testosterone and although the levels in their blood may not be raised, they still experience the unwanted facial and body hair growth, which are the symptoms and signs of hyperandrogenism. At least one-third of women with polycystic ovaries are overweight and there is some evidence to suggest that women with polycystic ovaries are more prone to gaining weight. If you have symptoms from your polycystic ovaries and are overweight, the first step in your treatment will be to encourage you to lose weight because this will help to improve the hormonal imbalance. Most importantly, if additional treatment with drugs proves to be necessary to help you ovulate or get rid of unwanted hair, it will be much more effective after you have lost weight.

Such treatments include the use of metformin and clomiphene to help induce ovulation, antioestrogens such as tamoxifen or letrozole and also the use of laparoscopic ovarian diathermy to improve ovarian function. Some of these treatments are discussed in more detail in Chapter 14.

Polycystic ovaries and recurrent miscarriage

It must be evident to the reader that polycystic ovaries can cause a wide spectrum of problems. At one end of the spectrum you may have no symptoms at all. At the other end of the spectrum, you may suffer from infertility, absent periods and hirsutism. Of course, like most other spectrums in life, the majority of people are in the middle and they do not have all the problems, just one or possibly two of them.

This is the point at which we must return to the subject of recurrent miscarriage. Polycystic ovaries are very common in miscarriage sufferers. So common that we perform an ultrasound scan on every woman who attends the recurrent miscarriage clinic at St Mary's just before their first consultation. We find that approximately 40% of our patients have the pearl necklace sign on the US scan, whereas the incidence in the general population is only 22%.

As we noted earlier in this chapter, high LH is a risk factor for miscarriage and high LH levels are only found in women with polycystic ovaries. So the finding of polycystic ovaries alerts us to the possibility that this recurrent miscarrier may have high LH levels, even though she may have no obvious symptoms of the polycystic syndrome. However, so long as her menstrual cycles are regular and there have been no significant delays in her conceiving, I really do not feel that more detailed testing for LH levels in either blood or urine need to be performed routinely, since the results usually do not influence how we manage that particular woman with regard to her recurrent miscarriages.

One further point needs mentioning here. In a small but very significant group of women who present to us in the recurrent miscarriage clinic also complain of perimenopausal symptoms, such as hot flushes, night sweats or light, irregular or even absent periods. In these women, testing for the levels of follicle stimulating hormone or FSH in their blood needs to be performed urgently. If the FSH levels are persistently raised over several different cycles then sadly, this suggests that the woman is starting to become menopausal. However, it is unwise to rely on the results of a single blood sample since these can fluctuate between different cycles or they may merely be a reflection that the blood test was taken on the wrong day of the cycle and has inadvertently picked up the normal surge that occurs in the mid-cycle.

When the FSH levels are raised repeatedly over several cycles, the chances of becoming pregnant and staying pregnant start to dwindle. This is because when the ovary has no more viable follicles, the oestrogen levels are so low that the pituitary gland responds by pumping out more and more FSH in a vain attempt to get the ovary to respond. If it is unable to do so, the FSH levels remain raised. If there are no eggs left in the ovary, then no amount of ovulation induction and miscarriage treatment will achieve a successful pregnancy. The only option available in this situation is IVF treatment using donor eggs. It is better to appreciate this situation earlier rather than later.

Possible treatments

If high LH levels are an important factor in determining whether a woman with polycystic ovaries can become pregnant and stay pregnant, suppressing the LH levels would be expected to improve fertility and lower the miscarriage rate. Since we now have drugs (the gonadotrophin releasing hormone analogues) that are capable of preventing the pituitary gland from producing LH and FSH, we can effectively suppress the high LH being produced by the polycystic ovaries to very low levels. Of course, this treatment also shuts down the normal cyclical activity in the ovary. In order for the woman to become pregnant, we therefore need to give her drugs to produce eggs and help her to ovulate these eggs.

This type of treatment was first tried in women with infertility. Several large studies of women attending fertility units which have demonstrated that about 50% of these women have polycystic ovaries. Although not all of them have high LH levels, we do know that the fertility treatment is less successful when the LH levels are high. Some fertility units have reported improved treatment outcomes, including both higher numbers of pregnancies and fewer early miscarriages, when they use drugs to suppress high LH levels before the woman starts her ovulation induction treatment.

The possibility that this treatment would help women with recurrent miscarriage, prompted us to set up a controlled research trial to see if there was a real benefit offered by this method of treatment. We recruited over 100 women with a history of recurrent miscarriages, polycystic ovaries and high LH levels, and divided them into three groups. If there was any suspicion that the woman had another cause for her recurrent miscarriages, such as antiphospholipid syndrome or a genetic problem, or if she had experienced any subfertility in the past, she was excluded from the trial. It took a lengthy three years to complete and I would like to express my appreciation of the research fellows and patients who participated in this trial. The results have had a major impact on our understanding of the problem and the way that recurrent miscarriage women with high LH levels have been managed ever since. This is why carefully conducted research studies are so critically important.

The first group were given the LH suppressing drug for several weeks until we could show that their LH levels were very low. This drug is often called the 'sniffing' drug because one of the ways of giving it is by sniffing it up your nostrils several times a day. It can also be given by injections in the skin. When we were sure that the ovaries were completely shut down, low doses of the follicle-inducing drug were given and when the follicle had reached the correct size, an injection of HCG was given to make the egg ovulate. After ovulation, these women were all given progesterone pessaries twice daily.

The second group were allowed to get pregnant naturally with no drugs, but they were monitored by scans and blood tests so that we knew when ovulation occurred. After ovulation they too were given progesterone pessaries. The third group were treated in exactly the same way as group 2, but instead of progesterone pessaries, they received dummy pessaries.

Of course, the best treatment trials are 'double blinded', which means that both the patient and the doctor are unaware of which drugs the patient has been given. This is the only way to completely eliminate bias. The problem for us was that it is impossible to 'blind' the effects of the LH suppressing drug, since it gives the woman menopausal symptoms, such as hot flushes, which are immediately recognisable to both her and her doctor. Even if we had given one of the groups of patients a 'dummy' suppressant drug, we and she would have known who was taking what. So we did not try to 'blind' this arm of the trial. However, we were able to 'blind' the treatment received by the women in groups two and three. Only the pharmacist who sealed the envelopes of pessaries knew whether the women received real progesterone or dummy pessaries. Groups two and three were an essential part of the trial because we needed to know whether the progesterone pessaries were having an effect of their own. Without these arms to the trial we would have been unable to assess the treatment given to group 1 accurately.

The results of this trial showed that the live birth rate in the women who were given pessaries only was slightly higher than the live birth rate in the women who were given LH suppressant and ovulation induction. Furthermore, there was no difference in the number of miscarriages experienced by the women who received progesterone or dummy progesterone pessaries. All of the treatment groups enjoyed a live birth rate in the region of 70%. These findings convinced me that the use of a complicated, labour intensive, expensive and emotionally stressful treatment with drugs to firstly suppress the LH and then to induce ovulation cannot be justified for women with recurrent miscarriages and high LH levels. It is important to remember that pituitary desensitisation and ovulation induction treatment take a toll on the patient and her doctor. This treatment involves numerous visits to the clinic for ultrasound scans and blood tests. The menopausal symptoms from the LH suppressant drug can be very troublesome and the risk of multiple pregnancy should never be underestimated. We had three sets of twins in group one, and we were lucky that none of them had any severe complications of prematurity.

Perhaps most importantly, the results of this controlled trial demonstrated that even if women do have high LH levels, polycystic ovaries and a history of recurrent miscarriage, they can still look forward to a 70% chance of a healthy baby if they are prepared to spend time visiting a dedicated clinic. I take my hat off to all the women who participated in this trial since it cost them a lot of physical and emotional effort. Their efforts were rewarded, however, since they all did so well in their future pregnancies. Their willing participation in a 'new venture' has ensured that we have uncovered the answer to an important clinical question. This treatment does not improve the miscarriage rate and not only do we no longer subject recurrent miscarriers to this type of treatment in our clinic, I don't know of any other clinics that still persist in using it. So the results of this research trial really have changed clinical practice because when we started the trial, there were numerous clinics recommending LH suppression followed by ovulation induction for women with miscarriages and high LH levels.

You will not be surprised that I am unable to finish this section without telling the reader that the results of this trial have again confirmed my belief that all miscarriage sufferers do much better if they join research programmes and are looked after by staff who have a special interest and expertise in their particular problem (see Chapter 22).

Our attention has now shifted to focus on the possible connections between polycystic ovary syndrome and insulin resistance, since insulin resistance is common in women with recurrent miscarriage and has been associated with an increased risk of miscarriage. Furthermore, since insulin resistance may be alleviated by treatments such as metformin which is often used for patients with Type 2 diabetes, it may be that this simple treatment can be helpful for some women with recurrent miscarriages (see Chapter 14 on fertility). However, it has also been proposed that the mechanism linking PCOS, insulin resistance and pregnancy loss is nothing to do with hormones and instead reflects a slowing down or impairment of the normal fibrinolytic response in our blood clotting mechanisms. Since this results in the blood developing a prothrombotic tendency, it is possible that the miscarriages in women with PCOS are a result of problems in the way that tissue remodelling occurs at the site of embryo implantation in the endometrium or decidua. There is accumulating evidence to support the hypothesis that hyperinsulinaemia is associated with impairment of fibrinolysis, which in turn is associated with miscarriage. This hypothesis is examined in greater detail in Chapter 13.

Androgens and recurrent miscarriage

Many researchers have explored the possibility that high androgen levels – specifically testosterone and androstenedione – are a useful predictive tool for identifying women with polycystic ovaries who were likely to have miscarriage problems. The results have been variable. Some of the data have suggested that recurrent miscarriers have higher androgen levels and that these increased concentrations lead to the endometrium being retarded in its development during the luteal phase, when it must go through a process of decidualisation in order to make it more receptive to any embryo that tries to implant. As a result, implantation is suboptimal and both a failure to conceive or a pregnancy that goes on to miscarry very early are more likely.

Certainly the initial results from the St Mary's clinic database identified that both serum LH and testosterone levels were raised in a minority of the recurrent miscarriage patients. But when we looked at a much larger population sample, the LH and testosterone levels among our PCO recurrent miscarriers were in the normal range for the laboratory assay that was being used. However, it may well be relevant that the LH and testosterone levels were higher overall in our PCO patients when compared to non PCO miscarriage sufferers, even though the average levels of these hormones remained within the normal range.

We need more detailed studies to explore the effect of androgens, both those produced by the ovary and by the adrenal glands, on the endometrium. We still do not really understand the effects of androgen on the endometrium in the normal luteal phase and in the decidua of normal early pregnancies, which makes interpreting results gained from failed pregnancies even more difficult. Nonetheless, I think there is much to be learnt about the causes of adverse pregnancy outcome, from a better understanding of the action of androgens on the endometrium in the second half of the luteal phase of the menstrual cycle.

Prolactin and recurrent miscarriage

Women with hyperprolactinaemia (raised prolactin levels) usually visit gynaecologists because of irregular or absent periods or because they cannot become pregnant. The symptoms are all interrelated and secondary to the fact that the secretion of high levels of prolactin from the pituitary gland invariably stops the woman from ovulating and hence the period and conception problems follow. When I first became interested in the field of pregnancy loss, I remember looking into the miscarriage rates that were experienced by women who had become pregnant as a result of fertility treatment. What I recall vividly was that several very eminent fertility experts at that time were stating categorically that when women with hyperprolactinaemia were treated with bromocriptine (the drug that suppresses prolactin secretion) and became pregnant, their miscarriage rates were no different from the sporadic miscarriage rate in the general population.

However, there have been subsequent studies suggesting that marginally elevated prolactin levels may be more common in women with a history of recurrent miscarriage. One Japanese group of researchers went on to correct the marginally raised reported prolactin levels with bromocryptine treatment. They reported that the subsequent live birth rate was significantly higher among the recurrent miscarriers with high prolactin who received treatment compared with those who were left untreated. This too is an area that probably warrants further investigation.

Endometrial receptivity

During the luteal phase of every normal menstrual cycle, the endometrial lining is transformed into 'decidua'. This change is essential to prepare the endometrium to become receptive for the implantation of an embryo. The human endometrium is unique in being able to undergo spontaneous decidualisation. Under the influence of progesterone hormone, the cells of the womb lining become swollen with nutrients that are secreted into the cavity to support any developing embryo. The supporting tissue around the cells (called the endometrial stroma) also undergoes complex changes. The stromal cells proliferate (increase in number) and secrete cytokines (special chemicals) and angiogenic factors (growth factors which promote new blood vessel formation) all of which are essential for decidualisation to be successful. We have known that this transformation is under hormonal control for many years.

Uterine natural killer cells

What has not been appreciated until relatively recently is that successful implantation also requires the presence of specialised immune cells in the decidua, which produce cytokines that help to control and modify this structural change. These cells were originally called 'endometrial lymphocytes' because they were identified by the characteristic cell surface label CD56 that they express. However, they have now become known as uterine natural killer cells (uNK). This is an unfortunate misnomer since these cells are not capable of killing anything and instead produce important cytokines and angiogenic factors that play a crucial role in helping to make the endometrial decidua receptive for implantation.

These uNK cells increase in number dramatically during the luteal phase of the menstrual cycle where they can be found surrounding the spiral arteries and glands. It is not understood whether the increased numbers of uNK cells start the process of decidualisation or whether they are the result of decidualisation, but everyone is agreed that they are there to play an important role in making the endometrium more receptive in readiness for an embryo to implant. The implantation process is a series of carefully orchestrated events. The outer cell mass of the tiny blastocyst makes contact with the decidual cells and then attaches to and subsequently invades the endometrial stroma. If implantation occurs, the outer cell mass differentiates into trophoblast or early placental cells which then start to secret HCG hormone, which in turn becomes detectable in the mother's blood and urine, giving rise to a positive pregnancy test.

When a pregnancy occurs, the uNK cells remain in high numbers in the decidua until the end of the first trimester of pregnancy. They amass in greatest numbers at the placentation site so that they are in close proximity to the invading trophoblast or placental cells and the spiral arterioles and glands. Although there are some uNK cells still present at term, they are most abundant in early gestation when the placenta is being established. This is a time of rapid placental growth before the period of accelerated fetal growth starts in the second half of pregnancy.

If no pregnancy occurs, their numbers start to dwindle just before the next menstrual period starts. These cyclical changes suggest that the uNK cells are also under hormonal control, but we know that they do not have the right cell surface receptors to be able respond directly to progesterone. Instead, the actions of progesterone on uNK cells have to be transmitted by another steroid hormone called cortisol, which in turn is enhanced by all the progesterone in the decidual bed. Cortisol has a direct effect on the preparation of the endometrial stromal cells in readiness for implantation and we now know that progesterone also binds to the cortisol receptors on uNK cells. What is so extraordinary about these uNK cells is that they are able to help the trophoblast cells burrow into the decidua and gain a foothold, but at the same time they prevent the process of invasion of the embryo from going too deep into the uterus. Exactly how they manage to do this remains a mystery and is the subject of much ongoing research.

All we can definitely say, at the present time, is that implantation involves a complex interplay of hormonal and immune factors in the decidua. A fine balance is needed for the invasion process to proceed to the right depth and no further. Many cases of infertility and miscarriage result when the invasion is too shallow or faulty in some other way. Indeed, we also know that some late pregnancy problems, such as pre-eclampsia, stem from events dictated by the quality of implantation at a very early stage in pregnancy. At the other end of the scale, when invasion is too deep, the placenta becomes so deeply embedded that it can actually grow through the deeper levels of the uterine wall. This situation is called placenta accreta. In the most extreme case, which is fortunately very rare in this country, the placenta actually behaves like a tumour and grows out of control – a choriocarcinoma or hydatidiform mole, as described in Chapter 3. In the future, when we have worked out the controlling mechanisms, we hope to be able to prevent abnormal cases of implantation. It is likely we will find that hormonal imbalances have a part to play when the decidualisation process is abnormal, but it is too early to say whether high levels of LH, FSH, testosterone, prolactin or any other hormone contributes directly to an unreceptive endometrium, or whether they are just downstream markers of other hormonal abnormalities that we have yet to discover.

Peripheral natural killer cells

I should mention at this point that the original interest in the role that NK cells may play in pregnancy loss was borne out of the old and now largely discredited hypothesis that rejection of the genetically dissimilar fetus occurs at the materno-fetal interface leading to miscarriage or recurrent implantation failure (see Chapter 12 for more details). Natural killer cells play a vital role in the innate immune response which is central to our host defense mechanisms. The primary function of the NK cells found in peripheral blood is to recognize any foreign antigens that are potentially harmful to us. Recognition of the foreign antigen initiates a whole chain of events in the blood that results in destruction or removal of the foreign antigen. Having heard this explanation, it is not difficult to understand how the term natural killer cell was born. If NK cells are capable of cytotoxic and cytolytic activity (which means killing cells and then dispensing with them) then it was proposed that this would have an adverse effect on the fetus.

However, we now recognize that peripheral NK cells and uterine NK cells are completely different types of cells and have very distinct functions. Although the peripheral NK cells circulating in our blood are so called because they have the innate ability to kill some leukaemia cell lines in laboratory conditions, the uterine NK cells have no capacity to kill these cell lines and, as noted earlier, they have a special function in the uterus to produce important cytokines to help the human implantation process. Regrettably, this name has been a driver for the myths that uNK cells can kill the embryo and are responsible for the reproductive failure in women with recurrent miscarriage and failed IVF treatment. The actual contribution of these maternal immune cells to success or failure in women with infertility and recurrent miscarriage is still largely unknown, but there is certainly no evidence that they kill trophoblast (placental) cells in these conditions. Nevertheless, a large industry has grown up to treat women who supposedly have high levels of these killer cells in their blood or their uterus. Apart from the lack of an evidence base for these treatments, they are not without risk to young healthy women. More details of these treatments can be found in in Chapter 12 on immunological treatments for recurrent miscarriage.

The Superfertility Hypothesis

More recently, a link between super fecundity or super fertility and repeated miscarriages has been proposed. An important study carried out by my colleague Professor Jan Brosens when he was working with us at Imperial College some years ago, looked at the time-to-conception intervals for women with recurrent early miscarriage. He noted that there is a subgroup of women with repeated miscarriages who appear to be able to conceive in a very short period of time – effectively in every cycle that they attempt to get pregnant. In the general population the statistical chance of this happening is extremely small, which prompted Jan to go on and undertake some laboratory experiments on tissue samples taken from the endometrium or womb lining of these women. He carefully obtained the endometrial samples in the second half of the cycle and was able to calculate how the sample date correlated with the time that implantation of the embryo can occur. This is frequently referred to as the human implantation window. He found that these women had much higher levels of implantation markers in their endometrium when compared to infertility patients and normally fertile controls. He also found that the normal markers of decidual change that should occur in the second half of the cycle were abnormally low compared with those found in woman with infertility and normally fertile controls.

He concluded that these women have 'superfecundity' because their endometrium had lost the ability to distinguish between normal embryos and abnormal embryos and as a result their endometrium allows any embryo to implant that arrives in the uterine cavity, even those embryos that are so genetically abnormal or disordered that they have no chance of developing into a viable pregnancy and are destined to miscarry very shortly after implantation.

Not surprisingly, these results and the media coverage that accompanied them led to much excitement that this was a new explanation for some cases of recurrent miscarriage and would be amenable to treatment. Furthermore, that having treated the women with recurrent miscarriages due to this problem, that many more successful pregnancies would be possible. Sadly, however, this has not proven to be the case and I think it is important for me to explain to the reader why this is so. Identifying a treatment that can make the endometrium or womb lining cells more effective at recognising which is a good or a bad embryo is not going to improve the live birth rate because that is going to be far more dependent on the genetic make-up of the embryo. And as we saw in Chapters 4 and 7 of this book, humans produce a large number of genetically abnormal embryos. It is likely that chromosomally normal embryos give out hormonal or immune signals that result in cross talk between the embryo, ovary and endometrial lining that allows the normal embryo a better chance of implanting successfully. Conversely, chromosomally abnormal embryos are less likely to be able to orchestrate this dialogue and are less likely to implant successfully and, if they do implant, they cannot develop very far and go on to miscarry early in pregnancy.

Hence, finding a treatment that normalizes the disordered endometrium in women with 'superfecundity' or 'superfertility' will mean that they have fewer positive pregnancy tests than they did before. This is because the improvement in the way that their endometrium functions means that they will be better able to differentiate between good and bad embryos arriving in the uterus. And this is why I predict that when future treatments are developed to improve this, disordered endometrium or abnormal decidualisation process will not mean that there are more live take-home babies. Instead it will mean that there are fewer pregnancies declared.

Uterine stem cells hypothesis

One of the most exciting new developments in our understanding of why some women suffer recurrent miscarriages must be the recent discovery that in some cases this may be due to a deficiency in the uterine stem cells they have present in their endometrial lining. As noted earlier in this chapter, decidualisation in the human endometrium is not dependent on embryonic implantation. Instead, the process is started during the luteal phase of each menstrual cycle and is driven by the rise in progesterone levels that are present after ovulation occurs. So, the decidualisation process is a repetitive one that depends on the successful activation of stem cells in the uterus, which can then differentiate into mature stromal endometrial cells. These stromal cells then serve as biosensors for an embryo that starts to invade the luminal epithelium. The decidualised endometrium then responds to embryonic signals in a manner that either supports further development or leads to a rapid demise by starting menstrual shedding of the endometrium. From an evolutionary point of view, this increases the likelihood of future human reproductive success by safeguarding the woman's resources and ensuring that her womb lining recovers swiftly in readiness for the next occasion when an embryo presents. Recent evidence suggests that abnormal decidualisation causes a loss of the selectivity checkpoint and makes the endometrium overly permissive to the implanting embryo but unable to sustain the pregnancy for any length of time.

Put more simply – in a healthy uterus, stem cells enable the endometrial lining to build up by about 10 millimetres over the course of 10 days after each menstrual period finishes. Some cells in the endometrium then become senescent, which means that they stop dividing and trigger an inflammatory response. The next step is for the uterine NK cells to flock to the scene and clear out the ageing cells. And in so doing the process creates a sort of honeycomb mesh in the endometrial lining, which contains holes just the right size for the tiny embryo to embed. It appears that something goes wrong in women who miscarry repeatedly.

Jan Brosens and his colleague Siobhan Quenby in Warwick have done some experiments to show that if you take samples of endometrium from the uteri of women with normal histories, that the number of NK cells keep cycling in a predictable manner throughout the month. But in the women who have miscarried several times, the numbers of NK cells varied every month, continually rising for several months in a row before disappearing and then beginning to re-accumulate. He believes that this is because they have too few stem cells and has identified that 40% of the recurrent miscarriage group he investigated had no stem cells at all. As a result, more cells enter the senescent state that attracts larger numbers of NK cells, which leads to bigger holes developing in the endometrium. This may explain why some women who frequently miscarry find it very easy to get pregnant because the large holes make it easy for the embryo to start implanting but then there is no stable structure to support ongoing development and the endometrium collapses. However, by deliberating inflicting an injury or a 'scratch' on the endometrium, it may be possible to kick start the recruitment of more stem cells into the uterine cavity in order to help with the tissue repair response that follows the injury.

Endometrial scratch technique

Endometrial scratching, also known as endometrial injury, biopsy or trauma, has been suggested as a technique that may be helpful in increasing the probability of successful implantation in women undergoing IVF treatment or those who have experienced multiple early miscarriages. The scratch procedure can be performed in the outpatient clinic with a plastic pipelle biopsy stick, without the need for a woman to undergo an admission to the day surgery unit and have any form of analgesia or anesthesia to obtain the sample. Usually the scratch procedure is scheduled for the luteal phase of the cycle immediately prior to the planned embryo transfer cycle with the idea being that the woman's endometrium would repair in time for the next treatment and improve the stem cell population and decidualisation response in readiness to receive the embryo.

There have been many anecdotal reports from private IVF units across the world suggesting that there may be a small increase in the ongoing pregnancy rates and live birth rates in women who undergo the procedure in the cycle prior to their embryo transfer. However, there are other researchers who remain sceptical about the supposed benefit of this further intervention and believe that it represents yet another unnecessary cost for a couple to bear during their distressing attempts to achieve a live baby. Several multicentre intervention trials have been funded to explore whether there is any true benefit and we await their results eagerly. We also need studies to try and better understand what the underlying mechanisms might be in the endometrial lining as it undergoes its repair following the injury.

Summary

Well-controlled diabetes, thyroid and parathyroid disease are only rarely a cause of miscarriage and routine screening tests for these disorders are not helpful. We still do not understand why polycystic ovaries are so prevalent among recurrent miscarriage sufferers. Although previous research suggested that high LH and testosterone levels could be used as markers of risk for future miscarriage, these data are no longer considered to be good predictors. Certainly, we can now state that suppressing high LH levels in recurrent miscarriers before they become pregnant does not improve the live birth rate over and above that of women with PCO who undergo careful monitoring before and during the early stages of their next pregnancy. We must now change the direction of our research and start to focus on other factors controlling the receptivity of the endometrium at the time of implantation. In the case of women with PCO it may be that they have an impaired fibrinolytic response, which contributes to the risk of miscarriage.

The exciting developments in our understanding of the factors which control endometrial receptivity and the success or otherwise of the implantation process have opened many new doors for the investigation and treatment of women with recurrent miscarriage. Studies of how the function of natural killer cells in our peripheral blood and uterine lining are so different has been a major step forward and will hopefully ensure that women with recurrent miscarriage are not advised to undergo expensive tests and non-evidence-based treatments that do not improve their chances of successful pregnancy outcome. The recent research into 'superfertility' promises to reduce the number of women who experience repeated very early losses because they have lost their ability to detect and prevent the implantation of highly abnormal embryos. Lastly, the knowledge that the uterus requires a supply of stem cells to help it go through the monthly cycle of regeneration and repair and that inflicting a deliberate injury on the endometrial tissues may help to recruit more stem cells and kick start a better response in future cycles, offers the promise of another avenue of treatment.

12

RECURRENT MISCARRIAGE – IMMUNOLOGICAL CAUSES

The human immune system plays several very important roles in reproduction. A woman's ability to become pregnant, remain pregnant and go on to deliver a healthy baby are all affected by a complicated jigsaw of immune factors. Many of these immune factors are still not clearly understood and much medical research is still needed to find the missing pieces to this fascinating puzzle.

Over the last thirty years, our understanding of reproductive immunology has increased enormously. We now recognise that there are many complex immunological adaptations that occur in the mother's immune system during pregnancy. As a result, there have been many attempts to understand whether some cases of miscarriage are the result of abnormalities in the different types of immune response to a woman's pregnancy. The two that have received most attention are alloimmune and autoimmune abnormalities and these are discussed in detail below. However, we now know that the alloimmune and autoimmune factors we can measure in the mother's general bloodstream are only part of the story. There is also a local and highly specialised immune system that develops during pregnancy at the materno-fetal interface. This interface or contact point is in the decidual bed – the part of the endometrial lining into which the placenta implants. The study of decidual immunity is now an active area of research since we know this immune response plays a key role in making the endometrium receptive to an implanting embryo (see Chapter 11 on hormonal causes). Hopefully a better understanding of the immune mechanisms that occur at the materno-fetal interface will help us to appreciate how the successful implantation of a genetically normal pregnancy is achieved and lead us on to find out what goes wrong in pregnancies that miscarry.

When we first recognised that women with Systemic Lupus Erythematosus (SLE) and other generalized connective tissue disorders, such as rheumatoid arthritis and scleroderma were at risk of pregnancy complications, they were classified as maternal disorders (Chapter 9). Further studies identified that the underlying problem was an autoimmune problem since it was only those SLE women who carried antiphospholipid antibodies (APL) that were at risk of miscarriage and later pregnancy complications. Hence, it was felt that they warranted their own section and they moved from maternal disorders into a separate chapter on immune causes of miscarriage. As we will see later in this chapter, a significant number of recurrent miscarriage sufferers have this problem.

By the time that the second edition of this book was written, we had come to realise that the antiphospholipid antibody syndrome, as well as being an autoimmune abnormality, is also an acquired type of prothrombotic disorder. This means that, having developed or acquired the antibodies, the woman becomes more susceptible to miscarriage because she is at greater risk of developing a blood clot (thrombosis) in the narrow blood vessels of her placenta. There are many different types of prothrombotic abnormality – some are acquired, and others are inherited, by which I mean they are genetically determined. The discovery that there is a variety of genetic mutations which place an individual at greater risk of developing a blood clot (venous thrombotic event, VTE) is a field of medicine that has been the focus of intensive research over the last 20 years or so. Subsequently, it was discovered that some of the women who carry these gene mutations (but by no means all of them) also appear to be at greater risk of developing a wide variety of complications during their pregnancies. And since those women who are carrying a specific genetic mutation will continue to do so for the whole of their lives, it was suggested that some of these mutations may be a cause of recurrent episodes of miscarriage. This is why in the previous edition the title of Chapter 12 was 'Immune and Prothrombotic Causes of Recurrent Miscarriage'.

As I predicted, our understanding of the important role that prothrombotic disorders play in many areas of reproduction has increased significantly over the last 10 years. I therefore think they now warrant consideration as a separate entity rather than remaining lumped in with the immune factors. This is why I have given them a separate chapter in this third edition of *Miscarriage*.

The immune system in pregnancy

I have received many requests from readers of the previous editions of *Miscarriage* for more details about the immunology of pregnancy, which is why I have included this next section. However, I need to emphasise that the theories I have tried to summarise below are exactly that – theories. At the present time there are no investigative tests that can reliably identify whether a pregnant woman has the correct immune response to 'protect' her pregnancy. Nor are there any established tests available with which we can identify potential miscarriage sufferers, and no miracle treatments, either. However, there are many websites and clinics that suggest undertaking expensive immune tests and then advise women to take a variety of unproven treatments when the results of these tests are considered to be 'abnormal'. I hope the information I have included below will help you understand why I am so concerned that you could be misled into having tests and treatments that are simply not going to help you and may in some cases cause additional harm.

The immune system is designed to protect our bodies from foreign invaders. There are two levels of immune response – innate and acquired. Innate immunity is present from birth. It is non-specific and forms a first line of defence against foreign invaders. The main cell types involved are white blood cells (lymphocytes) and natural killer cells (NK). These NK cells were originally called large granular lymphocytes because of their characteristic appearance under the microscope. The second line of defence is provided by our acquired or adaptive immunity. This is a specific response and it takes time to develop. The acquired immune response involves a variety of cells that are capable of a) attacking foreign material entering the body (cell-mediated or cytotoxic responses) and b) producing antibodies and developing a memory to the specific invaders in the body (humoral immunity).

Human pregnancy is a unique immune challenge to the mother and her baby. The baby develops in a specialised organ within the woman's body – the uterus. It is protected by a special barrier called the decidua – the name given to the endometrial lining which undergoes an extraordinary sequence of changes when the woman becomes pregnant. As the pregnancy increases in size it also exerts progressively more and more influence on the mother's body. For example, it produces many products, such as hormones and chemicals called cytokines, which are capable of altering the way that many of the mother's body systems work. Furthermore, cells from the baby and placenta float off into the mother's bloodstream on a daily basis. She has to deal with these cells which, as we will see below, is no small feat, since they are genetically different from her own. Indeed, at first glance we might be concerned that the mother's immune system would recognise them as a foreign invader and try to get rid of them.

Many theories have been suggested to explain the enigma of the mother's immune relationship with her baby. We know that both the innate and acquired systems are involved but we still do not fully understand the exact mechanisms. Many eminent scientists have worked on this puzzle for many years and numerous theories have been suggested. However, I think they can be broadly divided into two main hypotheses which are diametrically opposed to each other.

Some believe that in order for pregnancy to continue successfully, the mother's immune response must be completely suppressed during her pregnancy. But this cannot be the whole story since pregnant women do not become obviously susceptible to infections and other illnesses during pregnancy, although their response to some everyday infections may be modified or altered by being pregnant. For example, they are not at greater risk of actually catching influenza, but they do have a tendency to develop a more severe form of influenza if they are infected by the virus during pregnancy. Similarly, pregnant women are at greater risk of developing the more severe type of malaria (cerebral malaria) if they are infected during pregnancy. This is why I always tell my patients who are travelling to malaria zones or may have been exposed to the risk of catching malaria, how important it is to continue to take their anti-malarial drugs if there is any chance that they may become pregnant and to continue them during pregnancy.

The alternative hypothesis is that pregnancy requires the mother's immune system to be activated in a very specific way. Again, the details are not fully understood but it appears that there is an alteration in the balance between her innate and adaptive immune responses that allows her to tolerate the baby, but at the same time preserves her capacity to fight off any infection she meets during her pregnancy. In brief, it appears that the innate (non-specific) immune system becomes relatively active and the adaptive (specific) immune system shifts to a less aggressive type of immune response during pregnancy. The reader may have heard this alteration in balance described as a shift from Th-1 (T helper-1) immune responses to the less-damaging Th-2 (T helper-2) immune responses.

I mentioned earlier in this chapter that it is probably far too simplistic to consider the mother's systemic (bloodstream) immune response to pregnancy in isolation. Certainly, our experience in trying to pinpoint reliable and consistent alterations in her blood during pregnancy have been unsuccessful. As a result, much clinical and research effort is now being directed towards the specific localised immune responses that occur at the materno-fetal interface (or decidual bed) during pregnancy. This is why I have included a specific section on decidual immunity in this chapter and have already given the reader some details regarding endometrial receptivity in Chapter 11.

Alloimmune miscarriage

Alloimmunity is the immune reaction which occurs between the tissues of different human beings. When a tissue is taken from one human being and placed into another human being, for example during a kidney transplant, the transplanted tissue is called an allograft. Although the transplant has occurred between two humans, the genetic makeup of the donated kidney and the genetic makeup of the body into which it has been transplanted are different. In order to reduce the chances of rejection, the transplanted kidney and the person receiving it are carefully matched so that they are as genetically similar as possible. But they are not exactly the same – only identical twins have exactly the same genetic makeup. This is why drugs to suppress the alloimmune reaction are necessary to prevent the transplanted kidney from being rejected.

The amazing thing about pregnancy is that the developing baby (or fetus) is genetically different from the mother in which it develops. The fetus carries genetic material inherited from the mother and the father. As such, it has a unique genetic 'code' and is effectively a foreign transplant in the mother's uterus. The question that no one has been able to answer is: why is the baby not rejected immediately by the mother's immune system? We know that the baby is in close contact with the mother's blood supply. We also know that the uterus is not protected from immune attack. If skin from another person is placed in the uterus, it is rejected like any other foreign tissue. For many years, it was supposed that the fetus had not developed an immune system of its own, but we now know that even tiny embryos have a complex genetic structure. Furthermore, although the mother's immune system may be altered during pregnancy, it is not dampened down sufficiently to explain why she does not reject her foreign transplant – the baby.

The possibility that some cases of recurrent miscarriage are due to an abnormality in the immune relationship between mother and fetus has been an attractive one for many years. If we understood how the baby avoids rejection, we might be able to develop treatments which prevented some miscarriages. The most popular explanation that has been suggested is that successful pregnancy depends upon the mother's ability to develop a special protective response towards her baby.

This theory has undergone numerous alterations over the years as researchers have tried, in vain, to identify the exact nature of this 'protective response'. Since some women seem to miscarry repeatedly with one partner but are able to carry a pregnancy successfully with a different partner, the genetic makeup of these couples was studied. Surprisingly, some researchers reported that miscarriage occurred more frequently in couples who shared more genetic similarities (not dissimilarities) than would be expected by chance.

As a result of these findings, it was suggested that in order for the mother's body to form the appropriate protective response towards her baby, her immune system needed to recognise the 'foreign' nature of her baby. Furthermore, if the mother shared many genetic similarities with her partner, then there was a likelihood that her body would not make an adequate response, and miscarriage might result. However, subsequent research does not support the view that genetic similarities between parents increases the risk of miscarriage.

Immune therapies

Despite the lack of specific data to support the hypothesis, many clinicians still advise couples to undergo various forms of immune therapy in an attempt to reduce their risk of a further repeated miscarriage. This is why I feel that some details on these types of immunotherapy are needed here, even though there is no evidence base for their use. Let me start by telling you the story of how white cell immunotherapy came to be used in clinical practice.

White cell transfusions

White cell immunotherapy or leucocyte transfusions was one of the first immune treatments proposed for women with unexplained recurrent miscarriages. In simple terms, the woman is immunised or vaccinated with a transfusion of white blood cells taken from her partner. The idea is that this infusion of foreign white blood cells will prime her immune system to make a protective response in a future pregnancy. When she becomes pregnant again, her immune system will recognise the same foreign genetic material (contributed by the father) in her baby. As a result, the correct immune response will be 'remembered' and reinforced and the baby will be protected from rejection.

The drawback to this simple and apparently magical cure is that there is considerable doubt that it actually works. Since the first exciting reports of its use were published back in 1985, a lot of doctors have tried immunotherapy, but the results have been very variable. Some thirty years after its introduction, only one small randomized controlled trial of immunisation treatment has demonstrated a significant benefit to miscarriage patients. Several similar controlled trials have concluded that the treatment is of no benefit at all.

This is a very important point because, as you will read in a later chapter of this book, unless a treatment trial is controlled (by including patients who receive the new treatment and patients who are given placebo, or dummy, treatment) it is impossible to know whether the successful outcome is due to the treatment itself or the 'special care' that every patient involved in a trial receives. Another important issue that can no longer be ignored is that doctors who support the use of immunisation treatment are still unable to explain exactly why it should work. For the sake of completeness, I should also mention that immunisation treatment using infusions of placental tissue, white blood cells from unrelated (third party) donors and purified immunoglobulin preparations have also been tried. None of them have been shown to improve the live birth rate.

By now you will have gathered that I feel very sceptical about immunisation treatment for recurrent miscarriage, and it is interesting that most doctors feel very strongly either for or against it. Such divided opinion usually reflects the fact that those involved have developed a prejudice due to their research or clinical interests. I want, now, to give you a brief explanation of why I believe this treatment should not be used. You will then be in a position to make up your own mind, should it be offered to you in the future.

When I first became interested in the reasons why women miscarry repeatedly I felt very excited about immunisation treatment. The women I treated with white cell infusions did very well – 65% had a live baby following treatment. But when I reviewed the outcome of pregnancy in the patients who did not receive any treatment, I found that 70% of this group had a successful pregnancy. Effectively, both groups had identical pregnancy outcomes – the difference between 65 and 70% is not different statistically. So I then turned my attention to the possible differences that there may have been between these two groups of patients. I could not find any. All of the women had attended the same clinic, been offered the same investigative tests, and received the same specialised care before and during their pregnancies.

Next, I had to consider whether the test that we used to decide who was suitable for this treatment was valid. At that time, all miscarriage sufferers who were interested in having immunisation treatment had their blood tested for the presence of antipaternal cytotoxic antibody (APCA). The APCA test examined the response of the mother's blood to her partner's white blood cells. A positive APCA test result suggested that the mother was not suitable for immunisation because the presence of APCA in her blood showed that her immune system had already recognised the foreign nature of her partner's contribution to the pregnancies and responded to it. A negative APCA test result suggested that she was suitable for immunisation because she had not mounted the protective immune response to her partner's genetic material.

Helped by colleagues in Cambridge, where I was working at that time, I set up a prospective study to examine the natural history of APC antibodies in normal pregnancies. We recruited women before they became pregnant and measured their APCA levels every month throughout their next pregnancy. The results of this study, which involved over 400 women in the general population, showed that it is rare for any pregnant woman to develop APCA in her blood before the 28th week of pregnancy. If the antibodies developed in later pregnancy, they usually disappeared in the interval between pregnancies. So, in short, the absence of APCA in a non-pregnant woman is to be expected and I had to conclude that the APCA test should not be used to identify women as suitable for immunisation treatment.

Over the years, I have met many miscarriage patients who have told me that they have had a negative APCA test result and that immunisation treatment was presented to them as the answer to their problem. I used to think that although this was not correct, at least the negative result suggested that these women would not suffer side-effects if treated with white cell infusions. With the passage of time, however, I found it more difficult to try not to dissuade patients from undergoing this treatment because the evidence was accumulating that the side-effects in some cases can be serious.

Problems with white cell transfusions

Transfusion reactions, anaphylactic shock (a potentially life-threatening allergic reaction to foreign blood cells) and viral infections such as hepatitis were all reported after this treatment was first introduced. They were followed by some reports from colleagues working in infertility centres who identified that some women who had previously been miscarrying repeatedly, then became unable to conceive after the immunotherapy. This was particularly noticeable in older women who had undergone white cell treatment. Furthermore, these white cell transfusions also led to the development of many cases of chronic hepatitis later in life.

Some of the supporters of immunisation treatment have argued that as a result of small patient numbers in trials, the true benefit of immunisation treatment has been missed. However, even after pooling the results from many centres, the benefit of immunisation is very small, if it exists at all. Despite the lack of concrete data to support this treatment, it continued to be offered in some centres and I suspect that one of the reasons that immunotherapy has remained an option for so long is the extensive publicity it has received on the Internet. If I was a recurrent miscarriage sufferer I would be impressed by the adverts, too. I just hope that someone would have explained to me that the data published on the worldwide web are not subjected to peer review and that the majority of immunotherapy results reported did not offer comparisons of the pregnancy outcome among control groups because they were never performed. Many years ago, a colleague of mine in the US published a frank account of immunotherapy for recurrent miscarriage entitled 'Standard of care or buyer beware'. I think the title of his article sums up the problem for the readers of this book.

Finally, I should add that uncontrolled treatment studies using white cell infusions continued until finally a group of American and Canadian doctors performed a randomized controlled treatment trial which concluded that immunotherapy has no place in the management of women with recurrent miscarriage. This definitive conclusion effectively closed the door on the widespread use of white cell immune therapy and a few years later the US Federal Drug Administration bureau banned this type of treatment. Sadly, I have to report that other immune treatments have been proposed using a variety of different drugs. However, they are all based on the unproven theory that the recurrent miscarriage mother needs help to prevent her tiny fetus from being attacked or rejected by her own body. A brief summary of the many immunosuppressant treatment regimens that are currently available can be read later in this chapter.

Peripheral blood natural killer cells

Despite the absence of a clear immune hypothesis for recurrent episodes of miscarriage, many centres have developed increasingly more complex sets of immune investigations to identify those women who will supposedly benefit from immune therapies. Most of these clinics recommend blood tests measuring the number and type of special white blood cells in the woman's blood. These were originally called large granular lymphocytes and are now referred to as natural killer cells or NK cells.

As I mentioned in Chapter 11, these NK cells play a vital role in the innate immune response, which is central to our host defence mechanisms. The primary function of the NK cells found in peripheral blood is to recognise any foreign material (called antigens) that are potentially harmful to us. Recognition of the foreign antigen initiates a whole chain of events in the blood that results in destruction or removal of the foreign material. Having heard this explanation, it is not difficult to understand how the term natural killer cell was born. If NK cells are capable of cytotoxic and cytolytic activity (which means killing cells and then dispensing with them) then it was proposed that this would have an adverse effect on the developing embryo or fetus.

However, we now recognize that peripheral NK cells and uterine NK cells are completely different types of cells and have very distinct functions. The peripheral NK cells circulating in our blood are so called because under laboratory conditions they can be shown to have the capacity to destroy other cells which they perceive them to be harmful invaders. Uterine NK cells have no capacity to kill cells, but they do produce large quantities of important chemicals or cytokines to help the human implantation process, which is described later in this chapter in the section on 'Decidual Immunity'.

The NK cells that can be counted in the woman's circulating bloodstream are completely different to the NK cells that are active at the materno-fetal interface. I regularly see women in my miscarriage clinics who show me the results of the NK cell testing that they have undergone elsewhere – frequently at very significant expense. Often, they have been told that the results from their blood are high which indicate that they need to have some form of immune suppression treatment to dampen them down and that this will help them to protect their next pregnancy from attack. I need to mention here that the normal range for peripheral NK cell numbers and activity in blood varies widely from 5 to 30%. In any individual, the results will depend on the time of day that the blood is taken, the sex or gender of the person, and whether they are a smoker or have been exercising, to name just a few variables. Many clinics have chosen an upper cut off limit of 12%, telling their patients that any figure over 12% means that their NK cells are abnormally high and warrant treatment. However, the NK cell scientists that I have sought advice from tell me that this figure is a completely arbitrary or random choice of cut-off.

Furthermore, since there is no clinical useful information to be gained from peripheral blood NK cell testing, these tests are not routinely available in most hospital laboratories in the UK. As a result, many couples are charged to have their bloods sent abroad for a range of expensive 'special' immune tests including NK cell typing and ratios and the equally questionable T helper-1/T helper-2 ratios in peripheral blood. I have already mentioned that the human adaptive immune response is altered during pregnancy. In short, there are only ever very sparse numbers of T cells at the normal implantation site and B cells or plasma cells are completely absent from the decidua, which must raise the question of why anyone could suggest that these Th-1 and Th-2 tests on peripheral blood samples could be useful to perform in any circumstances.

Of course, some patients will take the view that blood tests are not dangerous and that they want to take every possible step to prevent a future miscarriage. However, not only do these non-evidence-based tests cost a lot of money, but perhaps more importantly they raise expectations that are frankly impossible to fulfil and, in my experience, may lead to bitter disappointments. For example, I often find myself having to explain to one of my patients that it is pointless to measure the NK cells in their circulating blood, since these cells bear no resemblance and have no correlation with the NK cells in their uterus. Indeed, in an attempt to explain this point, I wrote an article with my colleagues Ashley Moffett and Peter Braude many years ago in which we used the analogy that making the assumption that uterine NK cells were the same as peripheral NK cells was like estimating the number and activity of black cabs in Trafalgar Square by analysing the number of red minicabs circulating on the M25 motorway.

The next problem is that even if the woman has had her uterine NK cells analysed, there is still no evidence that suppressing her immune response with drugs is the answer. Indeed, it seems counter-intuitive to me to give women drugs that circulate everywhere in the body with the intention of suppressing a population of cells in the uterus that we know play an important role in allowing the embryo to implant. More recently, studies have suggested that overly inhibited uterine NK cells may cause the early placenta or trophoblast cells to prematurely halt the re-modelling of maternal blood vessels in the implantation site, which is an established characteristic of women who go on to develop pre-eclampsia in later pregnancy. The same researchers have also raised the possibility that these inhibited uterine NK cells may be the cause of many cases of unexplained recurrent miscarriage.

Despite all of these disturbing concerns, a large industry has grown up to identify and treat women who supposedly have high levels of these NK cells in either their blood or their uterus. Apart from the lack of an evidence base for these treatments, many of them are associated with potentially dangerous side effects. Brief details of some of the treatments which are being suggested to modulate the woman's immune system during pregnancy are included below.

Intravenous immunoglobulin (IVIG)

The intravenous immunoglobulin (IVIG) story turned out to be a mirror image of the white cell story. IVIG is made from antibodies extracted from the plasma component of blood from many different donors. It is usually given by an intravenous drip or infusion as treatment for severe immune deficiencies and a variety of auto-immune diseases. The theory behind treatment with IVIG was that the immunoglobulin infusions helped the mother's immune system to mop up any foreign antigen material in her body, presumably produced as a reaction to her developing baby. As a result, the immune rejection of her genetically different fetus was prevented. Once again, the theory was interesting but the data to support the actual events going on in her immune system were impossible to pinpoint. There are no specific tests to identify those women who may be most suitable for this treatment and no accepted methods for monitoring the progress of the treatment.

The initial reports of IVIG, which were uncontrolled, suggested that regular infusions of immunoglobulin during pregnancy were of benefit to some women with a history of unexplained recurrent miscarriage. The details of the treatment differed between different centres. Some used multiple doses in early pregnancy only; others advised that the infusions should continue at variable doses and intervals throughout pregnancy. Next came a couple of controlled studies of IVIG therapy which cast doubt on the benefits of this treatment.

At this point several clinicians started to query whether it was possible to justify such a high expenditure on a treatment without any proven benefit. Several financial analyses were performed and it was estimated that this treatment could cost up to forty thousand pounds per pregnancy, but there was no guarantee of success. Just like with white cell immunisation, it was then decided that a meta-analysis of all the treatment studies available be performed. This proved disappointing – no definite benefit could be identified. But this was not the end of the story and a further multi-centred controlled treatment trial of IVIG was commenced only to be abandoned when it proved difficult to recruit women to the study. It is difficult to understand why it was necessary to attempt another trial when the previous trials and the meta-analysis had already demonstrated that IVIG does not significantly increase the number of live take-home babies for recurrent miscarriage sufferers.

IVIG treatment has been associated with a variety of unpredictable risks and side-effects. Since immunoglobulins come from donor blood, there is the possibility of introducing blood-borne infections such as hepatitis and HIV. Since IVIG contains antibodies there is a theoretical risk that these antibodies could cross the placenta during pregnancy and enter the fetal bloodstream and possibly react against some of the baby's body cells. Most importantly, IVIG blocks receptors on other immune cells, alters cytokine production and neutralizes complement, thereby interfering with maternal immune defence mechanisms during pregnancy. As many as 40% of women who are given this treatment experience some sort of side effects which can range from mild to life threatening and include headache, muscle pains, fevers, chills, low back pain, thrombosis or blood clots, aseptic meningitis, kidney failure and anaphylaxis – a severe adverse drug reaction. It is important for me to mention here that the Royal College of Obstetricians and Gynaecologists, the Human Fertilisation and Embryology Authority and Public Health England have all published statements warning against the dangers of using IVIG treatment in reproduction.

Intralipid emulsions

This is a much cheaper, synthetic alternative to IVIG infusions and I have often wondered whether this was why it was first suggested as a substitute immune therapy for women with recurrent miscarriage and failed IVF treatment cycles. It is a form of intravenous nutrition which contains lipids or fats in the form of a thick liquid emulsion composed of 10% soya bean oil, 2% egg yolk and 2% glycerin. This is why many people refer to it as intravenous mayonnaise. It is said to decrease NK cell activation and for many women undergoing private fertility treatment, they are advised to have a transfusion, 7 to 10 days before their embryo transfer procedure and if they then have a positive pregnancy test they are advised to have the infusion repeated. The recognised side-effects of intralipid treatment include enlargement of the liver and spleen, jaundice, low blood platelet and white cell levels and fat overload syndrome. There has never been any evidence that intralipid improves pregnancy outcomes, but there have been several tabloid newspaper articles about women who have taken this treatment and refer to their successful pregnancy outcome as 'my miracle mayonnaise baby'.

Corticosteroids

These are a synthetic type of hormonal or steroid drug that at high doses can suppress the whole of the body's immune responses. Steroids suppress inflammatory responses and allergic disorders and are regularly used in the treatment of rheumatoid arthritis, inflammatory bowel disease, asthma and other autoimmune disorders. Steroids are a relatively cheap medication when compared to many of the other immune therapies described in this section and their usage has become widespread in miscarriage and fertility clinics over recent years. This is despite the fact that there has never been any proven advantage to the use of steroids before conception and during the first three months of pregnancy for women with a history of recurrent miscarriage or IVF failure. However, they can give rise to significant side-effects. One clinical trial in Canada demonstrated that steroid treatment increased the risk of the mother developing high blood pressure, diabetes and premature birth. Certainly, the Committee on Safety of Medicines in the UK states that corticosteroids taken in pregnancy should always be avoided unless absolutely necessary to control a previous chronic disease. There is a small risk that the baby will have its growth compromised as well as the maternal side-effects of stomach ulceration, water retention, thinning bones, fragile skin and exposure to the risks of overwhelming infections.

Anti-Tumour Necrosis Factor blocking drugs

Tumour Necrosis Factor (TNF) is a chemical produced by cells of our immune systems such as NK cells. The TNF promotes an inflammatory response and thereby allows the immune system to attack the source of the infection that is presenting to it. TNF-alpha blocking agents are drugs used to block the effect of TNF and stop the inflammatory response and thereby reduce the effectiveness of the response to the infection or agent that provokes the TNF response.

The stated rationale for using anti-TNF drugs as adjuvant or additional treatment for women with recurrent miscarriages and repeated IVF failure, is that they have NK cells in their uterine lining which are secreting TNF which in turn damages the chances of the tiny embryo from implanting successfully. Some clinics claim that in addition to making the endometrial lining thin and disordered, the TNF also damages the DNA in the embryo and it then fails to grow, divide and implant although the evidence for these assertions is lacking. Nevertheless, some women are advised to undergo an endometrial biopsy in the late stage of their cycle (such as day 26) and if the presence of

NK cells is confirmed, the anti-TNF drugs are prescribed for a period of 30 days before they try to become pregnant again. The problem with this theory is that there are always going to be NK cells in the endometrium on day 26 of the cycle – that is when they are present in the uterus at their highest number and, as we have already noted, they have an important role to play. Hence, I question the value of this type of treatment and certainly do not feel that the potential benefits are likely to outweigh the very significant side effects of these anti-TNF agents.

These TNF-blocking drugs, such as Enbrel and Remicade, have been used very successfully in the treatment of rheumatoid arthritis, asthma, ankylosing spondylitis, psoriasis and other auto-immune disorders. However, they carry significant potential side-effects, which need to be considered carefully if they are to be used in pregnant women. The clinics that prescribe them usually continue to do so until the woman is pregnant, and a viable pregnancy is confirmed on ultrasound scan. The consent form that the women are asked to sign, stating that they understand the risks and side effects of the drug they are consenting to use, is another source of worry to me. Animal studies have not shown specific fetal abnormalities associated with these drugs, but since TNF plays a role in organogenesis and the suppression of genes causing cancers, there are understandable concerns about the wide adoption of this form of treatment before properly controlled studies have been undertaken.

TNF-alpha is recognized to increase the risks of severe acute infections or septicaemia, chronic infections such as tuberculosis (and there have been case reports of TB reactivation in women treated with these drugs). In addition, cancers of the lymphatic system have been reported, together with liver problems and white blood cell disorders. These are all high prices to pay by young, fit, healthy women for receiving treatment with a drug that has never been shown to have any benefit in improving early implantation and pregnancy outcome.

Granulocyte colony-stimulating factor (GCSF)

This is another interesting new immunomodulatory option, which it has been suggested could play a part in the treatment of miscarriages and recurrent implantation failure. GCSF has been shown to stimulate neutrophilic granulocyte (white blood cell) proliferation and differentiation. It is found in reproductive organs, including ovarian follicles and the endometrium where it is tightly regulated throughout the menstrual cycle and produced by the decidual cells. The receptor for GCSF is expressed on the trophoblast (early placental) cells and we know that it is produced in large quantities during normal pregnancy. In an animal model experiment, GCSF has been shown to increase materno-fetal tolerance and reduce damaging cytotoxic activity, which is why a recombinant or synthetic human form of GCSF (rhG-CSF) has been developed for use in reproductive medicine. It is hoped that it will optimize maternal–fetal tolerance for successful implantation and maintenance of pregnancy.

GCSF has been safely used in the treatment of neutropenia (low white blood cell counts) during cancer chemotherapy, and there have been no embryotoxic effects of this substance reported. There is an ongoing randomized controlled trial called the RESPONSE trial which has been exploring the possibility that a synthetic form of GCSF called NT100, may be of help in the treatment of women with unexplained recurrent miscarriages by improving endometrial receptivity. However, we will need to await the results of this trial before we can decide whether the benefits outweigh the risks of treatment. Reported side-effects of GCSF include inflammation of mucous membranes, enlargement of the spleen and liver, anaemia, low blood pressure, nose bleeds, bone thinning and exacerbations of rheumatoid arthritis.

Decidual immunity and uterine NK cells

In Chapter 11 we looked at the factors which transform the endometrial lining into 'decidua' during the luteal phase of every normal menstrual cycle. This change is essential to prepare the endometrium for the implantation of an embryo. The cells of the womb lining become swollen with nutrients, which are secreted into the cavity to support any developing embryo. The supporting tissues around the cells (called the stroma) also undergo complex changes. We have known that this transformation is under hormonal control for many years. What had not been appreciated until more recently is that successful implantation also requires the presence of specialised immune cells in the decidua, which produce cytokines (special chemicals) that help to control and modify this structural change. These cells have been variably called endometrial leucocytes (white cells) or large granular lymphocytes (because they contain granules visible under the microscope giving them a distinctive appearance).

More recently they have become known as uterine natural killer (uNK) cells although, as I explained in Chapter 11, this is a complete misnomer since these uterine NK cells are incapable of killing anything. These NK cells increase in number dramatically during the luteal phase of the cycle. If a pregnancy occurs, they remain in the decidua until the end of the first trimester of pregnancy. If no pregnancy occurs, their numbers start to dwindle just before the next menstrual period starts and these cyclical changes suggest that they are also under hormonal control. These NK cells have special properties to ensure that the embryo, or rather the trophoblast cells of the early placenta, are able to burrow into the decidual lining and gain a firm foothold during the process of implantation. However, at the same time, the NK cells must prevent the trophoblast or early placental cells from burrowing too deeply into the uterine lining and somehow ensure that they know when to stop their invasion process. It appears to be a very delicate balance.

What we do know is that the NK cells found in the endometrium at the time of implantation have highly specialised surface markers that are only occasionally seen on the surface of the white cells or lymphocytes that are circulating in the rest of our body. Once again, this points to the likelihood that these uterine NK cells have developed specifically in order to facilitate human implantation and, of course, this function is not needed anywhere else in our bodies. This is why I mentioned earlier in this chapter that I think we need to move away from looking at and measuring the cells and immune responses in peripheral or circulating blood and concentrate more on the events that occur at the materno–fetal interface in the early weeks of pregnancy. This is easy for me to say but I am sure the reader will recognise that it is extremely difficult to obtain tissue samples from this site and undertake experiments, except when we know that the woman is not pregnant.

Nevertheless, there have now been many studies of endometrial NK cells in women with either a history of recurrent miscarriage or infertility or recurrent implantation failure following assisted fertility treatments. Several studies looking at women with a history of recurrent miscarriage who had endometrial samples (biopsies) taken in the luteal phase of their menstrual cycles, have reported an increase in the number of CD56 NK cells when compared to normal control samples taken from women with successful pregnancy histories. However, having followed these women through to their next pregnancies we now understand that these high pre-pregnancy uterine NK cell levels are not predictive of future pregnancy success or failure. The women with high levels of uterine NK cells were no more likely to miscarry than the women with so called 'normal' levels.

What is important for me to emphasise here is that many clinics are still advocating the use of systemic immunosuppressant drugs such as steroids, TNF alpha drugs, IVIG and Intralipid infusions (for details see earlier in this chapter) in order to 'suppress' the high NK cell levels. This is due to the mistaken belief that uterine NK cells are attacking the tiny embryo and threatening successful implantation and I hope the reader now recognises that this theory is seriously flawed. Sadly, the media reports of uncontrolled anecdotal treatments followed by a live birth and headlines stating, 'My body tried to kill my baby' and 'The killer cells that robbed me of my babies' has only served to heighten the demand for these immunosuppressant treatments.

The fact that some 70% of all the immune cells in the endometrium during the first trimester of pregnancy are NK cells suggests that they have an important role to play in the establishment of pregnancy. Exactly what they do is still not completely clear but they certainly contribute to endometrial growth, remodelling and breakdown on a cyclical basis. And when pregnancy is declared, their numbers increase and are maintained throughout the first trimester, so there is no reason to consider them as harmful – all of the evidence points to the fact that they play a crucial role in controlling the extent and depth of placental invasion and hence the allocation of maternal resources to the fetus. Furthermore, it is important to remember that there is emerging evidence that the suppression of NK cells may be harmful to the outcome of pregnancy. Recent studies have shown that when uterine NK cells are inhibited (for example with steroids or other systemic or generalised immunosuppressant drugs) that the trophoblast or young placental cells ceases remodelling of the uterine spiral arterioles too early in pregnancy. Premature cessation of remodelling of these maternal blood vessels is the hallmark of pre-eclampsia.

The scientific mystery which has earned human pregnancy the name of 'nature's successful transplant' has never been resolved satisfactorily. Perhaps more importantly we now recognise that considering pregnancy as an example of transplant biology is too short sighted a viewpoint. In many ways, human pregnancy has more biological characteristics in common with a tumour model which is capable of invading the mothers uterine blood vessels in order to establish successful implantation. The real scientific challenge will be to establish how the pregnancy manages to put brakes on the invasion process and knows how to stop at a certain point. When we understand that piece of the jigsaw we will be able to use the knowledge in the fight against cancers.

Inherited immune deficiencies

I mentioned in an earlier chapter, that there has been considerable interest in the possibility that inherited immune deficiencies may be a cause of some repeated miscarriages. A human being's ability to mount an appropriate defensive action against a foreign invader is very complex. Doubtless, it is designed this way, involving many different mechanisms, so that we can mount a successful defence and do not succumb to life threatening infections. Recently, it has been found that a mutation (abnormality) in the gene which is in charge of producing a protein called mannose binding protein (MBP) results in low levels of this protein in the blood. A low MBP-level in some infants makes them susceptible to severe infections during the first few years of their lives. Interestingly, there is also some evidence to suggest that some couples who experience recurrent late miscarriages have low levels of MBP in their blood, when compared to couples with a normal pregnancy history. Although only a theory at the present time, it is possible that these couples could pass on a double dose of the MBP mutation to their fetus, which makes their fetus susceptible to overwhelming infection while still in utero.

We have been considering looking into this possibility in the miscarriage clinic at St Mary's and looking for the MBP gene mutations. If we can show that a mutation is more common in these couples, we will then be able to extend the research by trying to identify the in utero infections that may be associated with this inherited immune deficiency. Of course, there is a long way to go before this type of research can be translated into a potential treatment. At the present time, the data do not show that this genetic mutation is more common in recurrent miscarriage couples than in couples with several successful pregnancies. However, there is a suggestion that the MBP mutation may be present more frequently in women who have had a previous premature delivery – another piece of evidence to support the hypothesis mentioned in earlier chapters of this book, that it is not just the presence of a bug that causes preterm labour to start. Instead, several adverse factors have to be working together to allow the bug to get a hold and one likely candidate is the capability of the host (mother's) immune system to deal with the problem.

Autoimmune miscarriage

Autoimmunity is the term used to describe immune reactions in the body, caused by the production of antibodies which act against our own tissues (anti-'self' antibodies). Our bodies are capable of producing autoantibodies which work against many different tissues and organs. In general, these autoantibodies are destructive and cause a variety of diseases. Why these immune reactions develop in some people is not fully understood, although they are often passed on from generation to generation. They are more common in women and tend to develop in middle age, although they can also occur at earlier ages. Common examples are rheumatoid arthritis and certain types of diabetes and thyroid disease. The possible links between diabetes and autoimmune thyroid disease with infertility and recurrent miscarriage have been included in the earlier chapter on hormonal causes.

It has been known for many years that women with the autoimmune disorder called systemic lupus erythematosus (SLE), often referred to as 'lupus', experience a variety of complications in pregnancy. SLE is the most common autoimmune disorder in women of reproductive age. Although SLE sufferers appear to have no trouble falling pregnant, they have a high rate of miscarriage, and are also at greater risk of a variety of later pregnancy complications. However, not every woman with SLE develops pregnancy complications. Many of them have completely normal pregnancies. The realisation that it is only the women with SLE who have circulating antiphospholipid antibodies (or APL) who experience the miscarriages and later pregnancy problems, prompted doctors to move this disorder out of the maternal disease section (see Chapter 9) and instead classify it as one of the immunological causes of miscarriage (see Chapter 12).

We now recognize that the mechanism that causes women with APL antibodies to suffer recurrent miscarriages is due to the prothrombotic tendency that these women develop. Since our understanding of this important area of medicine has grown dramatically since the last edition of this book was published, it now warrants a section of its own. The interested reader should now turn to Chapter 13 where I have included much detail about APL pregnancy complications, their treatment and many other prothrombotic disorders that have an effect on pregnancy outcomes.

Chronic histiocytic intervillositis (CHI)

This is a relatively rare autoimmune condition and is poorly understood. Since I have been asked to review an increasing number of cases recently from different regions of the UK, I think it is worth mentioning here. CHI is characterized by a dramatic infiltration of the placental intervillous space by massive numbers of white cells – monocytes, lymphocytes and histiocytes from the mother's blood. The presence of these maternally derived cells in the intervillous space underpins the hypothesis that an immune mechanism is responsible for the placental damage that occurs. However, it is recognized that malaria and cytomegalovirus infection is sometimes the precipitating cause. In the absence of finding any organisms or evidence of the mother having diagnostic symptoms of these infections, it is assumed that the problems are due to an abnormal immune response to the pregnancy.

CHI is known to have a very high recurrence rate of around 70–80%. In severe cases, the placental damage includes complete infarction of a section of the placental bed. By infarction I mean that an area of tissue dies because the feeder blood vessels are completely blocked by thrombosis or blood clot. To the naked eye the placenta can be seen to have sections or wedges of very pale tissue and the adjacent maternal surface of the interface between mother and baby is covered in fibrin deposits and copious white cells. In addition, CHI is frequently accompanied by perivillous fibrin deposits – tiny blood clots being deposited around the trophoblastic villi. Not surprisingly the condition is recognized to be a cause of intrauterine growth restriction (IUGR), oligohydramnios (low liquor volume) and fetal loss.

The diagnosis is made by examining the placenta histologically after delivery. It is important to perform a detailed thrombophilia screen for women who suffer CHI, since a small proportion of cases are associated with phospholipid syndrome and other pro-thrombotic disorders.

Whatever the test results demonstrate, most clinicians would agree that offering the woman treatment with a combination of aspirin and heparin during her next pregnancy is important. In very severe cases, the additional use of steroids may be beneficial, in an attempt to dampen down the aberrant immune response at the materno-fetal interface. However, there is no evidence that using IVIG or intralipid infusions is of any benefit and has the downside of being extremely expensive and associated with significant side effects.

Blood group incompatibilities

Blood group incompatibilities between mother and father may cause miscarriage, but this is a reassuringly rare occurrence. Evidence that parental incompatibility in the ABO and the P blood group systems, reported in the 1960s as an occasional cause of miscarriage, has never been substantiated. Detailed testing of blood groups in couples with a history of miscarriage is of no practical help.

The classic example of blood group incompatibility is severe rhesus disease, which occurs when a rhesus D negative mother and rhesus D positive father have a rhesus D positive fetus. If blood cells from the baby enter the mother's bloodstream, she recognises the rhesus positive fetal blood cells and produces antibodies which travel back across the placenta and destroy the baby's blood cells. Since fetal red blood cells usually only enter the mother's circulation after haemorrhage from the placenta, most cases occur at the time of delivery, which is why rhesus disease usually affects second or later pregnancies with greater severity.

This problem can be avoided if rhesus negative mothers are all given an injection of anti-D at the time of delivery of their rhesus positive baby. The anti-D then 'mops up' any rhesus positive cells from the baby and prevents the mother's immune system from recognising these foreign cells and developing antibodies to them, which will cause problems in a future pregnancy. Fortunately, rhesus disease is now very rare in this country, thanks to the introduction of routine treatment for rhesus negative mothers after delivery and miscarriage. Although the risk to a rhesus negative mother is low at the time of an early complete miscarriage, most doctors still advise a dose of anti-D when the miscarriage has to be dealt with surgically, whatever the age of the pregnancy, to ensure that no antibodies are produced in the future.

Anti-D is also given after ectopic pregnancies, prenatal diagnostic procedures such as amniocentesis and chorion villus biopsy and all cases of antepartum haemorrhage (bleeding in pregnancy after 28 weeks). Furthermore, many hospitals have now introduced routine injections of anti-D at 28 and 36 weeks of pregnancy for all rhesus negative women, in the hope that we will be able to eradicate rhesus disease in the newborn baby completely.

Anti-sperm antibodies

There have been a few studies suggesting that men and women who develop antibodies to sperm in their blood, or in the case of some men on the sperms, have an increased risk of miscarriage. I am not very convinced by these reports. They are usually based on small numbers of patients undergoing infertility investigations and treatments and normal control groups are lacking. The apparent increase in the miscarriage rate is just as likely to be due to the infertility problems and their treatment, as to the sperm antibodies. We do not recommend testing for anti-sperm antibodies in couples with recurrent miscarriage.

Conclusions

It is very important to ensure that future research effort into alloimmune miscarriage is focused on theories for which objective evidence is available. I believe that miscarriage sufferers deserve better than to be offered 'treatment' which no one can explain or monitor effectively, and which comes without guarantee that no serious side-effects will result.

Sadly, the myth that uterine NK cells can kill the embryo and are responsible for the reproductive failure in women with recurrent miscarriage and failed IVF treatment has persisted and proven difficult to displace. The actual contribution of these maternal immune cells to success or failure in women with infertility and recurrent miscarriage is still not completely understood, but there is certainly no evidence that they kill trophoblast (placental) cells in these conditions.

13

RECURRENT MISCARRIAGE – PROTHROMBOTIC CAUSES

It has been known for many years that women with systemic lupus erythematosus (SLE) or 'lupus' disease, experience a variety of complications in pregnancy. SLE is the most common auto-immune disorder in women of reproductive age. Although SLE sufferers appear to have no trouble falling pregnant, they have a high rate of miscarriage, which can occur at any stage during the pregnancy. They are also at greater risk of developing pre-eclampsia (toxaemia), growth restriction in the baby and placental abruption – severe bleeding behind the placenta causing the placenta to shear away from the wall of the womb, cutting off the blood supply to the baby. However, not every woman with SLE develops pregnancy complications. Many of them have completely normal pregnancies. We now recognise that it is only the women with SLE who have antiphospholipid antibodies (or APL) who experience the miscarriages and later pregnancy problems.

Primary antiphospholipid syndrome (PAPS)

Antiphospholipid antibodies may also be found in women who do not have obvious symptoms or signs of SLE but consult their doctor for the first time complaining of recurrent episodes of miscarriage. This led to the identification of a distinct clinical condition called the Primary Antiphospholipid Syndrome, which described the association between APL, and recurrent miscarriages in women who do not have full-blown SLE. Indeed, we now realise that in addition to women with three or more miscarriages, the antiphospholipid syndrome should also include those women who have suffered a single unexplained late miscarriage or very early preterm delivery or who developed severe pre-eclampsia or delivered a baby with severe intrauterine growth restriction (IUGR) in a previous pregnancy.

Antiphospholipid antibodies (APL)

Antiphospholipid antibody is the collective name used to describe a large family of autoantibodies. They are strongly associated with recurrent miscarriage and the development of thrombosis (blood clots). Historically, the most popular explanation as to how these antibodies exert their damaging effect on a pregnancy has been that they cause clotting in the blood vessels of the placenta. The steady accumulation of tiny clots results in parts of the placenta being unable to function (placental infarction), which eventually leads to the death of the baby.

We now know that these antibodies can also attack the cells of the placenta directly. By causing inflammation and turbulent blood flow, they disturb the normal pattern of invasion of the placenta into the maternal tissues, which is an essential step in achieving successful 'implantation' and a continuing pregnancy. This explains how APL can cause miscarriage at all stages of pregnancy. It also explains why early pregnancies which have developed a fetal heartbeat suddenly fail, why late miscarriages are often associated with small, gritty placentas, blood clots behind the placenta and an under-nourished baby, and why pre-eclampsia and premature labour are more common in these women. All these pregnancy complications may result from the effects of APL on the blood flow to the placenta.

Recurrent miscarriage patients may have other symptoms to suggest that the antiphospholipid syndrome is the cause of their pregnancy losses. I find that the miscarriage and obstetric problems which these women have experienced are frequently accompanied by evidence of thrombosis (usually a blood clot in their lower leg), arthritis, skin rashes, migraine, headaches and occasionally epilepsy. Furthermore, there is often a history of thrombosis, heart attack or stroke occurring before the age of 50 years in a member of their close family. These are all useful pointers suggesting that the diagnosis may be antiphospholipid syndrome. As one doctor who visited the clinic commented to me: 'The more you look, the more you find these APL!'

This is certainly the case. In the recurrent miscarriage clinic at the St Mary's Clinic we screen every patient we see on at least two occasions for the main types of APL, which are known as lupus anticoagulant (LA), anticardiolipin antibodies (ACA) and beta 2 glycoprotein-1 antibodies. We have established that one in every five or six recurrent miscarriers we see has the antiphospholipid syndrome. This incidence of 15–20% may not seem very impressive at first glance, but when you consider that only 1–2% of women with no previous history of miscarriage have APL, it becomes clearer that these antibodies make a significant contribution to the problem of recurrent miscarriage. In my experience, the Lupus anticoagulant is found more commonly than ACA or B2GP-1 and very few women are positive for all three tests. This is why it is important that all three tests are routinely available. Many women I see in the clinic tell me that they have already been tested for the 'lupus factor' but frequently the records show that only one of the tests has been performed (usually the ACA, which is more readily available). Testing for only one type of these antibodies will mean that many women with APL will escape diagnosis.

I need to mention here that the lupus anticoagulant, anti-cardiolipin and B2GP-1 antibodies are just three of the many APL and other autoantibodies that can be tested for. Extensive research has shown that it is only the lupus anticoagulant, the three subclasses of anticardiolipin (IgG, IgM and IgA) and B2GP-1 that are associated with recurrent pregnancy loss. This is an important point for the reader to understand since there are many services advertised on the internet which suggest that women with recurrent miscarriage will benefit from undergoing many more autoantibody tests. These tests are costly and yet they do not help in the diagnosis or identification of women at risk of recurrent miscarriage who will benefit from treatment.

The medical textbooks used to suggest that APL were only the cause of late miscarriages. Certainly, they can be found in a larger percentage of women whose pregnancies miscarry after 13 weeks and in whom complications such as pre-eclampsia and growth restriction have occurred. However, it is important to remember that the vast majority (75%) of women with recurrent miscarriages have only experienced early losses (see Chapter 6). Our research studies have demonstrated that antiphospholipid syndrome is also an important cause of early miscarriages and since early miscarriage is so much more common than later losses, it follows that if only late miscarriage sufferers are screened for APL, then the majority of patients with the syndrome will remain undetected and therefore unable to benefit from treatment.

The next issue is the accuracy of the laboratory tests used to detect these antibodies. This is an important point and explains why international guidelines were established to avoid the laboratory variation that bedevilled this field in the past. Several tests are available for the detection of lupus anticoagulant but the 'dilute Russell's Viper Venom Time' or dRVVT test is the most accurate for women with recurrent miscarriage. When testing for lupus anticoagulant, it is important that (a) the blood sample is taken without using a cuff, (b) it is a free-flowing sample, and (c) it is processed in the laboratory swiftly. If these guidelines are not followed, the test for LA may be reported as negative.

I am often asked by patients how they can have a negative test for either LA, ACA or B2GP-1 at one hospital and then be told they tested positive at another hospital. The problem is that, as with many other antibodies, the levels of APL fluctuate over time. This has been shown both in women with recurrent miscarriage and with SLE. It is therefore important that, before making the decision as to whether a woman has APL or not, she is tested on several occasions, as a single test cannot determine her APL status – either positive or negative.

The final point to remember about APL tests is that, apart from false negative results (due to incorrectly performed laboratory tests), a number of women will have temporarily positive tests. These test results are not thought to be of significance and are most commonly caused by viral or other infections (such as the common cold). Before a woman can be said to have the antiphospholipid syndrome, she should test positive for either LA, ACA or B2GP-1 on at least two occasions more than four to eight weeks apart. As you can see, testing for APA and the interpretation of results is not straightforward. The best way to achieve accurate results is to have the tests performed in laboratories with particular expertise in the detection of these antibodies.

Pregnancy outcome in untreated phospholipid patients

I have put much emphasis on the importance of performing the right tests for APL on all miscarriage patients. The reason why I am so 'picky' is simple. Undetected recurrent miscarriers with APL syndrome can be expected to have a dismal outcome in future pregnancies. When we started to look for APA in the miscarriage clinic, we followed a group of women with APL during their next pregnancy and compared their outcome with another group of women who were APL negative. In the

APL positive group, only 10% had a live birth, whereas 65% of the APL negative women had a successful pregnancy. A cynical person might argue that any treatment must be better than nothing for this unfortunate group of women!

Steroid treatment

Not surprisingly, this high miscarriage rate in women with APL has led to a variety of treatments being used in an attempt to improve the outcome of future pregnancies. Since steroids have long been used to treat women with active SLE, this was the first line of therapy tried for APL syndrome. The results were disappointing, not just in terms of live births achieved, but also because the steroids had side-effects for both the mother and baby. In one study, it was clearly shown that women with autoantibodies who were given steroids during pregnancy had a significantly higher incidence of pre-eclampsia, gestational diabetes and premature delivery, with all the attendant risks to the baby associated with these problems. Most doctors have now abandoned the use of steroids in women with APA syndrome. However, there are some medical problems which necessitate treatment with steroids even when the woman is pregnant. If you are one of these women, please do not worry. Your doctors will know that you are at risk of later pregnancy complications and will ensure that you and your baby are carefully monitored. You may have to be delivered early but as long as the delivery is planned and carried out in a centre with the experience and facilities to look after you, both you and your baby will be safe.

How do phospholipid antibodies cause pregnancy complications?

This is a complex question and has been the subject of considerable clinical and laboratory research effort over recent years. Earlier in this chapter, I mentioned that for many years it was thought that miscarriage in women with APL was due to thrombosis (or the development of blood clots) in the placenta and in the blood vessels leading to the placenta. This certainly explains many cases of late miscarriage, but it does not explain the very many miscarriages that occur early in pregnancy long before the placenta has grown to a significant size and when there is only limited blood flow in the placental villi in order to protect the embryo or fetus from being exposed to too much oxygen. Compelling evidence now exists to show that these APL also have a direct effect on the cells of the young placenta or trophoblast, resulting in inflammation and turbulent blood flow, probably because they disrupt the normal anticoagulant mechanisms that the placenta uses to combat the formation of clots on the surface of its cells.

If this seems a strange explanation, then just think about what a complex job the placenta has to do. The placenta has to invade the maternal decidual bed in order to implant in the womb. It must secure a position that allows the development of the pregnancy, but the invasion process has to be carefully controlled. It cannot be too aggressive because this would result in the placenta behaving like a tumour or cancer behaves – taking over the host body and destroying it. No, the placenta has to invade up to a point that allows the baby access to all the blood and nutrients that it needs from the mother. But it must not invade past that point because this would endanger her ability to control the situation. Most of the time the invasion is not too aggressive since, as we noted in an earlier chapter in this book, placental tumours, or hydatidiform moles as they are called, are quite rare.

The mechanisms that control this fine tuning are complex and many eminent researchers have been involved in trying to put together the many pieces of this jigsaw puzzle. Advances in our understanding of early pregnancy development and the biology of APL has allowed us to recognize that APL interfere with the signalling mechanisms between the cells which control the decidual change in the endometrium. The APL effectively incresase the levels of programmed cell death or apoptosis and reduce the ability of the placental layers to fuse together, which in turn means that the invasion of the trophoblast cells into the blood vessels in the mother's womb lining is impaired. Many of these studies have been carried out by researchers attached to our unit at St Mary's and I would like to take this opportunity to thank them all for their hard work. Importantly, the adverse effects of APL do not seem to be an all-or-nothing mechanism. If the APL are present they do not necessarily lead to an early miscarriage or end of the pregnancy, they can also store up problems leading to later miscarriages or pregnancy complications such as pre-eclampsia in the mother and growth restriction in the baby at a later stage.

Treatment with aspirin and heparin

The most effective treatment for women with APL is the use of low-dose aspirin in combination with the anticoagulant drug heparin. When we first started using this treatment for miscarriage sufferers I used to explain to my patients that these two drugs improved the outcome of pregnancy for women with APA because aspirin and heparin are both capable of thinning the blood and improving the blood flow through the placenta, albeit using different mechanisms. With more experience we now know that this is far from being the whole story. Although aspirin affects blood thinning directly by making the platelets in our blood less sticky or adherent to each other, heparin has a beneficial effect on the way in which the young placenta manages to invade the maternal uterine blood vessels. Effectively, heparin treatment can be thought of as a means of salvaging or protecting the trophoblast or young placental cells which would otherwise be damaged by the APL.

In 1997 our team at St Mary's published the results of the first large randomised controlled trial comparing the use of aspirin with aspirin in combination with heparin. The results from this trial were very exciting. They showed that the miscarriage rate in women with APL can be reduced dramatically with this combination of treatment. We found that in the women taking aspirin alone, the miscarriage rate fell from 90% to 60%, meaning that 40% of these women had a successful pregnancy. For the women who were taking heparin as well, the live birth rate rose to over 70%. Many clinics have published similar excellent results allowing us to definitely conclude that low-dose aspirin in combination with heparin has very beneficial effects in treating recurrent miscarriage in women with APL syndrome. Since we introduced this treatment into our routine clinical practice many thousands of women have benefited from this treatment at St Mary's and the therapy has been adopted as the gold standard by clinics all over the world.

I am often asked by both patients and doctors about this treatment, so I want to include details here for the interested reader. Only those women with a definite diagnosis of antiphospholipid syndrome (two positive APL tests more than four to eight weeks apart) identified in the non-pregnant state are suitable for this treatment. As soon as the next home pregnancy test is positive we ask the women to start taking low-dose aspirin tablets, 75mg daily, and contact us immediately. We then give them an appointment to attend the very next week's early pregnancy clinic. At this clinic we perform an ultrasound scan and as soon as we can see a pregnancy sac in the uterine cavity we teach the woman how to start the low-dose heparin injections. We used to use unfractionated heparin which has to be injected twice daily, but we soon switched to low molecular weight heparin preparations when they became available since these offer the great advantage of only requiring a once-daily injection. They are just as beneficial as the twice-daily unfractionated alternative. I should mention here that there are several different types of low molecular weight heparin on the market and they are all as good as each other. The only down side to the low molecular weight heparins is that they are more expensive and some hospitals and GPs may be reluctant to prescribe them.

Although many women coming to our clinic are worried about whether they will be able to cope with learning how to inject themselves with heparin, I can tell you that I have never known a miscarriage sufferer with APL who has not been able to conquer the technique quickly and satisfactorily. It is true that some women suffer bruising at the injection sites, but they invariably weather this side-effect with very little complaint and soon become expert at avoiding sites on their tummy or upper thighs which make them more prone to bruising.

Most women attending our early pregnancy clinic like to return fortnightly to see us until they reach approximately 12 weeks. At this point we make arrangements for them to attend the antenatal clinic either at St Mary's or at their local hospital. We call the 12-week visit to the miscarriage clinic the graduation visit and use it as an opportunity to make sure that all the medical records for that woman are summarised and sent to the doctors who will look after them for the remainder of the pregnancy. Many of my patients used to look very amused when they hear me dictate a letter to myself summarising the care that she had received to date and making suggestions about what monitoring tests are appropriate over the next six months. But I think it is important to continue to do so since most pregnant women carry their own antenatal notes with them, which do not always include copies of all the pre-pregnancy investigations. Important facts about their particular case may get forgotten unless a summary letter is written. We also give the women a pregnancy questionnaire at their last visit and ask them to fill in all the details and return it to us after their baby has been delivered along with a photograph for our 'Rogue's Gallery'! Indeed, the departmental walls are covered in happy pictures and the numerous photo albums sport an enormous collection of further pictures and grateful letters of thanks to the St Mary's team.

We sometimes advise regular ultrasound monitoring of the babies' growth and the Doppler scans in later pregnancy. These scans can be very helpful in identifying that small group of women who, despite receiving treatment, still experience later pregnancy complications including pre-eclampsia, growth restriction or preterm delivery. Of course, for those women who have previously suffered a blood clot or thrombosis in pregnancy we continue the treatment until at least six weeks after the delivery of the baby in order to reduce their risks of another thrombosis or VTE. But for the vast majority of women we stop the aspirin and heparin treatment at the end of the 34th week of pregnancy. I am frequently asked why we stop the treatment at this stage and the answer is quite simple. When we first introduced this treatment our ethics committee were worried about the potential risks of heparin in pregnancy and requested that we limit the duration of the treatment to the shortest possible time. We felt that after 34 weeks most babies would not require specialist neonatal care if it became necessary to deliver them and that they could be safely delivered at the woman's local hospital. We now know that heparin is quite safe to use for long periods of time in pregnancy which is very reassuring (see safety issues below). However, there is no evidence that continuing the heparin until the time of delivery further improves the outcome of pregnancy. Every woman in the original trial who reached 34 completed weeks of gestation went on to have a live take-home baby and obviously we cannot improve on this! Please do not be worried by the advice to stop the heparin at this stage. The benefit of the heparin on how the placenta has implanted has all been achieved in the first trimester and during the second wave of placental invasion that occurs between 20 and 26 weeks, so your pregnancy is perfectly safe from this point onwards.

Safety of aspirin and heparin in pregnancy

If aspirin and heparin are capable of changing the outcome of pregnancy for women with APL syndrome, we must understand how these drugs work and ensure that they have no serious side-effects for either the mother or her baby. Aspirin is a drug which combats inflammation and also prevents blood from clotting. It has been tried and tested in pregnancy and found to have no side-effects upon the baby, although it does cross (i.e. enter) the placenta. A large European study (called the CLASP study), which looked at whether aspirin treatment could reduce the risk of pre-eclampsia, was published some years ago and fortunately the investigators went on to follow up all the babies who were exposed to aspirin during their time in the womb. Happily, I can report to you that the physical and neurological development of these babies was entirely normal – all of the children were followed to the age of seven years, and many to much later ages, and no problems were identified.

Heparin is an anticoagulant drug which at high doses actually thins the blood. This is why it is used to treat patients who have already developed a blood clot or thrombosis. However, at low doses (such as those used in our APL treatment), heparin does not affect the clotting of blood directly, although we have known for a long time that small doses of heparin can prevent the development of a thrombosis. This is why many hospital patients are given heparin injections before and after major surgery. It is not entirely clear how low-dose heparin prevents the development of blood clots in the body, but it is probably by similar mechanisms to the ones we have discovered in the placenta. Namely, that the heparin acts as a salvage factor that mops up inflammatory cells that if left unchecked would then be the focus that attracted platelets and other blood cells to form a clot in a blood vessel. As I explained earlier, our research work on placental tissue suggests that heparin actually binds to the surface of the placental cells and also to some of the cells lining the maternal blood vessels in close contact with the placenta and prevents the APL from damaging the placenta or causing inflammation of the blood vessel walls.

The reader will be interested to hear that when we analysed the original trial data it became apparent that the beneficial effect of heparin was greatest during the first 13 weeks of pregnancy. After that time, it was extremely rare for a pregnancy to miscarry. This finding raised two important questions which are closely linked. The first was whether we could stop the heparin and aspirin much earlier, at about 15 weeks. We did try to answer this question by stopping the heparin earlier, but the results were alarming. Several women who had managed to get through the first 12 to 16 weeks of pregnancy went on to suffer a late miscarriage, and although the results of a few pregnancies should not dictate future protocols, I confess that I stopped this treatment trial before we had randomized more than a handful of women to it. I felt that we could not continue with this trial knowing that the 34-week treatment protocol resulted in such a high live birth rate and so few late miscarriages.

The second question we asked ourselves was: how is the heparin working? We know that until 10 to 12 weeks of pregnancy the blood flow through the young placenta is minimal and hence it is difficult to conclude that the heparin is preventing the formation of blood clots if there is no significant blood flow going on at this stage. This question is a lot more difficult to answer but brings us back to the points made earlier in this chapter, namely that heparin must have additional effects on the cells of the placenta and the decidual lining of the womb. These include reducing apoptosis or programmed cell death, promoting fusion of the syncytia placental cell layers and also promoting invasion into the maternal blood vessels in the decidua and thereby gaining access to the maternal circulation.

My personal view is that heparin probably works in two different ways. In the early weeks of pregnancy it must act on the placental and decidual cells to prevent the adverse effects of APL and after the blood flow to the placenta becomes fully established, it then helps to prevent the formation of blood clots in the placental vessels – which may be why we found that those few women who stopped the heparin at 15 weeks went on to suffer later miscarriages.

Heparin has no side-effects on the baby because it cannot cross the placental barrier and therefore never reaches the baby. However, heparin can occasionally cause complications in the mother and should always be used with caution and closely monitored. I have already mentioned that bruising at the injection sites can occur and may be troublesome. Rarely, heparin has been reported to cause a catastrophic fall in the mother's blood platelet count, resulting in generalised bleeding. Although we have never encountered this problem in any of our miscarriage patients, we usually take the precaution of checking the mother's platelet count soon after starting heparin treatment.

When we first started using heparin for the treatment of APL-positive miscarriage sufferers the most serious potential complication to consider were reports that women taking heparin during pregnancy may develop thinning of their bones, similar to that seen in osteoporosis. A few very frightening accounts of young, healthy women developing fractures of their spine after long-term heparin use in pregnancy needed to be considered before we could freely recommend this treatment for all APL-positive miscarriage patients. So we set up another large research study to measure the bone density of all our patients taking heparin on several occasions during their pregnancy. The results were fascinating and also very reassuring. We showed that women do lose about 3 to 4% of their bone density when taking heparin throughout their pregnancy. However, our study also included pregnant women who were not taking heparin and their bone density losses were almost identical. In summary, we can now confidently tell you that being pregnant means that your bone density will decrease by a factor of about 4%, but that taking low-dose heparin for the APL syndrome does not put you at greater risk of osteoporosis over and above the normal risk for any pregnant woman.

Interestingly, our study also showed that there are a few women who start their pregnancies with borderline osteoporosis and I suspect that it is these few women when treated with heparin who developed the fracture complications. These results make a good case for women at risk of osteoporosis (thin women, smokers, those with a family history of oesteoporosis or a medical history of long-term steroid drug use) to be offered bone density scans before pregnancy. If they are found to have low densities, they should be offered calcium and vitamin D treatment during pregnancy.

Further prothrombotic causes of miscarriage and later pregnancy complications

The discovery of APL syndrome as a cause of recurrent miscarriage and the knowledge that aspirin and heparin treatment is an effective remedy opened our eyes to the importance of prothrombotic disorders as a cause of miscarriage and later pregnancy complications. It also opened exciting new doors for future research.

Why is it, for instance, that some women still miscarry after treatment with heparin? They may experience a sporadic miscarriage due to a fetal chromosomal abnormality that is entirely unrelated to their APL syndrome, which is why it is always so important to analyse the miscarriage tissues of any future pregnancy that goes on to miscarry. Alternatively, it may be because they have another type of clotting or prothrombotic disorder that at the present time we do not have a specific name for, but that in the future we will be able to diagnose and offer different treatment for. In several chapters of this book I have referred to the molecular revolution that is changing our understanding of many different areas of medicine.

The prothrombotic disorders are one of those fields in which the discoveries are occurring extraordinarily fast and in which our understanding is expanding all the time. For example, in 1993 we knew that there were a couple of very rare blood disorders that placed individuals, both male and female, at greater risk of developing thrombosis, usually a blood clot in their legs or lungs, during their lifetime. We had also recently come to understand that the APL syndrome was a particular problem for pregnant women because they were at greater risk of miscarriage and other later pregnancy complications. What happened in 1993 was a real milestone in our understanding of prothrombotic abnormalities. It was discovered that resistance to the effects of activated protein C is a powerful cause of blood clotting. Protein C is a natural anticoagulant that is produced by the lining of our blood cells when they realise that a blood clot is being deposited on their surface. This protein C needs to be activated by other factors in the bloodstream in order to be able to start the fibrinolytic (or clot dissolving blood pathway) and prevent the formation of a blood clot or thrombosis. However, the tests for activated protein C resistance which became available at that time relied on special laboratory assays of coagulation. Similarly, we knew that protein C and protein S deficiency, together with the rarer Antithrombin III deficiency, which were all considered to be acquired prothrombotic disorders and had to be diagnosed with labour intensive coagulation assays, had all been associated with an increased incidence of venous thrombosis. Immediately the presumption was made that these disorders would increase the risk of miscarriage and later pregnancy complications. In short, our ability to diagnose acquired prothrombotic defects had outstripped our understanding of the mechanisms whereby they might give rise to fetal loss and later pregnancy complications.

Prothrombotic gene mutations and the risk of venous thrombosis

The very next year a clever scientist who worked in Leiden, Belgium, discovered that 90% of all cases of activated protein C resistance are due to an abnormality in the gene that produces factor V – an essential component in the blood clot dissolving process. This genetic mutation (inherited abnormality) at one point in the vast factor V gene was capable of making the whole of our body resistant to the effects of our natural defence against this part of our blood clotting system. In honour of its discoverer, the mutation was called the Factor V Leiden mutation. It did not take much longer for the experts to find that this mutation is very common – 5% of all Caucasians are heterozygous for the mutation, which means that they carry a single copy of the gene mutation which has been inherited from one or other of their parents. For reasons we do not understand, the prevalence of FVLeiden is much less frequent in African and Asian peoples. Carrying the FVLeiden mutation as a heterozygote is thought to increase an individual's lifetime risk of having a thrombosis four- to sixfold. Homozygotes who carry two copies of the gene mutation (one inherited from each parent) are less common in the population but it is estimated that being a homozygote increases an individual's lifetime risk of having a thrombosis eightfold.

So why do some people develop thrombosis and many others escape this problem? The answer must be that it is only when there are additional prothrombotic risk factors present that a thrombosis results. The search for these other factors has become a major medical quest. We do not have all the answers yet but the concept that multiple 'hits' are necessary before a man or woman develops a thrombosis is a very important one. Many studies have found that the risk of thrombosis continues to rise as the number of defects accumulates.

We now know that if we screen everyone who is attending a thrombosis clinic, some 40% of them will be carrying the FVLeiden mutation. But if being FVLeiden positive meant that the individual was definitely going to suffer a thrombosis then the incidence of thrombosis should be 5% (occurring in one in 20 people) and this is not the case. The overall incidence of thrombosis in the general population is much lower.

The search for other genetic mutations that predispose to thrombosis has been productive. Several more genetic mutations have been identified since the discovery of Factor V Leiden in 1994, such as the Factor II or prothrombin gene mutation which is present in approximately 2% of the general population and increases that person's risk of thrombosis some three- to fivefold during their lifetime. Similarly, homozygotes for the Factor II prothrombin mutation are less common than heterozygotes, but their lifetime risk of having a thrombosis is further increased.

The hyperhomocysteinaemia gene mutation (known as the MTHFR mutation) is found in as many as 40% of the general population. A further factor V mutation discovered in Cambridge was later reported and many other candidate mutations have since been investigated such as the 4G/5G polymorphism in the plasminogen activator inhibitor

(PAI-1) gene promoter. Since then, many publications have reported that individual coagulation defects are either as frequent or more frequent in women with recurrent miscarriage than they are in control women with normal obstetric histories.

Prothrombotic gene mutations and pregnancy outcome

Whether or not these genetic prothrombotic or thrombophilic mutations make a significant contribution to the problem of recurrent miscarriage and later pregnancy complications has been difficult to establish. There have been a large number of research papers published in the medical literature, based on retrospective groups of obstetric patients, which have claimed that these genetic throbophilic mutations account for almost every obstetric complication known. One large European cohort study found a 14-fold increase in the risk of stillbirth in those women who were identified with combined thrombophilic defects. Furthermore, the reader needs to understand that if we perform genetic tests on a group of women who have already had a serious pregnancy complication and recorded that the incidence is high, this does not mean that these gene mutations always lead to that particular problem. The only way that we can reach this conclusion is if we prospectively screen every pregnant woman for all of the different mutations, observe what happens to them during the rest of their pregnancy and can then demonstrate that the women who carry that particular mutation all suffer the pregnancy complications.

This appears to be far from the truth. For example, one large study suggested that 65% of women with serious pregnancy complications such as miscarriage, pre-eclampsia, growth restriction and stillbirth had one or more inherited or acquired prothrombotic or thrombophilic abnormalities. However, in the control group 17% of the pregnant women carried the same inherited or acquired abnormalities but suffered no complications. This prompts me to suggest that we need to remind ourselves that only 5% of all pregnant women are affected by serious pregnancy complications and this study reported that two-thirds of the women with serious complications carried a prothrombotic abnormality. This leads us to the conclusion that just over 3% of these complex pregnancies were to women carrying a prothrombotic mutation (since two-thirds of 5% comes to just over 3%). In contrast, 95% of pregnant women enjoy normal uncomplicated pregnancies and if 17% of these women carry the same prothrombotic defects we should expect that a much larger percentage of pregnant women would be suffering the same complications – and we know that they do not. There must be other factors that determine whether a pregnant woman with a known prothrombotic abnormality is at risk of developing pregnancy complications. Let me share with you a few examples.

When APC resistance was first described in 1993, we looked at a large number of our recurrent miscarriage patients and found that late miscarriage sufferers were more likely to have APC resistance when compared to early miscarriers and control women with normal obstetric histories. This data was exciting and suggested that there are a group of women with recurrent pregnancy loss who develop APC resistance during pregnancy which may place their baby at risk of miscarriage and later pregnancy complications. Soon after, we learnt that APC resistance develops progressively in normal pregnancy and is one of the reasons that pregnant women are at greater risk of thrombosis.

Next came the discovery of the Factor V Leiden mutation and the medical journals were soon full of confusing reports. Some said that the prevalence of FVLeiden was increased in women with a history of miscarriage and late pregnancy complications. Other studies reported that the prevalence was no different from the general population. The problem here is that most of the available studies have included insufficient numbers to allow us to draw meaningful conclusions. Furthermore, many of the studies have been performed in high risk groups of women who have been tested because they have suffered a previous thrombosis in pregnancy. The results from these women are unlikely to be representative of women presenting to doctors because they have suffered recurrent miscarriages.

So we set out to screen one thousand consecutive women attending our clinic. The results showed that just over 4% of them carried the FVLeiden mutation, which is no different from the general population prevalence. The next step was to follow some of these FVLeiden positive women through their next pregnancy and compare their outcome to recurrent miscarriers without the gene mutation. No woman in this study was taking any treatment apart from routine folic acid supplements in pregnancy. The results demonstrated that the FVLeiden positive women do appear to have a lower live birth rate and a higher incidence of preterm deliveries and other late pregnancy complications. However, nearly half of them had entirely uncomplicated pregnancies that delivered at term, which suggests to me that we now have to find ways of identifying those women who are at greater risk of pregnancy complications and protect those women who are not at risk of these complications from being subjected to unnecessary drug treatments.

Once again, just like with venous thrombotic events, we return to the important concept that it is multiple 'hits' and not a single prothrombotic or abnormal blood clotting test that leads to a pregnant woman increasing her risks of experiencing a pregnancy complication. The challenge continues to be finding novel ways to identify the additional 'hits' or risk factors and understand their implications. The thromboelastogram that I describe at the end of this chapter is one such test that may contribute to this.

Future pregnancy management of recurrent miscarriage women with prothrombotic gene mutations

This is a confusing and sometimes contentious area, by which I mean that many specialist doctors who are involved in the care of pregnant women who have been identified as carrying a prothrombotic gene mutation, hold widely differing views as to how they should be managed during pregnancy and the postpartum period.

I think it is best to address these differences of opinion by appreciating that they really depend on how it came about that the woman was found to be a carrier and which mutation has been found. If it was because she has experienced multiple miscarriages, or late pregnancy complications such as maternal pre-eclampsia, preterm birth or fetal growth restriction and she is carrying the Factor V Leiden or Factor II prothrombin mutation as a heterozygote or as a homozygote, it is likely that the doctors looking after this woman will advise her to start treatment with either aspirin and/or heparin in early pregnancy and continue through the pregnancy and also for six weeks after delivery. This is because we know that the quality and depth of placental implantation is determined very early in pregnancy and that the treatment may reduce the risk of early or late miscarriage and later pregnancy complications due to poor placental function. We also know that as pregnancy progresses, every woman's risk of thrombosis increases and that she probably requires treatment to ensure that she does not have a thrombotic event provoked by pregnancy. The same logic applies to the management of this woman during the six-week postnatal period, when every woman's risk of having a thrombosis is at its highest level and carriers of these two mutations will have another risk factor that needs to be considered.

On the other hand, I think that most doctors would consider that heterozygous carriers of the MTHFR gene mutation (and its various variants) are at much less risk of a prothrombotic event, indeed some doctors would say that they do not consider that there is a problem during pregnancy for these women. When they are homozygous for this mutation (by which I mean they carry two copies of the mutation, one copy being inherited from each of their parents), opinion is even more divided. However, recent discussions that I have had with haematological colleagues who specialise in genetic risk factors for thrombosis have convinced me that the thrombotic risks during pregnancy and the postpartum period for women with the MTHFR mutation have been overestimated. Perhaps more importantly, it is difficult to justify the potential gastrointestinal and bleeding tendency complications of aspirin treatment and the inconvenience and skin bruising from multiple daily subcutaneous injections of heparin treatment in these women.

The optimal treatment for a pregnant woman may be determined by another aspect of her medical history and the type of doctor who has been involved in her care in the past. For example, if a young pregnant woman has previously had a thrombotic event, whether it be linked to a previous pregnancy, provoked by taking hormonal contraception or following an episode of pelvic surgery, a prolonged period of immobility due to another illness, or even if the thrombosis was completely unrelated to any known provoking factors, she will undoubtedly have been seen by a haematologist with an interest in thrombosis. Since this haematologist spends all their time trying to prevent further episodes of thrombosis, they may well advise that since pregnancy is recognised to be a prothrombotic state, and that this woman is carrying an additional risk factor, it would be wise for her to have antithrombotic treatment throughout pregnancy. However, some haematologists will argue that the prospective studies justifying this course of action are lacking and that at most the woman should receive low dose treatment during the latter part of the pregnancy or alternatively only during the six-week postnatal period. Some will favour aspirin treatment and others will advise heparin treatment.

It is also important for me to mention here that there may be other previous medical problems that will require other groups of doctors to become involved in caring for a pregnant woman and their opinions may also vary as to whether antithrombotic treatment is required during pregnancy. For example, although relatively rare, if the woman has had a stroke or suffered transient ischaemic attacks, she will have previously been under the care of a neurologist and they too are likely to advise taking treatments during pregnancy to avoid a further episode of stroke. Similarly, women with rheumatological problems, such as rheumatoid arthritis or SLE (see Chapter 12) may well be judged at greater risk of a thrombotic event during pregnancy and be advised to have treatment with aspirin and or heparin.

For me, the most difficult dilemma as to whether a woman should receive antithrombotic treatment during pregnancy arises when women who have had no serious general medical or pregnancy problems ask for advice because they have undergone testing for genetic thrombophilic mutations and have been found to be a heterozygous carrier. Invariably they underwent screening because another member of their family developed a medical problem such as a thrombosis or stroke. In my experience, women in this situation immediately assume that they will have a problem during pregnancy and that they automatically require treatment. But there is very little evidence in the medical literature that an asymptomatic carrier is at significant risk of a thrombotic event during an uncomplicated pregnancy. Hence, opinions vary as to whether treatment should be prescribed during pregnancy and many clinicians rightly worry about the potential side effects that could result from unnecessary treatments when there is no medical evidence to justify them prescribing these drugs in the first place.

In this situation I often find it quite difficult to persuade my patients that we should not automatically assume they require antithrombotic treatment with aspirin and/or heparin and that instead we should try to carefully assess together whether they have additional risk factors that allow us to justify the side effects of these treatments. Good examples of such additional risk factors to take into consideration are whether they are overweight, have limited mobility, are older women (by which I mean in their late forties), or have had assisted fertility treatments with high doses of ovarian hormone stimulation. Women who have these risks, may well end up being considered in need of treatment. However, I think the majority of doctors would agree with me when I say that there are no hard and fast rules available in these situations as to whether to treat and with what they should be treated and that every individual woman and her pregnancy should be considered on its own merits.

The Thromboelastogram (TEG test)

By now I hope that the reader has understood that what is really needed in the clinic at St Mary's is a general test that can identify recurrent miscarriers who have screened negative for any of the currently known inherited or acquired prothrombotic markers or factors but may still be at risk of developing a prothrombotic problem during pregnancy. This is why our clinical and research teams have been exploring the potential of using thromboelastography (TEG testing for short) to find additional ways to identify these women.

Since individual genetic thrombophilic defects appear to offer us little value in predicting pregnancy outcome, we felt there was a need to develop a more general test that can be used as global markers of haemostatic function, in order to more accurately identify those women who present to us with recurrent miscarriage and who may have a prothrombotic or pro-inflammatory tendency that we could pick up either before or during her next pregnancy.

The conventional prothrombotic tests described earlier in this chapter can only measure the established abnormalities but the TEG test provides us with a general assessment of the woman's prothrombotic state. By definition this may include additional factors that have not been previously identified or given an official label. The TEG test measures the speed and the strength of the blood clot produced when a small sample of blood is placed into a special machine which mimics the physical conditions found in blood vessels in the body. The great advantage of this test is that it is quick – the results are obtained in a pictorial print out that includes a large number of separate measurements in just over one hour. It is also relatively cheap and reproducible, which means that the test can be performed repeatedly, and the same answers obtained. Of course, the low cost and the speedy reporting of the results means that we can also use the TEG testing in the early weeks of the next pregnancy. These are very important advantages over the conventional thrombophilia blood tests which were expensive to perform and often took many weeks to report the results. This meant that trying to get a woman tested quickly or to attempt to undertake testing in the early weeks of pregnancy was completely impossible.

Our TEG results are very exciting. We have been able to show that there are some women who present to our miscarriage clinic who are in a prothrombotic state or have a prothrombotic tendency that we can identify even when they are not pregnant. They may not have phospholipid antibodies, or any of the recognised genetic mutations that we are able to test for, but we now recognise two groups of women who have distinct abnormalities that we can detect on the TEG test in the non-pregnant state and can advise them of how best they should be treated during their next pregnancy.

The first group have an increase in the maximum amplitude (MA) of their TEG test. The MA measures the strength and speed at which the individual forms blood clots and these women produce blood clots more quickly and these clots are stronger than those produced by women with normal pregnancy histories. These women appear to benefit from treatment during pregnancy with aspirin at a dose of 150mg daily. Initially when we treated these miscarriage women, they were found to have a raised MA before pregnancy with 75mg aspirin but the TEG parameters remained unchanged. However, on treating them with this higher dose (150mg) of aspirin the MA moved back down into the normal range and the pregnancy outcome improved.

The second group have a reduction in their fibrinolytic parameters (as measured by the LY 30 and LY 60 values) on the TEG test. This means that they are slower to dissolve the naturally occurring tiny blood clots that we are all constantly producing in our blood vessels, with the overall result that they too are exhibiting a pro-clotting tendency but via a different pathway. We have found that this group of women respond well to low molecular weight heparin injections during their next pregnancy but that the use of aspirin does not improve their pregnancy outcome. Another interesting finding in this second group of women with reduced fibrinolytic parameters is that they very often have polycystic ovarian morphology. In Chapter 11, where I discussed hormonal causes, I mentioned that we now think that the over-representation of PCO in women with a history of recurrent miscarriage is more likely to be linked to abnormalities in the haemostatic pathways of women with PCO rather than being due to a hormonal imbalance alone. An impairment of the fibrinolytic response is also more likely to be identified in the TEG results of women who attend our clinic with a history of late miscarriages compared to women with early miscarriage.

In addition to be being able to identify recurrent miscarriers before their next pregnancy who may benefit from treatment to avoid pregnancy complications, we are now also able to identify that some women only develop the prothrombotic abnormalities that we are able to detect on the TEG testing when they become pregnant again. Since the TEG test is so quick and easy to perform, this means that we now have the opportunity to identify pregnant women who have proinflammatory markers or prothrombotic abnormalities during the first few crucial weeks of their pregnancy. By looking at the TEG results we can then decide whether they may benefit from taking either aspirin and/or heparin treatment and commence the treatments soon after the pregnancy has been declared or confirmed.

In Chapter 12 of this book, I mentioned that we recognise that there is a subtle but definitive switch in the immune system of the pregnant woman which occurs very early in pregnancy. Many researchers in this field have tried to determine exactly what does happen in a woman's immune system at this time, which in some way allows her to adapt to her pregnancy and the baby that is developing in her uterus in a mutually advantageous fashion. The answers remain unclear, but presumably are linked to the proinflammatory switch which occurs in early pregnancy.

These pregnancy TEG findings, together with the general medical clinical studies and drug trials that have shown that for some people, a small daily dose of aspirin offers them protection against heart disease, stroke and venous thrombotic events, has resulted in many women and their doctors to wrongly assume that taking low dose aspirin in early pregnancy is the answer for all women who have suffered miscarriages. I want to emphasise to the readers of this book that this is not the case and that choosing to take aspirin routinely when the clinic tests have failed to show a prothrombotic or proinflammatory abnormality may actually be counter-productive.

Indeed, an important study that we undertook in our clinic at St Mary's and published some time ago, clearly showed that in women with unexplained EARLY recurrent miscarriage, empirical aspirin treatment in the next pregnancy does NOT improve the live take-home baby rate – in fact it had the opposite effect and the miscarriage rate was higher. However, for the much smaller number of women with recurrent LATE miscarriages, particularly those late miscarriages in which there was evidence of poor placental function (such as maternal pre-eclampsia or fetal growth restriction) there did appear to be a benefit in them taking aspirin and also heparin treatment in low doses. These results suggest to me that the late miscarriage sufferers may well have some form of prothrombotic abnormality that currently we do not recognise or have a specific label or name for.

At the risk of repeating myself, I must state again that there are bound to be further new discoveries that reduce the pool of unexplained prothrombotic risk factors that pregnant women are exposed to in the near future. Having said this, I also believe that at the present time our ability to identify inherited prothrombotic abnormalities has outstripped our understanding of the natural history of venous thrombosis, and pregnancy complications. As previously mentioned on several occasions, we know that it is the presence of multiple hits or risk factors which determines who develops a systemic thrombosis. I suspect that we will conclude in the next few years that there are multiple hits and risk factors that decide whether a woman with a history of recurrent miscarriage is more likely to develop a pregnancy complication, such as a further miscarriage or pre-eclampsia and growth restriction in later pregnancy.

Long-term health issues for women with prothrombotic abnormalities

A major advance has been made by our relatively recent understanding that some women with recurrent miscarriage have an increased clotting tendency even when not pregnant. This finding has important implications for the long-term health of these relatively young women, who first come to the notice of doctors when they report recurrent miscarriages or later pregnancy complications such as maternal pre-eclampsia or fetal growth restriction.

For example, some of the third-generation contraceptive pills that have been developed to reduce unwanted cyclical hormonal swings and side-effects have been reported to marginally increase the risk of thrombosis in non-pregnant women. This concern has led to the suggestion that all young women should be screened for inherited APC resistance before they commence the contraceptive pill. The reality is that these women will be at greater risk of thrombosis if they become pregnant. But we do not know at the present time whether their lifetime risk of thrombosis or other general medical problems justifies the screening of all women, pregnant or not. However, I do hope that you the reader now recognise that routine screening is likely to result in more complications and confusion than it would resolve, bearing in mind the differences in opinion that I have shared with you as to whether we should be proactively treating women found to have genetic or inherited thrombophilic mutations or only treating them if they become symptomatic or develop a problem.

We definitely need to establish whether women with any of the problems discussed in this chapter should be offered long-term follow-up in an attempt to try and prevent other medical problems in later life, after the reproductive years have ended. My personal view is that it is very important that we set up long-term surveillance studies that can answer these questions. And that is exactly what we have started to do.

For example, every woman who comes to our recurrent miscarriage clinic and is diagnosed with antiphospholipid syndrome (APS), is encouraged to complete a detailed questionnaire about her health and invited to join a long-term follow-up study. This is aiming to track what happens to these APL positive women as they grow older and to document whether they are at greater risk of a thrombotic event in later life. We are hoping that it will not be too long before we can determine the answers to important questions such as 'Is it safe to take the contraceptive pill?' and 'Is it safe to take hormone replacement?' Although these studies will take many years of follow-up before we can answer these questions with authority, I would like to share with the reader some of the early observations that we have made about women that we diagnosed with APL many years ago and have managed to keep in contact with, since I think they are quite reassuring.

It does seem to be true that APL positive recurrent miscarriage women are at greater risk of having a thrombosis in later life. However, the data we have collected on them so far suggests that this increase in risk only appears to be a problem for those women who have a later exposure to an additional risk factor. For example, a future pregnancy that was not managed appropriately with a combination of aspirin and heparin. Women who become seriously overweight, obese or are persistent smokers are at particular risk of thrombosis in their later years. So too are those women who become relatively immobile either due to inactivity or prolonged illness, and exposure to pelvic surgery is also a major risk factor. In short, it appears that many of our recurrent miscarriage women who have subsequently had a venous thrombotic event were exposed to another provocation or risk factor in later life, in addition to being APL positive.

I should also mention here that many women have reported back to us that when they have alerted their local health carers to their past obstetric history and the fact that they are APL positive or carry one of the genetic thrombophilic mutations, it has been suggested that they take antithrombotic treatment prior to or during an episode of surgery or prolonged immobility, for example due to a general medical problem or a fractured limb. This group of RM women did not go on to experience a thrombotic event, which suggests that taking the caution of offering thromboprophylaxis at times when another risk factor for VTE is present, is the correct approach. Having said this, some clinicians do worry that we may be treating many women unnecessarily and that it would be difficult to justify the decision to treat them, given the lack of prospective randomized controlled trial data, if they were to suffer one of the rare but serious side-effects of treatment.

Some very important large scale epidemiological studies have now been carried out looking at the incidence of cardiovascular disease, both heart attack and stroke in populations of both men and women, with the aim of identifying risk factors that could help us to identify those individuals who might be helped to avoid these life-threatening problems with preventative healthcare measures. The results are extremely interesting and in all of the studies performed to date, predictably it is a poor-quality diet, obesity, lack of exercise and smoking that can be shown to significantly increase the risk of cardiovascular disease in later life.

However, for the readers of this book, I think the really important findings come from those studies that have also included an analysis of the risk of cardiovascular disease, based on past obstetric history. These have shown that the risks of a heart attack and or stroke in later life increase significantly in those women who give a history of repeated (meaning three or more consecutive) miscarriages, when compared to women whose pregnancy outcomes have all been successful. This adds further weight to the hypothesis that some women with RM suffer pregnancy loss because they have a proinflammatory or prothrombotic disorder even when they are not pregnant and that this disordered state is one of the factors that later provokes their early onset cardiovascular disease.

These epidemiological findings suggest to me that we should now be undertaking prospective follow-up studies of not just the RM women in whom we diagnose APL syndrome or in whom we identify the Factor V Leiden or Factor II prothrombin gene mutation, but also those RM women in whom we have identified TEG abnormalities – either an increase in their clot amplitude or a deficiency in their fibrinolytic parameters before or during the first few early weeks of pregnancy, in order to see whether they too have increased risks of cardiovascular disease in later life and need thromboprophylaxis when they find themselves exposed to further prothrombotic risk factors or lifestyle situations. What I am sure we can all agree upon is that being warned of risks that can be partially avoided by simple preventative lifestyle measures is greatly preferable to suffering a VTE, heart attack or stroke and then being told of the risk factors that have contributed to the event.

PART THREE

PRACTICAL ISSUES AND ANSWERS TO YOUR QUESTIONS

14

IS MISCARRIAGE MORE COMMON IN WOMEN WITH INFERTILITY PROBLEMS?

To miscarry after a prolonged period of infertility is devastating. Many women tell me that losing this long-awaited baby is even more distressing than not being able to conceive. I believe them – and I am sure that most individuals who have desperately wanted something in life can understand the pain of glimpsing the winning post before it is snatched away from them.

The theory that the risk of miscarriage is higher than normal in patients with infertility is not a new one. It was first suggested some 40 years ago and certainly predates our modern methods of treating infertility. The causes of infertility are many and diverse, but with the development of assisted conception techniques, it is now possible to overcome or at least circumvent the majority of problems presented by the subfertile couple.

As infertility treatment improves, it becomes increasingly important to ascertain how many miscarriages occur in women who have been successfully treated for infertility. If miscarriage is more common in women with infertility problems, is it related to all cases of infertility, or only certain types of infertility? Do the various therapies now available increase the rate of miscarriage or fetal abnormality? It may be that associated factors are responsible for the increased miscarriage rate, for example, increasing maternal age or the past pregnancy outcome. Alternatively, it may be that the early pregnancy monitoring and surveillance that women with infertility usually undergo, means that we are diagnosing more pregnancies which might have been missed in a woman with no infertility history.

Before we can attempt to answer these questions, we need to compare the miscarriage rate after a period of infertility to the miscarriage rate in women of proven fertility. In Chapter 2 we noted that the fate of a fertilised egg is an unhappy one – one in three conceptions miscarry before pregnancy is declared. Although we know that one in four women will suffer a sporadic miscarriage, the exact incidence depends upon whether we are looking at the clinical or subclinical miscarriage rate. So when we consider miscarriage in women with a history of infertility, we must specify whether we are looking at subclinical losses or clinical losses. Of all clinically recognised pregnancies, one in five or six will end in miscarriage. We also know that one in six couples seek treatment for infertility. Even worse, one in three recurrent miscarriers also has a degree or subfertility or experiences a delay in conception.

The next task is to remind ourselves of the recognised causes of miscarriage – genetic, anatomical, infection, maternal, endocrine (hormonal), immune and prothrombotic factors – in order to focus on factors which may be particularly important in subfertile women. For example, in the genetic category, we need to establish whether chromosomal abnormalities in the baby are increased by the use of fertility drugs, or by the laboratory techniques used to manipulate the eggs and the sperm in treatments such as in vitro fertilisation (IVF), intracytoplasmic sperm injection (ICSI) and all the other newly introduced techniques for sperm retrieval and egg maturation.

The presence of a fibroid near the cavity of the uterus may hinder implantation of a fertilised egg. A previous infection may have resulted in damage to the fallopian tubes or an infection of the womb lining, increasing the chance of an ectopic pregnancy. We know that women who suffer from thyroid disease experience difficulties in falling pregnant and many other hormonal disorders may prevent a potential pregnancy from implanting successfully. Disorders of the immune system may also be a cause of fertility problems (see Chapter 12).

Maternal age and infertility

It is a fact of life that infertility patients tend to be older and that chromosomal abnormalities in the baby increase with advancing maternal age. At least 50% of all sporadic miscarriages are due to chromosomal abnormalities, but an important Italian study reported that in women aged 40 years and over, genetic abnormalities were present in 83% of their miscarried pregnancies.

Delaying the age at which the first pregnancy is conceived also increases the risks of ovulatory disorders, endometriosis and the possibility that a woman may have undergone previous gynaecological or abdominal surgery, causing damage to the uterus and/or the fallopian tubes. Perhaps most importantly, increasing maternal age is accompanied by a natural decline in fertility. The number and quality of the eggs available for fertilisation falls dramatically after the age of 40 years and for some unfortunate women, this poor ovarian reserve occurs even earlier. Furthermore, the womb lining becomes progressively less suitable for the implantation of an embryo and thus places the pregnancy at greater risk.

Past obstetric history

In Chapter 5, we noted that a woman's past obstetric history is very important in determining the likelihood of miscarriage. Primiparous women (who have never been pregnant before) have a very low risk of miscarriage, as do women who have enjoyed successful pregnancies. However, women who have miscarried in the past have an increased risk of future miscarriage. If we now look at women who have suffered infertility, we can see a similar pattern emerging. In the Cambridge population study that I described in detail in Chapter 5, we were able to include a group of 90 women who were being treated for infertility. By following these women carefully, we discovered that women with primary infertility who conceived their first ever pregnancy following fertility treatment, have the same low risk of miscarriage as first pregnancies in women with no infertility problems. This was not the case for multiparous women (those women who have had a previous pregnancy) who had suffered a miscarriage or an ectopic pregnancy after fertility treatment. For these sufferers of secondary infertility, the risk of miscarriage was much higher if they had difficulty becoming pregnant again. Secondary infertility is therefore strongly associated with a poor obstetric history – 75% of these women have had previous pregnancy losses.

Recurrent miscarriage and infertility

Fortunately, women who suffer from recurrent miscarriages are relatively uncommon. However, they deserve a special mention in this chapter since they undoubtedly share some important characteristics with infertility patients. When I first became interested in the field of recurrent miscarriage, I was puzzled that so many of the women I talked to appeared to have difficulties in becoming pregnant, as well as staying pregnant. It occurred to me that there must be some important thread linking infertility and subsequent recurrent early miscarriage. In short, the only difference between the infertile women and the sufferers of miscarriage, was the result of the pregnancy test.

Years later, with more experience and a large recurrent miscarriage database to draw upon, I think my gut feeling was right. Infertility and very early miscarriage represent two points on the same spectrum of reproductive disease. At one end of this spectrum sits the infertility patient whose fertilised egg tries to implant in the womb lining but does not gain a strong enough foothold to allow it to produce enough HCG (pregnancy) hormone to turn the pregnancy test positive. At the other end of the spectrum sits the early miscarriage patient, whose embryo manages to implant sufficiently to start manufacturing HCG, but because the implantation process is faulty, cannot continue to develop. These explanations are no longer just fanciful ideas from an interested young doctor. There are now some robust research data to support these views.

By taking a careful history from all women attending the miscarriage clinic at St Mary's Hospital, we now know that one in three women with recurrent miscarriage have also experienced a degree of subfertility. The most useful question to ask them is how long it has taken them to get pregnant before each miscarriage. A delay of more than 12 months is an abnormally long period of time. Many of these women have undergone a variety of 'infertility' investigations in the past. Further questioning often reveals that these women have irregular periods, ovulation difficulties and have, in the past, been given drugs to help them ovulate. In Chapter 11 the links between recurrent miscarriage and ovulatory problems (in particular polycystic ovaries) are described in detail for the interested reader.

In summary, I think it is very important to identify recurrent miscarriage sufferers who also have difficulty in becoming pregnant, at the first clinic visit. If this association (which is present in just under one-third of miscarriage patients) is overlooked, the opportunity of identifying the root cause of the problem may be lost. As a result, the chances of achieving a successful pregnancy may be delayed or greatly reduced.

Early pregnancy surveillance

One of the main differences between pregnancies achieved spontaneously and after infertility treatment, is the intensity of the early pregnancy monitoring that occurs. It is customary to perform a pregnancy test towards the end of the cycle of treatment on approximately day 26 for those undergoing assisted fertility treatment such as IVF. In this way many women will know that they are pregnant before the time of the expected start of the next period. By contrast, it is more usual for the woman who conceives spontaneously to wait until the expected menstrual period is delayed and then perform a pregnancy test. As a result, biochemical pregnancies which do not continue into clinically recognisable pregnancies are identified more frequently in women undergoing assisted fertility treatment. Infertility patients are also more likely to have an ultrasound scan performed at the end of a cycle of treatment. Using vaginal ultrasound, an intrauterine sac will be visible between four and five weeks after the last missed menstrual period.

Types of infertility

It is beyond the scope of this chapter to provide a detailed classification of the causes of infertility. However, we need a simple checklist to work with. I find the most useful aide-memoire when talking to patients is to divide the causes of infertility very roughly into four groups; ovulatory problems, tubal problems, male factor (sperm) problems and unexplained infertility. Conveniently, these four groups each account for approximately 25% of all cases of infertility.

Lots of studies have looked at the incidence of miscarriage after infertility treatments. Overall the miscarriage rate ranges from 10% to 45% and this wide variation undoubtedly reflects the fact that the risk of miscarriage depends on the underlying cause of the infertility. For example, if the woman has high prolactin levels (hyperprolactinaemia), simple treatment with a drug called bromocriptine usually resolves the difficulty in conceiving very quickly and simply. Interestingly, the miscarriage rate after this treatment is very low, about 12%, which is similar to the incidence of sporadic miscarriage in the general population (see Chapter 11).

Similar results can be expected when a severe male factor problem is the only cause of infertility and the couple choose artificial insemination from a donor (AID). Donor sperm does not increase the miscarriage rate, but if other infertility factors are also present, the miscarriage rate rises. For example, when artificial insemination by the husband/partner is the chosen treatment method, the miscarriage rate can be much higher, because the root of the problem in this situation is often more complex than a low sperm count alone. There may be problems with ovulation as well, requiring treatment to induce the growth and release of an egg. For exactly the same reasons the risk of miscarriage following surgery to unblock fallopian tubes is very variable. If the problem is purely mechanical, the miscarriage rate is low, but when drugs are required to ensure that ovulation is regular, the miscarriage rate goes up.

Sperm abnormalities

Judging by the large number of anxious enquiries that we receive at the miscarriage clinic, it is important to make a few comments about sperm abnormalities and the risk of miscarriage. The use of donor sperm does not increase the miscarriage rate per se. As noted earlier in this chapter, it is only when there are additional fertility problems requiring treatment that the miscarriage rate increases.

There has been much discussion about the role of abnormal sperm and whether they affect the rate of miscarriage. Sperm may be classified as abnormal on the basis of their structure (morphology) as seen under the microscope, or they may be chromosomally (genetically) abnormal. A good example of the latter situation is found in couples with recurrent miscarriage, when the male partner is known to carry a certain abnormality called a 'balanced translocation' (see Chapter 7). Of all the sperm that this man produces, 50% will carry the translocation. If one of these genetically abnormal sperms manages to fertilise an egg, then a chromosomally abnormal fetus will result and the vast majority of these pregnancies are destined to be miscarried because the translocation has now become 'unbalanced'.

The situation is less certain when there is an abnormality in the numbers, mobility or physical structure of the sperms. Some doctors have suggested that there is an increase in the miscarriage rate in these situations, but I must emphasise to the reader that evidence to support this viewpoint is sparse. Sperm counts that are exceptionally high or low may result in delays in conceiving, but they have not been directly linked to an increase in the risk of miscarriage. However, there are an increasing number of studies to show that men aged 45 years or older have higher rates of structural sperm chromosomal abnormalities. Further, advancing paternal age is linked to an increased rate of autosomal dominant disorders, autism, schizophrenia and congenital malformations such as cleft palate and diaphragmatic hernias.

Fertility may be reduced when there are abnormalities in the shape, structure or motility of the sperm, but these problems are not thought to be accompanied by an increased miscarriage rate. Most of the currently available evidence suggests that sperm work to an 'all or none' rule. If they are capable of fertilising an egg, then the resultant embryo is unlikely to be abnormal. However, many abnormal sperm are incapable of successful fertilisation, and because they have lost their ability to fertilise the egg, no pregnancy occurs. Sadly, the same safety mechanism is not present in human eggs. An abnormal egg has no ability to avoid being fertilised by a normal sperm and in this situation a miscarriage may well be the result. Having said all this, I think it is important to remember that our understanding of sub-chromosomal mechanisms that may be the cause of miscarriages is still in its infancy. Abnormal sperm morphology may be reflecting that there are mutations present at the molecular level in the sperm that we are ignorant of at present. Small deletions or duplications are not detectable by conventional chromosomal analysis or even by the newer FISH (fluorescent in situ hybridisation) techniques (see Chapter 7 for further details).

Perhaps the most important new development in our understanding of the role that sperm abnormalities may play in causing miscarriages, is the realization that advancing paternal age is frequently accompanied by an increase in sperm DNA fragmentation. Sperm DNA fragmentation can be caused by a wide variety of environmental and lifestyle factors such as obesity, smoking, cannabis, alcohol, sexually transmitted infections (STIs), various medical disorders and their related drug treatments (for example steroids) and of course, paternal age as noted earlier in this chapter.

Since sperm DNA damage leads to an increase in the conception interval (the time it takes to get pregnant), poorer embryo development and increases the risk of miscarriage, it does also appear that the observed increase in the age of fathers in our society is also making a contribution to the increasing numbers of miscarriages that we are now documenting. Many male patients that I have seen recently in the St Mary's clinic have been advised by other clinics and websites to go and have their sperm tested for DNA fragmentation and then become extremely worried by their results. Not only are these sperm tests expensive, but these couples' anxieties are then made worse in my opinion, by the further advice that invariably follows the report of high sperm DNA fragmentation rates, namely that the next step is for them to purchase courses of expensive remedies to 'fix their problem'. These take the form of a wide variety of anti-oxidant therapies and vitamin supplements that have never been shown to significantly improve the situation. Nevertheless, these couples are then encouraged to undergo repeat sperm DNA fragmentation testing after a three-month course of so called 'treatment' to reassess the sperm quality with predictably variable results. When the prospective randomized trials have been undertaken to show that one of these anti-oxidant or vitamin combi-nations does improve sperm DNA fragmentation rates then I will be happy to include them in our clinic. But at the present time, I really do feel that many couples who are already feeling very vulnerable are being exploited to spend significant sums of money on expensive tests and treatment packages that are difficult to justify.

One last point needs to be mentioned here. There has been much concern expressed about the possibility that the newest high-tech assisted fertility treatments may cause an increase in the numbers of miscarriages or abnormalities in the babies born. For example, intracytoplasmic sperm injection (ICSI) involves injecting sperm from men with very low abnormal sperm counts into the woman's eggs using a microscopic technique. This procedure could potentially allow a grossly abnormal sperm to fertilise an egg. Reassuringly, I can state that many thousands of pregnancies have now been achieved as a result of this ground-breaking technique, but there have been no reports of a significant increase in the miscarriage rate. The number of major congenital abnormalities in babies born after ICSI treatment does not appear to be higher when allowance is made for the increased numbers of multiple pregnancies and premature births that occur, both of which are independent risk factors for congenital abnormalities. However, there is an increase in the incidence of hypospadias (when the urethral opening or urine hole does not reach the end of the penis) in male infants, but since this is easily correctible by surgery, it is considered a minor abnormality. Overall,

I think it is fair to say that ICSI treatment has proved to be one of the most important breakthroughs in assisted fertility therapy since the technique of IVF was first described in 1974.

Influence of fertility drugs on the miscarriage rate

There is no doubt that drugs which improve ovulation carry with them a penalty of an increased miscarriage rate. What is not so clearly understood is whether it is the drugs themselves or the underlying ovulation problem which determines this increase in the miscarriage rate.

We noted earlier that ovulatory failure (anovulation) accounts for at least 25% of infertility. In about three-quarters of all cases of anovulatory infertility, the problem is due to the presence of polycystic ovaries. Furthermore, we know that polycystic ovaries are associated with a higher rate of miscarriage when compared to the miscarriage rate in women with normal ovaries (see Chapter 11). So any increase in the number of miscarriages experienced by women with polycystic ovaries and infertility could be due to the effect of the drugs used or it may reflect that the drugs are forcing an egg to be ovulated which, if fertilised, is already at greater risk of miscarrying.

Over the last 30 years, a variety of drug treatments have been used to induce ovulation. Regular ovulation can be achieved in the vast majority of women with polycystic ovaries using modern drug therapy. However, ovulation does not guarantee a pregnancy or a successful birth. Broadly speaking, there are four groups of drugs that can be used singly or in combination, depending on the type of fertility treatment undertaken. These are the anti-oestrogens (clomiphene citrate or tamoxifen), the insulin sensitizing agents (metformin), the gonadotropins (human menopausal gonadotrophin or pure follicle-stimulating hormone) and the gonadotrophin releasing hormone (GnRH) agonists (buserelin).

Ovulation induction with clomiphene citrate

This was the first drug used to induce ovulation and is still the most widely prescribed. It is cheap and has fewer side-effects than HMG, hence it has an important place in first line therapy for anovulation. Clomiphene has anti-oestrogenic effects and it is thought to promote ovulation by stimulating the release of natural follicle-stimulating hormone (FSH) from the pituitary. FSH acts upon the ovaries to produce follicles. There have been many studies undertaken to examine the effect of this drug and very variable miscarriage rates have been reported ranging from 9 to 50%. Before ultrasound was routinely used to watch the growth of the ovarian follicles, it was often very difficult to monitor the individual's response to the clomiphene. The diagnosis of pregnancy was usually not made until the period had been delayed, and so the true rate of miscarriage for these patients was never really determined.

If we look at the results from more recent studies, most doctors would agree that when clomiphene is used, the miscarriage rate is in the region of 20 to 30%. Many patients I meet have been alarmed (I would say unnecessarily so) by suggestions that the miscarriage rate increases even further when pregnancy occurs during the first cycle of clomiphene treatment or after six cycles of treatment. There is no truth in these assertions.

One of the concerns about the use of clomiphene has been whether it increases the incidence of chromosomal abnormalities and congenital abnormalities. Several reports have suggested that there is an association between the use of clomiphene and neural tube defects, such as spina bifida. However, most studies have concluded that there is no evidence for concern on this issue. Indeed, it is now generally agreed that babies born after the mother has been treated with clomiphene are no more at risk of being malformed than if they were conceived spontaneously.

Many doctors believe that the increased risk of miscarriage after clomiphene treatment is because the drug causes an abnormal hormonal environment, which in turn has an adverse effect on the developing egg and or the development of the womb lining. Clomiphene increases the secretion of FSH and LH in the early part of the menstrual cycle before ovulation. The effect of these high levels of LH during the time at which the egg is undergoing maturation may result in the ovulation of an egg which is 'over-ripe' and which, if fertilised, is less likely to be able to implant successfully and miscarries early. Equally, if the endometrium is less receptive, any embryo that is created is less likely to implant successfully.

The most common cause of persistently high LH levels is polycystic ovary syndrome (see Chapter 11) and, in such cases, clomiphene probably exaggerates the already high LH levels, leading in turn to miscarriage problems. The best approach to ovulation induction in women with PCOS is aimed at preventing the high LH levels from occurring. To this end, some doctors use tamoxifen or letrozole as an alternative to clomiphene citrate because this drug has been shown to induce ovulation without increasing LH concentrations.

I frequently meet patients in the miscarriage clinic who, despite the fact that they ovulate spontaneously, have been given clomiphene (or ask me to prescribe it) in the mistaken belief that this drug will 'improve their fertility'. It is important for me to emphasise that this use of clomiphene is unhelpful and frequently leads to problems. Because clomiphene may also have some anti-oestrogenic effects, it can lead to thickening of the cervical mucus and prevent sperm from penetrating. It can also interfere with the development of the uterine lining, preventing the embryo from implanting easily. Furthermore, the ovaries may develop persistent cysts after clomiphene treatment and interfere with the woman's normal ovulatory pattern.

Lastly, clomiphene is invariably unsuccessful in treating women over the age of 40 years when there is no evidence to suggest that they are not ovulating. Indeed, in this situation it is likely that the only result will be the occasional release of an abnormal egg, which if it does get fertilised, will not implant or will miscarry soon after. These are all good reasons why clomiphene should only be taken when there is a genuine problem with ovulation and only when its use is supervised and carefully monitored to prevent complications developing.

Insulin sensitising agents to improve ovulation induction

Women with PCOS may develop insulin resistance, which means that their body stops reacting appropriately to normal levels of insulin in the bloodstream. To compensate for this, they start to produce more insulin hormone (which comes from the pancreas gland) than their body needs and this in turn leads to them having higher levels of androgen hormone which adversely affects their ovulatory function. Strictly speaking, metformin or Glucophage is not an ovulation induction drug, but because it is an insulin sensitizing agent and used very successfully in people with Type 2 diabetes mellitus to control their blood sugar levels, it can be used in women with PCOS who are not ovulating properly.

By reducing the circulating high levels of insulin, metformin reverses the hormonal abnormality in PCOS and effectively normalizes their endocrine, metabolic and reproductive functions. When the metformin treatments make the insulin levels return to normal, this allows the ovulatory process to be reset and normalize. Several small retrospective studies have shown that the use of metformin in the early weeks of pregnancy is associated with a reduction in the miscarriage rate for women with PCOS. However, larger studies have not confirmed these findings but nevertheless, many women that I see in the clinic at St Mary's have been started on metformin therapy because they have PCOS and have had problems in conceiving recently or alternatively because they are obese and have been told that the metformin therapy may help them to lose weight.

Currently, the best advice to offer women who conceive while taking metformin is that they should continue taking the same dose of medication until the end of the first trimester. However, some doctors consider that it is better to continue the drug throughout pregnancy since it does not appear to be associated with any side-effects and there are some anecdotal reports to suggest that ongoing therapy may reduce the risk of the woman developing gestational diabetes mellitus or GDM.

Ovulation induction with gonadotropins

For those women who do not respond to clomiphene citrate, gonadotropin treatment may be needed to induce ovulation. There are a variety of preparations available, either human menopausal gonadotropin (HMG) which contains equal quantities of both FSH and LH, or purified FSH, which is more expensive to produce. Although it was previously thought that preparations containing low levels of LH would benefit women with polycystic ovaries, by minimising circulating LH levels, experience has shown that the use of purified FSH offers no advantage.

Whatever preparation is used, the main problems with gonadotrophin treatment are the multiple pregnancy and miscarriage rates, two problems which are often related to each other. The miscarriage rate after gonadotropin-induced ovulation ranges from 10 to 48%. There is no difference in the miscarriage rate if conception occurs in the first or the subsequent treatment cycle. However, the miscarriage rate following HMG therapy is dependent on the outcome of previous pregnancies. This is in keeping with the miscarriage pattern seen in natural conceptions (see Chapter 5). For example, one very large study reported a miscarriage rate of 24% in the first treatment cycle, which rose to 48% in those women whose first HMG pregnancy had ended in miscarriage. By contrast, if the first HMG-induced pregnancy had been successful, the incidence of miscarriage in the second HMG pregnancy was only 7%.

It is very important that HMG treatment is carefully controlled. Some women overreact to the gonadotropins and develop ovarian hyperstimulation syndrome. Their ovaries become grossly enlarged and cystic, and large quantities of fluid are produced, which then leaks into the peritoneal cavity (the space surrounding all the organs in the abdomen). Not only is this complication extremely painful, it is also potentially life-threatening. There is also a serious risk that HMG treatment will result in the production of many follicles, each containing an egg, all of which may be released if careful monitoring is not performed. By watching the growth of the follicles using ultrasound scans and performing regular hormone measurements, this problem can be limited. Where necessary, the doses of the drugs given can be adjusted and the injection of HCG (human chorionic gonadotropin), which triggers ovulation, can be withheld in cases when too many follicles have been produced.

Several theories have been proposed to explain why the miscarriage rate is high after gonadotropin therapy. We know that the miscarriage rate increases with maternal age and also when the mother is very overweight or obese. Approximately one-third of patients with polycystic ovaries suffer from moderate obesity and it is important to advise women who are overweight that their chances of a successful pregnancy will be better if they lose weight before undergoing treatment. High levels of LH, as we know, definitely have an adverse impact: numerous studies have reported that women with infertility, polycystic ovaries and high LH have a far poorer outcome of pregnancy after gonadotropin treatment than women with infertility, polycystic ovaries and normal LH levels.

In summary, the babies conceived following treatment with gonadotropins do not suffer from any increased risk of abnormality. They have the same incidence of congenital abnormalities as the general population.

Controlling the ovaries

In recent years, there has been a definite move towards using gonadotropin-releasing hormone (GnRH) agonists in order to control the number of eggs produced. The agonists effectively shut down (desensitise) the pituitary gland and impose a temporary menopausal state upon the woman, allowing us to take over the control of egg development. Having suppressed the pituitary gland, the ovaries are also suppressed, and they are then very receptive to gonadotropins such as HMG, and not affected by any spontaneous hormonal changes. Using this method to down regulate the ovary has improved pregnancy rates in IVF programmes and has been adopted widely. This type of treatment is particularly useful for women with polycystic ovary syndrome, since it allows the doctors to actually suppress the high levels of LH. Eggs produced in this way appear to fertilise better than those from other treatment cycles. However, it is important to mention that the use of this treatment for women with recurrent miscarriage and high LH levels does not improve the miscarriage rate (See Chapter 11 for more details).

The influence of IVF and related procedures on the miscarriage rate

The number of pregnancies that miscarry after IVF and related procedures varies widely. Overall, the miscarriage rate is in the region of 25%, but in older women the figure is certainly higher. Many patients are concerned that the laboratory techniques involved in IVF treatments may increase the risk of miscarriage, but this does not seem to be true. Nor is there any increase in the numbers of congenital malformations in the babies born as a result of IVF (mentioned earlier in this chapter).

Multiple pregnancy

For every 80 pregnancies that are conceived naturally, one will result in the delivery of twins. The delivery of triplets is much rarer, only occurring once in 6000 spontaneous pregnancies. When fertility drugs are used, the number of multiple pregnancies is much higher. After clomiphene treatment, more than one in ten pregnancies are multiple, and when gonadotropin treatment is used, the figure rises to one in five pregnancies, even when the treatment has been carefully controlled. Indeed, the UK regulatory body for assisted fertility treatment, the Human Fertilisation and Embryology Authority (HFEA) website advises that women are 11 times more likely to have a multiple birth following IVF than if they conceive naturally.

Now that early ultrasound scans are so widely used in pregnancy, we know that many pregnancies start with more than one pregnancy 'sac' in the uterus and that many potential twins and triplets are miscarried very early. Indeed, some doctors think that as many as two-thirds of twin sacs seen on the scan during the first eight weeks of pregnancy 'vanish' and result in a single baby being delivered at the end of the pregnancy. It is reassuring to note that when one of the sacs vanishes very early, the pregnancy usually continues without complications.

Multiple pregnancies involving more than two embryos are often associated with disastrous outcomes. There is a much higher risk of early and late miscarriage, stillbirth and an inevitable risk of premature delivery, not to mention the long-term complications of being born too early in babies who survive the neonatal period. If this sounds frightening, then I have succeeded in making my point. I cannot overstate the importance of ensuring that fertility treatment does not result in a multiple pregnancy of triplets or more, which is why I think it is so important to promote the use of single embryo transfer or SET.

In the UK, the HFEA has done much to help reduce the multiple pregnancy rates in women undergoing IVF and other related procedures, by enforcing their recommendations that no more than two embryos are ever transferred into the uterine cavity at the same time. Any UK clinic will have its licence to practice IVF revoked if an inspection by the HFEA identifies that they have not been adhering to this ruling. As a result, most of the multiple pregnancies that are now conceived in the UK are secondary to the use of clomiphene and other ovulation induction agents, which are not subject to the same legal regulatory rules. However, many clinicians who have had to deal with the complications associated with multiple pregnancies now argue that undoubtedly the best way to safeguard against these disasters is to allow the transfer of only one embryo at a time. In a memorable quote, one fertility specialist that I know was quoted as saying: 'Transfer as many embryos as you like – so long as you do it one at a time.' Now that the facilities for embryo freezing are freely available, there is really no excuse for SET not to be a part of routine good practice in every UK clinic, although there is no way that fertility clinics overseas can be subjected to the same strict regulations.

Antiphospholipid antibodies

I mentioned in Chapters 12 and 13 that antiphospholipid antibodies (APL) have been associated with previously unexplained infertility. In particular, they are reported to be more common in women who have had repeated IVF treatment failures. Not surprisingly, an increasing number of doctors and their patients have explored the possibility that treatment with aspirin and heparin may have the same beneficial effect in infertility patients that it offers women with recurrent miscarriage. However, the results have been disappointing and they warrant a brief description here, since many couples that I meet appear to believe that the aspirin and heparin treatment is the answer to their infertility problems. At the present time it is important that I state quite firmly that this is not the case.

There have been several studies published, mostly originating from private fertility units in the United States, that have shown a high prevalence of phospholipid antibodies in their patients. The figures quoted have varied enormously but some units have reported prevalence rates of over 50%. I hope these variable figures raise as many queries in the reader's head as they do in mine. I think the only reasonable explanation can be that the assays used to detect the phospholipid antibodies have not been standardised and must therefore be regarded with suspicion.

In an attempt to answer this question, we undertook a large study in collaboration with fertility colleagues at my own London hospital some years ago. By ensuring that all the tests were performed in the same specialist haemostasis laboratory and that they adhered strictly with international laboratory guidelines, we were able to demonstrate that APA are present in 23% of women embarking on an IVF treatment cycle. However, the most important finding from our study was that the presence of APA did not affect the outcome of IVF treatment. The success rates in terms of pregnancies achieved and the ongoing pregnancy rates and live births were identical in women with and without phospholipid antibodies. These results convinced me that the use of aspirin and heparin in these women is quite simply unethical. If this sounds strong language, then I think the reader needs to reflect on the fact that no drug treatment is ever completely without side-effects and complications. Since our pregnancy outcome study has shown that the success of IVF treatment is unchanged by the presence of the APL, I would find it enormously difficult to have to look a couple straight in the eye who had experienced complications or side-effects and try to argue that I had used the treatment in their best interests. There is no evidence to justify this treatment.

Additional immunological therapies for infertility patients

My views are not shared by all fertility units and many IVF doctors are currently prescribing aspirin and heparin treatment for their patients along with complex cocktails of other so called 'add on immunological therapies' such as steroids, intravenous immunoglobulin, intralipid and anti-TNF alpha drugs. In Chapter 12, I explained the supposed rationale for the use of these drugs and add-on treatments and provided the reader with details of the potential side-effects, but a few points need to be re-emphasised again here. At best these so called immune modulating treatments are expensive interventions which raise false hopes and expectations in couples with subfertility who understandably feel quite desperate and often decide to accept their doctor's advice and take the drugs because they want to feel that they have done everything in their power to achieve a successful outcome. However, in the worst case they could be the source of significant clinical side-effects and litigation procedures.

If and when a properly randomized controlled treatment trial of aspirin, heparin, steroids, IVIG, intralipid, anti-TNF alpha and any other drugs which come onto the scene in the future, demonstrates that these therapies significantly improve the chances of conceiving and achieving a live take-home baby in women undergoing fertility treatment, then I will happily and humbly retract my comments and applaud the study. But at the present time this is not the case and, in my opinion, the widespread use of these treatments only serves to confuse and mislead couples who are seeking help from fertility specialists at an extremely vulnerable time in their lives.

Conclusions

There are specific factors that increase the risk of miscarriage in women who have had infertility. These are advancing maternal age, poor obstetric history, multiple pregnancy and obesity. I would argue that miscarriage is more common in women with infertility because of these associations. However, it is important to note that the treatments used to improve fertility do not in themselves increase the risk of miscarriage. Nor do they increase the risk of abnormalities in the babies that they help to produce.

15

HOW WILL I RECOGNISE A THREATENED MISCARRIAGE?

Miscarriage is a process, not a single event. A detailed account of the ways in which the woman and her doctor can diagnose the various types and stages of miscarriage was given in Chapter 3. In this chapter, I will mention some of these points again. However, the aim of this chapter is to talk about the questions that I am most frequently asked by women when they are threatening to miscarry or have just suffered a definite miscarriage.

One of the first signs of threatened miscarriage is vaginal bleeding. It can occur at any time after a missed period. The bleeding usually starts lightly and is much less heavy than a menstrual period. Often the bleeding is first noticed when going to the toilet. You may see a smear of pink, brown or red blood on the tissue paper. Bright red blood indicates that the bleeding is fresh, whereas brown blood suggests that the bleeding has occurred some time ago and that the blood is old. Sometimes the blood comes in a gush and can be very heavy with large clots. As a general rule, the older the pregnancy, the heavier the bleeding may be. But whatever the stage of pregnancy, it is sensible to report it to your doctor without delay.

Whatever the quantity or the colour of the blood, it is always very frightening and upsetting. I meet many couples who are quite simply devastated when they experience some bleeding in pregnancy. I think much of the distress is because we feel so helpless in this situation. Certainly, this was the feeling uppermost in my mind when I suddenly had an episode of heavy bleeding six weeks into my own pregnancy.

I found it difficult to believe that it was happening to me and since I was sitting quietly in a meeting with about 20 other gynaecologists, I can remember thinking that all the expert help in the world could do nothing to help. Happily, my twins did not bat an eyelid (so to speak), and the only casualty was the chair I was sitting on!

It is important for you to realise that bleeding in early pregnancy is extremely common. Most importantly, you need to remember that in most cases, the pregnancy continues safely. Every doctor who has cared for women with bleeding in early pregnancy will tell you that even when the bleeding is quite heavy, this does not necessarily mean that the pregnancy has been lost. There is still a good chance that the pregnancy will progress normally. This is one of the reasons that an ultrasound scan is usually performed before we assume that the pregnancy has ended. I never cease to be amazed by the amount of blood that can be lost and yet when I turn on the ultrasound machine, there is the beating fetal heart clearly visible on the screen.

Many women I see are worried that bleeding in early pregnancy may cause some damage to the baby. This is not true. Even if you bleed quite heavily, the baby will come to no harm if the pregnancy continues. In later pregnancy, bleeding may also occur and be a source of great anxiety. Once again, if the pregnancy does not miscarry, the baby will not be deprived of its oxygen and nutrient supplies, and you can feel reassured as long as the episode of bleeding has been carefully investigated by your doctor.

When lower abdominal pain occurs with or after the bleeding, the situation is more worrying. This is because cramping pain may be a sign that the pregnancy is about to miscarry. Sometimes women describe pain in the lower back or at the top of the vagina. Having said this, I must emphasise strongly to you that lower abdominal pain is common during early pregnancy and does not necessarily mean that anything is seriously wrong. If the pain becomes severe, resembling labour pains, and the bleeding becomes heavier, then it is important to see your doctor.

When lower abdominal pain occurs before any bleeding is noticed, it is possible that the pregnancy is ectopic. This is a potentially serious complication and the whereabouts of the pregnancy needs to be confirmed straight away (see Chapter 3).

Some women are extremely sensitive to the general symptoms of pregnancy such as nausea, breast tenderness and tiredness. Such women may actually be able to tell that their pregnancy has miscarried before they experience any physical signs such as bleeding or pain. It is true that the complete disappearance of these symptoms in early pregnancy is unusual, and that when they fade away, this might be a signal that the pregnancy is not continuing. It is also true, however, that some women do not experience the symptoms in the first place. It is important to understand that a lessening of these symptoms does not necessarily mean that a miscarriage has occurred. It is to be expected that these symptoms will pass away after 14 weeks, and in some women, even earlier.

So please do not panic if you do not feel as pregnant today as you did yesterday. Remember that for every woman who recounts her personal story of how she knew exactly when she lost her pregnancy, there are many more women who have also had this sensation, but have not turned this into a story – because everything turned out well. It is much more likely that your pregnancy is progressing normally. If you are worried that something is 'not quite right', then go and see your doctor. He or she will probably suggest that you have an ultrasound scan to assess the situation and hopefully provide you with the reassurance you need.

One further point needs mentioning here. I know that some women who experience a missed miscarriage (see Chapter 3) feel very distressed that they did not realise that their pregnancy had died until some time after the event. I make a special point of telling women that this in no way suggests that they have been negligent or insensitive, and assuring them that they will be every bit as capable a mother when their successful pregnancy does come about.

Perhaps the most painful question that I have to try and answer when I am talking to a woman who is threatening to miscarry is, 'What can I do to prevent it?' I am sorry to say that there is very little you can do in very early pregnancy. At this stage the outcome of the pregnancy has already been determined and you cannot change this outcome whatever you do. Of course in later pregnancy, there are some treatments that may stop the uterus from contracting or the cervix from dilating, such as bed rest and the use of some drugs. But in early pregnancy these remedies do not help. I mention this here, not to fill you with gloom but to make sure that you realise that retiring to your bed and wrapping yourself in cotton wool is unlikely to prevent a miscarriage. Although many women believe that the bleeding restarts only when they stop lying down, this is because the blood collects at the top of the vagina and only drains away when they get up to walk around or go to the toilet. If you feel that going to bed may reassure you, then go to bed. If, on the other hand, lying in bed thinking about the problem non-stop makes you feel even worse, then don't go to bed and get on with your everyday life.

16

WHAT TESTS ARE AVAILABLE TO DIAGNOSE MY MISCARRIAGE?

There are several methods which may help you and your doctors to diagnose that you have miscarried. We have already discussed the importance of a physical vaginal examination (Chapter 3). When the cervix is closed and the uterus is firm and of normal size, it is likely that the uterus is empty and the miscarriage is described as complete. When the cervix is still open and the uterus feels soft and bulky, it is possible that there are still products of conception (usually pieces of placental tissue) in the cavity. The diagnosis of an incomplete miscarriage can be confirmed with an ultrasound scan, although this is not always necessary.

If you have had a missed miscarriage, the physical examination will reveal that the uterus is smaller in size than would be expected for your pregnancy dates and the cervix is usually closed. An ultrasound scan will show that the baby has died and has started to be reabsorbed. In this type of miscarriage, the woman is often aware that her pregnancy symptoms have faded, because the hormones of pregnancy have stopped being produced.

Pregnancy tests

Although the pregnancy test is very useful to diagnose that you are pregnant, it is not always helpful in deciding that you have miscarried. This is because the human chorionic gonadotropin (HCG) hormone that is being measured in the pregnancy test takes time to completely clear from your body after the pregnancy is ended. This time delay is referred to as the 'half life' of the hormone and in the case of HCG the half life is about 36 hours. This means that the levels of HCG will fall by half every 36 hours that pass after the pregnancy dies.

If the miscarriage occurs very early and the HCG levels have never been high, the pregnancy test will become negative very quickly. A good example of this is a biochemical pregnancy (see Chapter 2), in which the woman may have no physical symptoms or signs of pregnancy. On the other hand, if the levels of HCG have reached a high level by the time the miscarriage occurs, it may take many days for the HCG to clear completely and for the pregnancy test to read negative. This applies to both blood and urine tests and explains why your pregnancy test may still be positive when the ultrasound scan shows that the pregnancy has miscarried. This can be a cause of great confusion and distress for women who have just miscarried.

Nowadays, the HCG pregnancy tests that are performed on blood samples can be 'quantified' very accurately. Instead of a yes or no result, the actual levels of HCG may be reported. Knowing the number of units of HCG present in the blood may be useful in certain situations. If the levels are increasing very slowly in the early weeks of pregnancy, this is often a sign that the pregnancy is not developing properly, but this is not a hard and fast rule. I do not use HCG tests very often for miscarriage patients because I find that they rarely influence how I manage my patient.

The exception to this is when I suspect that a woman has an ectopic pregnancy (see Chapter 3). In this situation it may be possible to avoid an operation if the levels of HCG start to fall with conservative management. Some ectopic pregnancies do stop growing before they reach a size which endangers the woman (due to the risk of rupturing through the wall of her fallopian tube). The ectopic may just shrivel up and be absorbed within the tube or it may miscarry out of the end of the tube into the abdominal cavity. If the woman is not experiencing abdominal pain and the HCG levels are starting to fall, it may be possible to keep a close eye on her, repeating the HCG test every couple of days until the levels reach zero.

Alternatively, it may be indicated to perform a laparoscopy (telescopic procedure through the navel) and remove the affected tube with the ectopic pregnancy. If the tube on the other side of the one with the ectopic also looks abnormal and dysfunctional, the gynaecologist may advise you that it would be better for you to undergo a laparoscopic salpingostomy instead of completely removing the affected tube, which is called a salpingectomy. The salpingostomy is a procedure whereby a hole is made in the tube and the ectopic sucked out of it. This leaves the woman with at least one potentially functional tube and the possibility that she may be able to conceive spontaneously. However, this more conservative surgical method does have a higher chance of the woman experiencing repeat ectopic pregnancies when compared to a complete removal of the tube. These procedures should only be carried out by doctors experienced in this method of treatment for an ectopic pregnancy.

Progesterone tests

It is true that your blood levels of progesterone hormone will usually be lower than normal if you are miscarrying, but this is not a helpful test. I always advise doctors not to perform it and explain to my patients why it is not useful for them to request this test. Very low progesterone levels reflect the fact that the ovary and/or the early placenta are not working properly. The production of hormone falls because the pregnancy has failed and is destined to miscarry. Since injections of progesterone (or HCG) cannot make the pregnancy come alive again (see Chapter 4), the information gained from a progesterone test is of no practical use.

I know that many women who have had fertility treatment are offered regular progesterone tests in early pregnancy. The reason for this is that high levels can be interpreted as showing that the pregnancy is off to a good start. While this may be comforting for some women, I think it is important to remember that progesterone levels may vary widely from individual to individual. A lower than average level does not necessarily mean that the pregnancy is in trouble, but the low result almost always causes anxiety and distress. I think progesterone tests in early pregnancy should be avoided and in later pregnancy they are of no help at all.

Development of future blood tests

The medical journals and the lay press are always very quick to report potential new tests which may help us to predict pregnancies that are at risk of miscarrying. The problem is that many of the new tests that are initially heralded as breakthroughs in miscarriage care, subsequently do not stand up to the test of time and longer-term evaluation of their benefit. Some of them are very sensitive, which means that they pick up a lot of possible abnormalities – but frequently they are then found to be poor in specificity, which means that they identify too many false positive results. Of course, the reverse can also be the case – the test may be a good one in terms of specificity but not sensitive enough to pick up all the potential abnormalities.

So the best advice I can give you is by all means investigate the possibility that the latest test described in your daily newspaper or favourite magazine is helpful, but make sure that you also find out how many false positive and false negative results this test is likely to produce. Trying to tease out the most useful test results has always been a difficult task, but now that most individuals have easy access to the Internet, I think the problems have escalated. The information that is placed on the world wide web does not have to be peer reviewed or formally critiqued by experts in the field in the same way that information published in reputable journals has been carefully scrutinised. So be wary and try to ensure that you don't rush off and undergo new tests that lead to untried treatments until you feel confident that there is enough sound evidence to justify your participating in potentially disappointing and possibly harmful procedures.

Oxidative stress

Although oxygen is essential for life, we now understand that as we use the oxygen it gives rise to very toxic waste products called free radicals, which cause all sorts of damage to our cells. This is known as oxidative stress and has long been known to be associated with some cases of infertility, miscarriage and pre-eclampsia. The media regularly offers us information, some useful, some not, about ways in which we can include antioxidants in our daily dietary intake to tackle or counteract these damaging free radicals. Red wine, a wide range of so called 'superfoods', together with most vegetables and fruits are great natural sources of antioxidants as are the vitamins C and E.

Initial studies on the use of vitamin C and E to prevent pre-eclampsia raised everyone's hopes that regular supplements of these everyday vitamins throughout pregnancy would be beneficial. However, the results of a large MRC randomized, controlled trial demonstrated that this simple intervention did not reduce the incidence of pre-eclampsia – indeed the control arm had better obstetric outcomes. Nevertheless, the idea that women with single or repeated miscarriages might benefit from taking high dose vitamins in the pre-conception period and during the first trimester of pregnancy to try to offset the oxidative stress that is known to occur in some miscarriages, is a concept that attracted much interest. The theory was that when the mother allowed placental perfusion with oxygen rich blood to occur too early in pregnancy, the tiny embryo would then be exposed to reactive oxygen species (ROS) and early exposure to the damaging effects of free radicals. While it may seem a reasonable assumption that high dose anti-oxidant or vitamin supplements could provide some protection against miscarriage, a meta-analysis of all the relevant studies which was later published as a Cochrane Review, failed to identify any significant benefit.

Kisspeptin testing

I will try to resist the temptation of including all of the potential new tests that have been reported in the last few years because I believe that the readers of this book need to receive information that is evidence-based and tried and tested. But I am going to mention the work that my colleagues Steve Bloom and Channa Jayasena have been undertaking on trying to identify hormones and proteins that will help us to predict both miscarriage and successful pregnancy outcomes. They have performed extensive studies on the kisspeptins, a family of proteins which are produced by and are present in the placenta. The fact that the KISS1 gene, which encodes for this protein, is so abundant in the placenta, gonads (both ovaries and testes) and hypothalamus (in the brain) led early researchers in this field to hypothesise that kisspeptin had an important role to play in reproductive health and is involved in several vital processes necessary for ensuring a successful pregnancy outcome.

Pregnancy levels of circulating kisspeptin increase dramatically during a normal pregnancy by several thousand-fold. The levels peak in the third trimester, reaching up to 7000 times that of non-pregnant controls, but by five days into the postnatal period they have fallen dramatically, which further confirms that the protein is produced by and is under placental control. Furthermore, circulating kisspeptin levels appear to correlate with placental function in ongoing pregnancies. Studies have shown that circulating kisspeptin values in the early part of the second trimester at 16–20 weeks' gestation are lower in the pregnancies of women who subsequently went on to develop pre-eclampsia and intra uterine growth restriction. Further reports have now been published of significantly lower circulating kisspeptin levels being found later in pregnancies affected by Type 1 diabetes, gestational diabetes, pre-eclampsia and gestational hypertension.

Most recently, evidence that kisspeptin levels are lower in pregnancies that go on to subsequently miscarry has emerged. Jayasena and colleagues showed that circulating kisspeptin levels at the antenatal booking visit correlated with the risk of miscarriage, being 60% lower in women who miscarried compared to those with healthy pregnancies outcomes. This offers us a novel predictive marker for assessing the risk of miscarriage and other later complications of pregnancy due to poor placental function, since low levels in the first trimester were also associated with small for gestational age babies in the neonatal period.

The predictive value of a single blood test for serum kisspeptin levels in the first trimester is much more accurate than for serum HCG levels measured at the same time interval. The relationship of kisspeptin with miscarriage has also been demonstrated in twin pregnancies, where death of one fetus was associated with lower kisspeptin levels than those without complications. In summary, low kisspeptin levels are reliably diagnostic of a pregnancy that is destined to miscarry and, by contrast, kisspeptin values that exceed a certain value can provide women with much needed reassurance that their pregnancy is safe, which cannot be said for HCG levels. Hence, kisspeptin measurements are now emerging as a predictive tool which will help us to monitor and best manage women with pregnancies at risk in the future.

Although much further research is needed to unravel the intricacies of the role of kisspeptin in embryo implantation, it seems to be clear that it does have an important role to play in successful pregnancy and the current evidence suggests that its importance continues throughout pregnancy and into the early stages of postnatal life.

Ultrasound scans

Without doubt the most useful method to find out what is happening to your early pregnancy is the ultrasound scan. I often wonder to myself how we used to manage when ultrasounds were not so freely available. Of course, the answer is that many women experienced long periods of worry and uncertainty about whether their pregnancy was safe or at risk.

A wide range of early pregnancy US signs and appearances have been studied in the hope that they will provide us with information as to whether the pregnancy is going to continue successfully or fail to progress. Several studies have suggested that an irregular shape to the gestation sac or yolk sac, a slow fetal heartbeat, slow growth of the early embryo and the presence of blood clots behind the placenta are indicative of a poor outcome or prognosis. I need to emphasise here that none of these signs are conclusive.

The first questions you will want answered if you experience pain or bleeding in early pregnancy are, 'Am I still pregnant?' and, 'Is my baby alright?' An ultrasound scan will be able to see whether the pregnancy sac is intact and whether there is an embryo present in the sac. It will also be able to tell you whether the pregnancy is in the right place. If there is no sac visible in the cavity of the uterus, it is important to find out whether you have had a complete miscarriage or whether the pregnancy is in an ectopic site, most usually the fallopian tubes. Ectopics are notoriously difficult to visualise on the scan, but there may be tell-tale signs suggesting that you are pregnant, even though no pregnancy sac can be seen. These are thickening of the uterine lining in the absence of a small round early pregnancy sac, and fluid in the space behind the body of the uterus – known as the Pouch of Douglas. The fluid which collects in this pouch is usually blood which has escaped from the fallopian tubes. These scan findings will alert your doctor to the fact that you may have an ectopic pregnancy.

If you have a vaginal ultrasound scan, it is usually possible to see whether there is a tiny embryo with a fetal heartbeat by six weeks into the pregnancy. If there is a heartbeat present, this is a very encouraging sign because many miscarriages happen before the baby has grown to a size that requires a proper circulation of blood with a heartbeat.

If there is no heartbeat, but a tiny fetal pole is visible, it is still possible that a heartbeat will develop by the seventh week. It is important to remember that sometimes your pregnancy dates will be wrong, or you may have a particularly long menstrual cycle which means that you became pregnant later than you thought! By seven weeks, if there is a fetal pole within a healthy-looking intrauterine gestation sac, then you should be able to see a heartbeat.

For women who have not had miscarriages, the likelihood of the pregnancy being successful after a fetal heart has been seen is over 95%. For women who have experienced several miscarriages, the prognostic value of a fetal heart is not so good. Some cases of autoimmune recurrent miscarriage due to phospholipid antibodies (see Chapter 13) are notorious for miscarrying after fetal heart activity has been seen, but this problem affects no more than 15% of all recurrent miscarriage sufferers.

If you have experienced some bleeding, you will want to know where it is coming from. The US scan may be able to see an area of blood clot behind the placenta (haematoma). It may also demonstrate that there is another sac in the uterus which is not developing and is starting to break up, which is the cause of the bleeding you are experiencing. Second sacs (twin conceptions) are actually very common. We did not realise this until US scans became so routine a procedure in early pregnancy. A further scan in a week or two will probably be able to show you that the blood clot is smaller in size or the second sac is being reabsorbed.

I think you will be comforted to hear about the results of a study we performed at St Mary's Hospital many years ago. We looked back into the miscarriage clinic database over a period of several years and collected together all the women who had attended our dedicated early pregnancy scanning clinic during their next pregnancy. When we analysed their early pregnancy scan reports we found that the presence of intrauterine haematomas was really quite common. 12% of our patients with a history of recurrent miscarriage developed a haematoma in their next pregnancy. We then looked at the final pregnancy outcomes of these women and happily we were able to identify that the presence of an intrauterine haematoma in early pregnancy did not predict a further miscarriage or later pregnancy complication such as fetal growth retardation, pre-eclampsia or premature delivery. Yes, it is true that the haematoma patients did experience more episodes of vaginal bleeding and they were also more likely to have phospholipid syndrome, but this did not affect the final pregnancy outcome. I think this is a reassuring finding and I hope that it will give you some comfort if you are told that you have a haematoma on the US scan during your next pregnancy.

Try not to worry if the scan does not identify any obvious cause for the bleeding. This situation is very common and in most cases the bleeding will stop and the pregnancy will continue safely. As mentioned earlier in this book, red bleeding indicates a fresh or recent loss, but when the blood is brown, this means that it is old. There is only one place for the blood to drain out of the uterus and that is through the cervix and into the vagina. It may continue draining for some time, so try not to worry about brown discharge if the pregnancy is continuing to grow on the scan.

I think one of the most valuable uses of early pregnancy US scans is to show you that the pregnancy is developing. At five weeks the pregnancy sac is small, but it will probably contain a small yolk sac, which looks like a thick-rimmed circle or balloon near the edge of the sac. One week later the sac will have doubled in size and the fetal pole will be visible. By seven weeks the sac will again have grown, the fetal pole will be longer and the heartbeat will be visible. By eight weeks the baby is starting to lose its comma-like shape and by nine weeks it will have a recognisable head and body. It may also be possible to see the baby's legs and the umbilical cord which attaches the baby to the placenta.

Week by week, the scan will be able to show you whether the baby is growing. Of course, if you find that the baby has not grown over a period of two weeks, this is a cause for concern. If the fetal heart is still visible there is still hope, but if the fetal heart disappears, then sadly, your doctor will have to make the diagnosis that the baby has died. This is always very distressing and some women will not be able to believe it at first. You may feel that you want to wait for a few more days and have another scan. Although the result will almost always be the same, this need for proof is very understandable. Which is why I never try to persuade any woman I see in this situation to have a medical or surgical evacuation (ERPC) until she is absolutely sure in her own mind that the pregnancy is truly over.

Having said this, I think the scan is enormously helpful in this situation, because it can avoid delays in making the diagnosis. For many women I meet, the most upsetting problem is being unsure of what is happening. If you have only had a scan at eight weeks and the result suggests that the baby is smaller than it should be, it is difficult for the doctor to know whether there is a problem with the pregnancy or whether it is simply that your dates are wrong and that the pregnancy is younger than you thought. In this situation, it is likely that your doctor will suggest that you wait for another week or two and then have a repeat scan to confirm what is going on. But if you have had an earlier scan, the doctor will be able to compare the two reports and will be able to make a much more accurate assessment of the situation.

In addition to the emotional trauma that delays in the diagnosis of a miscarriage may cause, the delay can also mean that the opportunity of obtaining fresh tissue for genetic analysis is lost. This is one of the reasons that I try and persuade my patients to undergo an ERPC as soon as they are confident in their own minds that the pregnancy has died. Although this is unlikely to be at the top of your priority list when you have just received the sad news, I can promise you that when the initial shock wears off, you will want as much information as possible about your pregnancy and why it miscarried.

Knowing the genetic makeup of the baby is of great value, as I have mentioned on many occasions in this book. If the baby was chromosomally abnormal, I think you will be surprised how much comfort this information will provide you with in the future. Of course, it does not bring back the baby you have lost, but it does allow you to understand why the miscarriage occurred. For so many women who have no knowledge of why they lost their pregnancy, this is a piece of information that they would dearly love to have.

Examination of the placental tissues can also prove to be very useful, as I discussed in detail in Chapter 3. In the short-term the pathologist can tell us whether the placental tissues were developing normally, whether there was evidence of infection or possibly a prothrombotic abnormality (see Chapter 13). However, the microscope slides can be stored for many years if required and this is potentially very valuable. As we improve our understanding of the causes of miscarriage it will be possible to go back to these slides and carry out newly discovered tests on the stored tissues. If this sounds fanciful, then let me give you an example. Many of the latest medical advances rely on extracting the DNA (genetic code) or RNA (message) from tissues and it is now becoming possible to do this with tissues even when they have been fixed in formalin, embedded in paraffin and stored for some years. As new genetic disorders are identified we will be able to go back and literally 'probe' the miscarriage tissues to find these molecular abnormalities. I believe that this is one of the most exciting avenues for future research into the causes of pregnancy loss.

I frequently talk to anxious couples in the miscarriage clinic who are concerned that their pregnancy is not the 'right' size for dates. What matters in this situation is not the actual size of the pregnancy, but whether the pregnancy is growing. For example, if the scan at seven weeks shows a small sac only, but two weeks later it shows that the pregnancy has increased in size by two weeks' worth of growth, then it really does not matter that the size of the baby is still smaller than the original dates would suggest.

Another source of concern is whether the repeated scans may cause any harm to the baby. About this issue I feel very confident in telling you: no, the scans will not harm your baby in any way. Several large studies have shown that repeated ultrasound scans have no adverse effects on the development of the baby (for further details see Chapter 9).

Doppler ultrasound

Most hospitals now have US machines which are routinely able to look at the blood flow through the vessels in the uterus and the placenta. This is called Doppler ultrasound and the patterns of blood flow can be translated into different colours on the scan picture. This technique has taught us a lot about the development of blood circulation in the uterus and placenta and has led to us now being able to identify blood flow problems in the uterus and early placenta and by recognizing these flow patterns we are better able to predict those pregnancies that are at risk of miscarrying. The results of these Doppler scans are also a helpful way for us to reassure women who have experienced problems of bleeding or pain in early pregnancy.

Investigations in later pregnancy

If you have suffered a late miscarriage, you will have noticed that this chapter has not offered you much information about the tests available in later pregnancy to diagnose a miscarriage or a pregnancy that is in trouble. There are no useful blood tests, but the ultrasound scan can provide useful information particularly about the rate of growth of your baby and the health of the placenta. Slow growth of the baby, a placenta which appears small and gritty and a reduced level of amniotic fluid (liquor) around the baby are all signs that the baby is in trouble.

The problem (or rather the limitation) with these US findings in later pregnancy is that even when they diagnose that the baby is at risk, there is nothing that can be done about it. It is only after 24 weeks when the baby has a chance of surviving, if it is delivered, that the results of these US scans can influence how we manage the pregnancy. Before this date the only thing we can do is cross our fingers and hope that the pregnancy will continue until the baby has reached a size that is potentially viable in the outside world.

At the present time Doppler blood flow scans in later pregnancy are much more useful than in early pregnancy. For example, they can identify that the blood flow to the baby is reduced before the baby's growth starts to fall off. This is an enormously important development and means that we can 'rescue' some babies before serious trouble develops, by making a decision to deliver them early. But this is only feasible after 24 weeks and, exciting as it is, I recognise that further details are beyond the scope of this book.

17

THE PHYSICAL PROCESS OF MISCARRIAGE – WHAT TO EXPECT

It is difficult to make generalizations about the physical events that may occur at the time of your miscarriage. They usually depend upon the stage in pregnancy at which the miscarriage occurs. And of course, they will vary from woman to woman and from pregnancy to pregnancy. What usually happens in early pregnancy is that you will experience some bleeding and will be seen by your GP or by one of the doctors at the local hospital. They will examine you and may suggest that you have an ultrasound scan if it is not clear what is going on.

You may actually see the miscarried pregnancy if the bleeding is heavy or occurs suddenly. If you pass a creamy coloured sac of membranes, with or without a tiny embryo inside it, then you will immediately recognise it. More often, you will be aware of passing large clots of blood but not be sure whether there is tissue in the clots. If the miscarriage starts at home, you may have tried to save the tissue you have passed so that the doctor can look at it. Many women I see worry about what happens to these tissues. If you have suffered several miscarriages, the doctors will hopefully arrange for them to be sent to the genetics laboratory for analysis. Alternatively, they may be sent to the routine pathology laboratory where they will be fixed in formalin (see Chapter 4) and examined under the microscope. This type of analysis may show that the embryo or the placental tissues are malformed in some way, but it will not establish the genetic makeup of the baby. This can only be done in the genetics laboratory.

If the miscarriage occurs before eight weeks and is complete (see Chapter 3) it may not be necessary for you to be admitted to hospital. If you are, and the physical examination or ultrasound scan shows that the uterus is empty, you will be able to go home without any treatment. Indeed, you may not even have to visit the hospital if your GP has been looking after you and has made the diagnosis of a complete miscarriage.

If you have experienced a lot of bleeding, which is continuing, and the physical examination or ultrasound scan suggests that there are still tissues present in the uterine cavity, then you will be advised to go into hospital and either undergo a short operation to clear out the uterus, called an ERPC (evacuation of retained products of conception) or take some medication that will help the uterus to expel the pregnancy tissues. However, the US scan and clinical examination may conclude that there is no need for you to have any further treatment.

Medical management to clean out the womb

It is now possible to use drugs to empty the pregnant uterus for women whose miscarriage has occurred before nine weeks. The drugs used are a combination of an anti-progesterone and prostaglandins. The anti-progesterone blocks the action of progesterone hormone, which maintains the early pregnancy in the uterus, and the prostaglandins can then act upon the cervix and uterine muscle to expel the pregnancy from the uterus. This method has become increasingly popular over the last few years since it avoids the need for an anaesthetic and an operation. It also reduces the amount of pain relief that is required by most women.

If you decide to have this medical evacuation of the uterus, you will be asked to attend the hospital where you will be given a tablet of mifepristone which is the anti-progesterone drug. You will be asked to wait in the clinic for about 30 minutes, until the tablet has been absorbed and then you can go home. Some women feel a bit sick after taking the tablet, but this usually settles quickly. You may have some period-like pain or bleeding the day after and if you feel uncomfortable you can take a paracetamol tablet.

Approximately 24 hours later you will return to the hospital and at this visit you will be given the misoprostol (prostaglandin) medication. This can either be administered as vaginal pessaries or given as oral tablets, following which you will be able to return home. You will probably experience some pain and bleeding and should take some painkillers if you need them. Most women will miscarry within four hours of having the misoprostol pessaries, but light vaginal bleeding may continue for up to 12 days after first being administered. However, for most women the vaginal loss has usually stopped before they return for their clinic follow-up visit two weeks later. Treatment with prostaglandin drugs is not recommended for women with heart disease, asthma, or kidney and liver disease, but your doctor will be able to advise you about whether this method is suitable for you.

Surgical management to clean out the womb

If you decide that you would like to have surgical management in order to be sure of obtaining all the pregnancy tissues for genetic analysis, you will be admitted to hospital and you will be asked to sign a form in which you give your consent to the operation. It is important that you do not have anything to eat or drink for at least four hours before the operation so that you will not have any complications with the anaesthetic. You will probably be taken into the anaesthetic room (which is just outside the operating room) lying on a trolley bed. Here you will meet the anaesthetist who will explain that you are going to have an injection in your arm to put you to sleep. The general anaesthetic is light and you will recover quickly from it.

During the operation your cervix will be gently dilated (opened) so that small instruments can be inserted into the uterine cavity to clear out any tissues that remain there. When the pregnancy is less than 12 weeks, the tissues are usually sucked out of the uterus using a type of small vacuum cleaner. All the tissues are collected in a clean sealed jar and can then be sent off to the laboratory for analysis, if needed. The advantages of this vacuum method of cleaning out the uterus are that it is very efficient, and it is much less likely that any pieces of tissue will be left behind. It also reduces the risk of the tissues becoming infected by organisms in the vagina and cervix. As we discussed in Chapter 4, this can affect the chances of genetic analysis on the tissues being successful.

Sometimes the diagnosis that the pregnancy has died will be made with the ultrasound scan, but the baby and the placenta are still intact within the uterine cavity. In this situation, it is usually advisable to have the pregnancy evacuated rather than wait for the pregnancy to miscarry spontaneously. If the pregnancy is more than 12 weeks, it may be necessary to use specific drugs to 'prime' or prepare and gently soften the cervix in order to minimise any potential damage to the cervix when it is dilated or stretched up. This is important because the size of the baby may necessitate the use of special forceps to remove some of the tissues before a final cleaning of the cavity is performed with the suction method.

When it is known that the baby is larger than 16 weeks' size, the doctors will probably advise you that they need to induce you to go into labour and for you to deliver the baby vaginally. This may sound very frightening to some readers but I think it is important for me to explain exactly what will happen so that you are prepared if you have the misfortune to be in this situation. The process of labour can take quite a long time because at this early stage in pregnancy the uterus is less prepared to contract and expel the baby. In order to make the cervix soften and start to dilate, a pessary is put into the vagina. It will probably be necessary for you to have several pessaries inserted at intervals of approximately four to six hours. The pessaries contain prostaglandins, which are chemical substances normally produced by the cervix at the time of delivery to 'prime' the uterus to contract. It is now possible to give this prostaglandin drug in tablet form which is often more acceptable to women. However, a small proportion of women may experience side-effects such as nausea, vomiting and other gastrointestinal symptoms with the oral form of the drug.

The pessaries can only be used one at a time because occasionally they have a strong effect on the uterus, making it contract violently. It is likely that you will think that nothing is happening for many hours after the first one or two pessaries are inserted. The cervix will be softening silently and when it starts to open gently you will probably experience some discomfort in the lower abdomen, similar to period pains. A bit later, the uterus will start to contract and eventually the baby will be delivered. This usually takes about 24 hours, but may be a longer or shorter period of time.

Many women are understandably very worried that they will experience a lot of pain. Let me reassure you immediately that you will not suffer much physical discomfort because you will be offered plenty of analgesia (painkilling drugs). The most commonly used painkillers are pethidine and morphine, which are given as an injection into a muscle in your bottom or upper thigh. The pain relief lasts about four hours, after which further injections will be offered to you. Some units will be able to offer you an epidural anaesthetic. This is an injection in your back which numbs your body from the waist downwards.

The great advantage of an epidural is that it can be 'topped up' at regular intervals to keep you pain-free without the need for further injections. Having said this, I must tell you that when a mother in this sad situation asks me for advice about the most suitable method of pain relief, I almost always suggest that she has pethidine injections. This is because the pethidine will make you feel a bit sleepy and gives you the feeling of floating on air. You will not be fully aware of events all of the time. An epidural anaesthetic will make you pain-free but you will be wide awake and conscious of everything that is happening to you physically and emotionally. Of course, you and only you must decide whether you want to be acutely aware or slightly numbed emotionally. However, I think most women will find some relief in the escape that pethidine can provide at a time like this.

There is one more physical hurdle to cross after this distressing labour and that is the delivery of the placenta. In very late miscarriages, after 20 weeks, the placenta may deliver spontaneously after the baby, or with the help of the midwife pulling gently on the umbilical cord. Before 20 weeks the placenta is usually, but not always, retained in the uterus. It needs to be removed to avoid further bleeding and later infection. If you have had an epidural for the labour this can be 'topped up' to allow the removal to take place. Otherwise you will need to undergo a light general anaesthetic.

A newer method of uterine evacuation is the manual vacuum aspiration. This can be performed in the outpatient setting without the need for admission to the day surgery operating theatre and a general anaesthetic.

Possible problems you may encounter in hospital

If you do have to go into hospital and have an ERPC the staff will try to arrange your operation as quickly as possible. But sadly, even the best laid plans can go wrong, and you may experience long delays which are extremely distressing. If you have had to fill up your bladder by drinking water for an abdominal ultrasound scan, the anaesthetist will insist that at least four hours passes before they give you a general anaesthetic. The operating theatre may be busy and, just as you think your turn has come, an emergency may claim your operating slot, forcing your ERPC to be delayed still further.

After the operation, the doctors may be so busy that no one is available to come and ensure that you are well enough to go home for some time. You may feel that no one cares about your problems and feelings and although this really is not the case, I understand how you may well feel this way. You are tired and distressed, and the staff are overworked. The doctors may be unable to answer your questions fully and appear to have no time for the explanations you are looking for. You may end up with the impression that you are 'just another routine miscarriage' and from this point onwards everything goes from bad to worse. I am not suggesting that you should be trying to understand everyone else's problems at this difficult time, but I think it is helpful for you to know that the hospital staff do care and they do want to sort out your problems as quickly as possible.

If the only bed available is in the postnatal ward, the sound of crying babies can be the last straw. Although we try hard to prevent this situation, it is sometimes unavoidable. Indeed, this is one of the reasons why we aim to discharge you from the hospital as quickly as possible but this in itself may make you feel that no one wants to spend time with you. If you have suffered a late miscarriage, you may find that you are starting to produce milk, and this is always very distressing after losing a baby. Tablets are available (called bromocriptine) to suppress milk production if this is very troublesome.

Your GP will be sent a summary of your admission and treatment as soon as you are discharged from the hospital. Sometimes the communications are slow – particularly at weekends – which is why we usually fax the report to the surgery these days.

Saying goodbye to your baby

Having gone through all the physical events of your miscarriage, you may then have to face some emotional traumas. Most couples find that the miscarriage, whether they have undergone medical management, a surgical evacuation of the uterus or labour, feels like a bad dream and that it is only after these have ended that the full realisation of what has happened hits them emotionally. Whatever the age of the pregnancy, you may want to seek advice about how you can say goodbye to your baby. If the miscarriage occurred early in pregnancy, then there will be no specific practical issues that require you to make a decision. You will be grieving and ways of coping with this very natural response are discussed in the next chapter.

If you have had a late miscarriage, a late termination for medical reasons or a stillbirth, you will be asked if you want to see your baby. I urge you to do so and more than that, hold and cuddle your baby, give him or her a name, and spend as much time with the baby as you feel you want to. You may initially be afraid to see the baby because you feel he or she may be deformed or look odd in some way. What you imagine is usually far worse than the reality.

I shall never forget listening to the thoughts of a woman who had delivered a baby 60 years earlier with severe spina bifida. She recalled how all those years ago it was not recognised how important it is for the mother to be offered the chance of seeing and holding her baby. The baby was whisked away and for 60 years she had experienced nightmares, thinking that the baby she had delivered was some sort of monster. When she eventually told her new young GP about these fears she showed her a picture from a textbook of a baby with spina bifida. It was only then that her nightmares stopped and she was able to think about this lost baby without fear.

Many women tell me how important it is to have had some time with their baby and they find it enormously helpful in dealing with their grief, later on. This is because spending time with the baby provides you with an opportunity to say hello and goodbye to him or her. Most importantly, it will remove the fear of the unknown. I am absolutely confident in saying to you that every woman's baby is beautiful and special. Please do not miss the opportunity of realising this fact.

If you feel that you do not want to see the baby, he or she will be taken out of the room as soon as you deliver. However, most hospitals will take a photograph of the baby which will be given to you or kept for you in the medical notes in case you would like to see it or have it at a later date. These records are kept for many years. If you find that you want to come back to the hospital a long time after the pregnancy loss, these photographs will have been kept in your notes.

There is little doubt that you will be feeling very distressed after your late miscarriage. Try to talk to the staff involved in your care and ask them questions if there are any problems troubling you. I have never worked with a doctor, midwife or nurse who does not feel saddened and distressed by the plight of a woman who loses her baby in late pregnancy. They may have seen the problem many times before, but this will not stop them from feeling great concern and sympathy for you. Talk to them, cry with them and be angry with them. They will understand, and they will also have useful advice to offer you.

The doctors may suggest that your baby undergoes a post-mortem examination (autopsy) to try and identify a medical condition that may have led to the death of your baby. I know that this can be a cause of great anxiety and distress for parents who have just lost a baby. I would like to explain to you what happens at the post-mortem in the hope that it will comfort you, allay your fears and encourage you to find out all you can about why your baby died.

The post-mortem will be carried out by a pathologist who has received specialist training in disorders of children and babies (paediatric or perinatal pathologist). At the post-mortem the baby's body and internal organs will be examined. This examination needs to be carried out as soon as possible after the baby's death and usually within 72 hours. The post-mortem will be carried out with great care and can take up to three hours. The pathologist will make sure that openings are made in places that are not visible when your baby is fully dressed. Your baby's face, arms and legs will not be affected by the post-mortem.

During the examination small samples of tissue and body fluids may be taken for special tests. The results of these tests may not be available for many weeks, but this will not affect the funeral arrangements. The pathologist will write a detailed report and send it to the doctors looking after you. Most hospitals arrange to see parents some four to six weeks later when the test results are all available to discuss with them.

At the end of the post-mortem, the baby's body will be carefully repaired so that you can see and hold your baby again if you wish. The hospital will have suitable clothing to dress your baby, but you may want to dress the baby in your own baby clothes. If you do not want to see the baby again after the post-mortem, the body will be stored in the mortuary.

Unless a coroner has legally authorised a post-mortem to be performed on your baby, the post-mortem cannot be carried out without your consent. Some couples become very concerned that the post-mortem will be against their religious beliefs. Many of these worries can be easily sorted out by discussing them with your doctor or religious leader. If you decide that you do not want your baby to have a full post-mortem, talk to your doctor about other tests which may provide some limited information about the cause of death.

There is a legal requirement for any baby born after 24 weeks to be buried or cremated. If your baby has died at an earlier date, before 24 weeks, you can make arrangements for a funeral, but you will not require a death certificate. Some hospitals will organise a funeral on your behalf or help you to arrange it yourselves. If you have had a very early miscarriage, it is likely that your baby will be disposed of by the hospital.

The funeral may be a way of helping you with your loss. Many couples find that it provides them with a dignified way of saying goodbye to their baby. If you do not want the formality of a full funeral service, you may want to arrange for the hospital chaplain or a religious leader of your own faith to give a short service or prayer for your baby, either during or after your stay in hospital.

Some hospitals organise regular memorial or remembrance services for parents who have lost babies. At my own hospital we hold a special service twice a year to which both parents and the staff involved in their care are invited. It is always extremely well attended, which suggests to me that these more formal acts of remembrance can be very helpful after your baby has died. Some cemeteries have special areas for premature or stillborn babies. The hospital chaplain, patient affairs officer or one of the midwives looking after you should be able to give you the information you need to find out what is available in your area.

There are many different ways of remembering your baby. For many parents, this will be extremely important and can play a significant role in their grieving process in the short and the long term. Giving the baby a name is particularly comforting and will help you to remember him or her as a 'real' person. You will probably find that other people find it easier to talk to you about your baby by name, instead of 'the baby', which can sound so anonymous.

Many parents find that compiling a book of memories helps them enormously in the years to come. It may include a photograph of an ultrasound scan, antenatal test results, a photograph of the baby, a lock of hair, a hospital name bracelet, a copy of the memorial or funeral service, a few pressed flowers, perhaps some letters of sympathy. Some parents may prefer to remember their baby by planting a rose bush or tree, or marking a bench with a plaque placed in the park. Of course, you may not find any of these things helpful and there is certainly no reason to feel that you are expected to create memories of your baby. You may feel that your private memories are the most comforting and the most precious and, if this is the case, this is the right course for you to follow.

18

IS IT NORMAL TO FEEL THIS WAY AFTER A MISCARRIAGE?

Yes, it is entirely normal. I promise you that whatever feelings you experience after a miscarriage, they are entirely normal. They may be different from the feelings that a friend of yours tells you she experienced, but you need to remind yourself that we all deal with grief, anger, despair, depression, guilt and self-blame in different ways.

The loss of a baby is a devastating experience. It doesn't matter how the pregnancy ended; all pregnancy losses, including miscarriage, ectopic pregnancy, stillbirth, neonatal death, or being forced to end the pregnancy because your baby is abnormal or your health is at serious risk, are equally heartbreaking.

It will be difficult for you, your partner and your family to come to terms with what has happened and you are likely to experience grief, anger and emptiness, not just immediately, but for a long period of time. No matter what kind of pregnancy loss you have experienced, you will probably be unprepared for the pain and anguish you feel. Instead of looking forward to the arrival of your baby, you are now left with a terrible sense of emptiness, frustration and even failure. All the love you were hoping to give this new person in your life has no outlet any more and this can give rise to very intense emotions. It is entirely normal for bereaved parents to feel isolated, angry with themselves, each other, the staff at the hospital, and jealous of other people who have healthy babies.

Grieving for your baby

It is quite normal for the shock of the pregnancy loss to numb all your feelings initially. With time, the process of grieving will start. Grief can be frightening and overwhelming especially if you think that it is abnormal to feel this way. Try not to fight it. Grieving is a natural way of expressing your feelings of loss and it needs to run its natural course.

The process of grief has different stages that may last for days, weeks or many months. It cannot be hurried up and if you try to skip one of the steps you will probably find that you have to revisit this stage at a later date. Undoubtedly, your feelings will change over time. The first feelings of shock, disbelief and denial are usually followed by severe emotional distress, including anxiety and depression. As the grieving process continues, you may experience feelings of anger, guilt and jealousy. Sometimes the yearning you may feel for your lost baby will be overwhelming. With time, these feelings will give way to a deep sadness. The acute grief will be replaced by feelings of mourning and regret for what has not happened. Eventually, you will feel resigned to what has happened, although this resignation will probably never take away the emotional pain entirely.

Even if you find it difficult, you should try to express your feelings and not bottle them up. By expressing them, you will find that it becomes much easier to understand these feelings and this will help you to deal with them. Easy for her to say, you may be thinking as you read this, but not so easy to do. I know that some people find it extremely difficult to express or share their grief. This is often because they are afraid of losing control if they let go of their emotions in any way. It does not matter if you lose control for a while. In fact, it is an essential part of the process you have to go through in order to recover from your loss.

If you are someone who is used to keeping your feelings to yourself, you may try to pretend – to yourself as well as everyone else around you – that you have recovered from the miscarriage. It may seem easier to try and brush aside or suppress your feelings of grief, in the hope that they will go away more quickly. They will have to come to the surface at some time. Let me say again that grieving takes time and there are no short cuts. Each one of us will need a different length of time to recover. I think it is also important to remember that the process of grieving does not always go in a straight line. Sometimes feelings you thought you had dealt with will return. You may think you have started to get over it and then suddenly you will be overwhelmed again.

Many women I meet in the miscarriage clinic tell me how distressed they feel by people who tell them that 'time is a great healer'. When you are grieving, you do not really want to hear that the acute feelings of pain and loss will fade with time. In some ways you do not want them to fade, at least for a while, because these feelings are the only part of your pregnancy that is still with you. You do not want to turn your back on your baby until you feel ready to do so. You should not feel guilty or fear that you are 'indulging' yourself. It is a perfectly healthy and normal response and an important part of coming to terms with your loss.

I have never been convinced that time heals completely, but I do believe that as time passes, the way in which we perceive grief changes. It becomes more manageable and less likely to catch us unawares. This does not mean that you will forget the pain and disappointment but, with time, it will become a part of your life that does not overwhelm you. You will be able to think about it and even revisit your emotions when you want to do so without feeling that you are helpless and out of control.

Similarly, you should not feel guilty if you feel strong and philosophical about your loss after the initial grieving period. You may find that you are ready to get on with your life quite quickly and I suggest that you do not allow other people's expectations of how long it should take you to recover to influence you. There are no right or wrong ways to deal with these important life events.

Depression

Depression is quite a common sequel to the acute phase of grief. You may feel tired or lethargic, with no energy and no desire to get on with anything. Changes in appetite and sleeping patterns, headaches and other aches or pains may develop, all of which can be symptoms of depression. Many women experience feelings of worthlessness and lose confidence in themselves. They often feel unable to cope with the daily routine of life or work. Other symptoms may be lack of concentration, irrational fears or behaviour, feelings of panic, or uncontrollable crying.

This type of 'reactive' depression usually passes of its own accord but it can last for weeks or months. If the symptoms continue, it is important that you are honest with yourself and recognise that you need some help. This is not a failure on your part, it is the only sensible way to help pull yourself out of the depression. Go and tell your doctor. He or she may be able to put you in touch with a bereavement counsellor, and occasionally it may be helpful to take some medication, either for depression or to help you sleep. Support groups have a very useful part to play in this situation.

Guilt

Guilt and self-blame are very common emotions after a miscarriage. 'What did I do wrong?' is a question that I hear regularly. This feeling is very understandable, particularly when there is no clear reason why the miscarriage occurred, but it is misplaced. You need to remember that it is highly unlikely that you did anything to cause the problem, so try not to punish yourself. You are not a failure. Nor are you a victim. You have had a miscarriage, which is a bitter disappointment, but it is not recompense for something that happened in your past. You will have a baby in the future and the quicker you start liking yourself again, the quicker a new pregnancy will end in success.

Your partner's grief

I think men have a particularly difficult role to play when their partner has a miscarriage. Remember that your partner will probably have had to watch you bleeding, in pain and, in many cases, undergo a general anaesthetic and an operation. It is very tough to see someone you love suffering and feel that you are powerless to help. It is also very frightening and this fear often leads to outbursts of anger. Distressed partners often ask me what will happen if something should go wrong in the operation, or if the bleeding cannot be stopped.

I meet many men who feel very frustrated and angry when their partner has to wait for an ultrasound, or for the doctor to see and assess the situation. If there is a further wait for an ERPC operation, the anger often bubbles over and explodes. This is an entirely understandable reaction which stems from the fact that he is trying to protect you. Many couples tell me that they later feel embarrassed if a scene developed during their hospital admission. Don't worry about it, no one will hold it against you. The hospital staff really do understand that your partner is concerned for your safety.

Your partner may find it difficult to express his feelings but he will be grieving too. He may well feel that he should hide his grief in an attempt to try and protect you from any more distress and help you through the physical traumas you have experienced. If this is the case, you will need to encourage him to talk to you about his feelings and not to keep them entirely to himself. Shared tears can be very therapeutic. When I see couples soon after a miscarriage, I often suggest to the man that he needs to do some crying too. I point out to them that he is also feeling the pain, and that they both need to accept that he cannot be the strong and supportive partner all the time.

For many couples, the experience of pregnancy loss brings them closer together. Sadly, for some couples the miscarriage raises feelings of resentment, guilt, self-blame and bewilderment, which can be very difficult to sort out. If you find yourselves in this situation, seek help – from friends, counsellors, a religious adviser – but don't allow the feelings to fester and get out of control. Throwing yourselves into work in the hope that it will all get better if you ignore your feelings seldom solves the problems and usually makes them much worse.

Telling your children

If you have other children, the pregnancy loss will almost certainly affect them too. However young they are, they will know that something is wrong. It is understandable that you may feel that you want to protect your children from something painful and difficult for them to understand. The reality is that the truth is usually less frightening for them than the things they may imagine are happening if you don't try to explain.

It is important that you tell them about the baby, and how you feel. You will need to listen carefully to what they say and ask them gentle questions to find out what they are thinking. Above all, answer their questions honestly, however painful it may be for you. There is no need to avoid using words like 'died' or 'death' as long as you try not to show them that you are frightened or anxious. They need to understand why you are feeling sad and in particular they need to be reassured that you love them and want to cuddle and kiss them even though you are distressed.

Many children may find it difficult to talk about their feelings immediately and you will need to be prepared for fears and difficult questions to emerge at a later date. Most importantly, you need to reassure them that they are not the cause of what has happened and try to stop them blaming themselves. They may feel lost and abandoned if you have needed to spend some time in hospital and they may be worrying about your safety in the future. Signs of emotional disturbances such as tantrums, sleeplessness, bedwetting and nightmares are all common. They will pass if you provide the children with love, support and constant reassurance that everything is going to be all right. Above all, encourage them to share their feelings with you.

Dealing with other people and their reactions

One of the most difficult things about having a miscarriage is dealing with other people and their reactions to your grief and distress. We human beings are not very good at coping with someone else's pain. We often take the easy way out and avoid talking about it. I am quite sure that this is not because we do not care but because we are frightened of saying the wrong thing, hurting feelings or reminding the sufferer of his or her pain. Embarrassment at the raw emotions that may be uncovered by a simple question is another reason. Few reactions in life could be so inappropriate. Most women who suffer a miscarriage positively want other people to talk to them about what has happened. Indeed, many women I meet tell me how distressing it can be when other people avoid the subject. Many feel resentful that someone they counted as a friend will not take the risk of asking them about the miscarriage. Worse, they may start to feel that their grief is unacceptable and should be hidden from public view.

One of the most important things I have learnt about miscarriage sufferers is the enormous comfort that you can offer by expressing your feelings of sadness for them. Of course, it does not take away the pain but a few spoken words or a brief note (however inarticulate) can make all the difference to someone who is grieving.

Losing a twin

Losing a twin or a triplet can be the start of a series of complex emotions. You may feel that you have a split personality for a while. One half of you will be mourning the death of the lost baby, while the other half will still be excited and relieved about the surviving baby or babies.

You may try to suppress your grief for the lost baby and put all your energies into thinking about the survivor(s). On the other hand, you may find it very difficult to cope with the remaining baby and be guilty that you feel this way. I think it is important for you to remember that just because you are still pregnant and can look forward to a baby being born, this does not mean that you feel the pain of your loss any less acutely. Once again, you need to allow yourself time and space to grieve properly. Remember, too, that you may need to find a way of explaining to the surviving baby what happened to his or her lost sibling.

Coping with anniversaries

When you have suffered a miscarriage, certain dates may suddenly take on great importance. As one patient explained to me, 'I could never remember dates without my diary before I lost my baby, and now I can tell you when I first missed my period, when I first started to bleed, when I miscarried and when my baby should have been born, right down to the last hour.' These anniversaries can be very painful and difficult to deal with.

I think the best way of tackling them is to give in to them and allow yourself to feel sad, robbed, disappointed, angry or whatever feeling they bring you. Just because the rest of the world does not recognise the anniversary is no reason for you to feel that you have to forget it or push it behind you. With the passage of time, the anniversary date will become much less painful. You won't forget it, but you will find that it becomes a wistful rather than a painful memory.

One of my miscarriage patients (who has subsequently had three healthy bouncing babies) tells me that she always takes a day off when her miscarried baby should have been born. She needs to spend a few quiet hours remembering the baby who 'did not make it'. When she first told me this, I was struck by how much comfort this had provided her with and asked her if she would share her idea with some other patients. She did and the letters I have received as a result of this 'self-help' suggest that it may be a very useful practice. Anniversaries for sadness can be as important as anniversaries for joy. The most important thing is that you recognise what you want to remember and remember it in your own way and in your own time.

Deciding whether to try again

This is a very individual decision. For some couples, there is no question – they want to embark on a new pregnancy without delay. There are no rules about when is the right time. If you feel emotionally prepared to embark upon another pregnancy, then it is likely that you are physically ready too. For others, it may take longer, particularly when the miscarriage was late. There is no doubt that losing a baby during the second and third trimesters of pregnancy is a particularly difficult blow to deal with. The emotional adjustments involved and the recovery time needed are often longer. Nonetheless, it will be you and only you who knows when and if you are ready to contemplate another pregnancy.

Most of the couples I meet decide that they do want to try for another pregnancy. The desire to have a child, whatever the obstacles met previously, is a strong and driving force. But there may come a time when you and your partner decide that you cannot expose yourselves any longer to the stress and trauma of repeated disappointments. I am often asked whether I think it is sensible to try again. I suspect that there will never be a correct answer to this question because it depends upon the couple, their history and their circumstances. The most useful advice I can offer is that you will know when you want to stop trying. Before this date, you will not want to give up because you believe that there may be a chance of reaching your goal.

The most important point here, I believe, is that whilst you still feel these emotions, you cannot and will not stop trying. The decision to put this quest behind you is rarely a sudden one. It comes after much soul-searching and heartache. There may come a time when you feel that you need to stop trying for a baby and put your energies into other parts of your life. I certainly meet couples who feel relieved after coming to this decision because their lives have become dominated by trying to have a baby and they feel that this drive has started to become destructive. At the end of the day, only you can make the decision to stop trying. As long as you feel confident that you have pursued all the possible options available to you and that you will not be consumed by regrets that you did not try 'once more', then I think that this is the right decision for you and you need to take it.

Summary

Grieving for a lost baby is a process. It goes in stages and it has no set pattern and no time limits. For some women, it will be relatively quick, for others it will be longer. You do not need to feel that you should be over it because other people expect this of you. Nor should you feel that a short period of mourning means that you are odd or unusual. Give yourself as much time as you need to come to terms with what has happened.

19

FINDING OUT MORE ABOUT THE PROBLEM OF MISCARRIAGE

Some hospitals are able to provide a counselling service for women who have suffered a miscarriage. If you think it may be useful, then find out whether this service is available to you and then use it for as long as you need to. If your hospital cannot provide help in this way, then go and see if your GP is able to help directly at the local surgery or can put you in touch with local organisations and self-help groups. A quick search online or a few telephone calls may provide you with some useful contacts that you never realised were available near you.

The Miscarriage Association is a very useful organisation to contact. They can offer support and information, including a whole range of leaflets. They can also provide you with contact details for telephone support volunteers who live in your area and who have suffered miscarriages themselves. Some areas have support groups where you can meet other people with similar experiences to your own and this can be enormously valuable. In addition, you may want to offer help to others in the future and this is another very positive way of coming to terms with your loss.

The Miscarriage Association also publishes a regular newsletter with information, articles and personal accounts from members who have experienced miscarriage or ectopic pregnancy. In addition to local support volunteers, the association also runs an annual conference which you may want to attend. The annual conference usually invites doctors who are particularly interested in miscarriage to come and speak to the members.

If you have suffered repeated miscarriages, your doctor may suggest that you are referred to a specialist miscarriage clinic. These clinics can provide more extensive investigations into your problem and usually arrange to help you during the first few anxious months of the next pregnancy. Since there are not many specialist clinics across the country, it may be necessary for you to travel considerable distances for clinic appointments.

I know that most of the couples we see at the St Mary's recurrent miscarriage clinic do not mind the travelling and often tell me that they are prepared to go to any lengths to try and sort out their problem. If you are referred to the clinic at St Mary's by your GP or your local hospital consultant, you will be asked to fill in a detailed questionnaire about your general health and your pregnancies before you attend the clinic. The information in this questionnaire makes it possible for us to contact your local doctors for any missing pieces of information before we see you. It also means that when you first come to the clinic, the time can be spent talking about your specific problems, instead of trying to piece together the dates, scan results, complications and other details about your previous pregnancies.

While you are waiting for a clinic appointment, we will also try to arrange for you to have some investigations (usually blood tests) performed. This can save a lot of time and means that we have some of the results to discuss with you at the first visit. We can then arrange for further investigations that are suited to your individual case. For example, about one-third of recurrent miscarriage sufferers also experience problems in getting pregnant. As I mentioned in Chapter 13, if these delays in conceiving are not clearly identified, then the chances of being able to sort out the problems are reduced. In other cases, complications in a previous pregnancy, which may have resulted in a live baby born prematurely, may provide clues about your particular problem.

Perhaps the most important function of specialist clinics is that they will also give you an opportunity to become involved in the most recent research into miscarriage (see Chapter 22). Joining a research programme is probably the most useful thing you can do to help yourself. Research programmes are crucial to the future development of successful treatments for miscarriage. As I frequently say to couples I see in the clinic, the treatment we can offer you today was an idea last year and the tests we want to perform today may result in a new treatment being available next year.

PART FOUR
THE NEXT STEP

20

GETTING READY FOR THE NEXT PREGNANCY

General health issues and pre-conceptual care

Every woman trying to conceive should be as healthy as possible. It is sensible to consider several general health issues which can affect the chance of getting pregnant, the risk of miscarriage and the health of the baby. Certain risk factors can be avoided or minimised by simple precautions taken before pregnancy and during the pregnancy. Some hospitals and doctors' surgeries have introduced special clinics for women before becoming pregnant. These 'pre-conception' clinics are very helpful, offering general medical advice about diet, drugs, exercise, what to do and what to avoid doing when you are trying to become pregnant. Most importantly, they attempt to answer many of your queries and concerns about pregnancy.

It is important that a woman who is trying to become pregnant has a healthy, well-balanced diet and is of normal weight. If you are either under- or overweight, this can affect your chances of becoming pregnant. If you are underweight when you conceive, you are at risk of having a baby who is smaller than is ideal for his or her health. If you are overweight, avoid crash dieting and follow a well-balanced low-fat, low-sugar, high-fibre diet of approximately 1500 calories a day.

The Department of Health advises all women trying to conceive to take 0.4 milligrams (400 micrograms) a day of folic acid before pregnancy and to continue this for the first 12 weeks of pregnancy, in order to reduce the risk of having a baby with spina bifida or other neural tube defects (the name for disorders in which the brain and/ or the spinal cord do not develop properly). It is likely that folic acid may also reduce the risk of other types of congenital abnormality and birth defects. Furthermore, it is useful to remember that there is some evidence to suggest that the levels of folate in our blood are increased more efficiently by the daily intake of 0.4mg in tablet form, rather than by eating an extra 0.4mg of folate in the diet each day. This dose of folic acid is available over the counter at chemists and can be taken on its own or as part of a multivitamin preparation. If you are taking a multivitamin tablet, do check that it contains 0.4–1.0mg of folic acid and not more than 5000 IU of vitamin A.

If a woman has had a previous pregnancy affected by spina bifida or another type of neural tube defect, it is recommended that she takes a higher dose of folic acid (a 5-milligram tablet) every day whilst trying to conceive, and for the first 12 weeks of pregnancy. This dose is available on prescription only, from your doctor. If you are epileptic, it is important that you discuss this with your doctor before starting to take folic acid, as it could alter the dose of anti-epileptic medication that you require. Women with epilepsy need to take the higher folic acid dose of 5 milligrammes each day because epileptics have a higher risk of having a baby with spina bifida (see further on in this chapter).

Alcohol can have a damaging effect on male fertility by a direct toxic effect which lowers sperm numbers. In heavy doses, alcohol can affect female fertility as well. It is sensible to restrict alcohol intake to 21 units per week for men and 14 units per week for women.

Smoking cigarettes may make both men and women less fertile. It has been reported that the chance of conceiving is reduced by one-third in women who smoke. Since smoking increases the risk of miscarriage as well, it is more than just a good idea to give up smoking before becoming pregnant. Passive smoking is also a risk – so if you live with someone who smokes as well, make an effort to give up together. There are several organizations which you can contact to help you, such as Quit and ASH.

Rubella (German measles) infection during the first four months of pregnancy can cause severe handicaps to the baby. Most adult women in the UK and all children born after 1988 will have been vaccinated against rubella as a small child and we have now abandoned routine vaccination of teenage girls at school. The vaccination does not always provide long-term immunity, so make sure that you have a blood test to check your immunity before you try to become pregnant. And if this test shows that you are not immune to infection, get vaccinated straight away. Since the vaccination could potentially cause damage in very early pregnancy, it is sensible to have it done early in your menstrual cycle, just after your last period and before you could have possibly become pregnant, and to take contraceptive precautions until a repeat blood test four weeks later shows that the vaccination has been effective. In the past, women were advised to wait for three months after rubella vaccination before becoming pregnant, but we now know that only one month is necessary.

During the last few years I have met several patients who have become pregnant almost immediately after having a rubella vaccination. Their distress and fears that their tiny embryo may have been damaged prompted me to contact several virologists with special experience in rubella. Happily, I can tell you that there is a UK registry for all women who have conceived at the same time or soon after their rubella vaccination and that no abnormalities have ever been detected in the babies who have been born.

If you are rhesus negative and need to have an injection of anti-D after your delivery because your baby is rhesus positive, your doctor will probably suggest that your rubella vaccination is left to a later date. This is because the anti-D (which is another type of gamma globulin injection) can interfere with your ability to develop the correct antibody response in your blood to the rubella vaccination. This failure to 'sero-convert' is important because the only way to ensure that you and your baby are protected from rubella in the future is to measure a strong level of anti-rubella antibodies in your blood. This is why you will be asked to have a blood test a few weeks after your vaccination date to ensure that you have sero-converted. Rubella antibodies will be present in your blood if you have had the infection in the past or if you have been vaccinated.

Exercise is obviously a good idea for general health and also in preparation for pregnancy. However, if you are an unfit 'couch potato', do not start a gruelling exercise programme on day one of your new fitness campaign. Regular, gentle exercise such as walking briskly for 30 minutes per day, cycling and swimming are all good ways to introduce regular exercise to your daily routine. If you are already used to more strenuous exercise like aerobics and working out in the gym, you are probably quite fit already and should continue exercising to remain so.

Serious medical disorders

If you have any long-standing medical condition, it is important to see your doctor when planning to become pregnant. It is also important to continue taking any medication that you have been prescribed for your medical problem until the doctor either changes it or stops it. If you are diabetic it is essential that your blood sugar levels are well controlled whilst you are trying to conceive. Poor diabetic control will reduce your chances of becoming pregnant and increase your risk of miscarriage.

If you suffer from epilepsy, it is particularly important that you are under close medical supervision when you are trying to become pregnant and during the pregnancy. Some anti-epileptic drugs can cause abnormalities in the baby, such as heart and limb defects, mental retardation, cleft lip and cleft palate, and are best changed to a different type of drug when trying to conceive. Pregnancy can change the way anti-epileptic drugs are metabolised in the body and you may need a higher dose. As noted earlier in this chapter, anti-epileptic drugs may reduce the mother's folic acid levels and it is very important that women with epilepsy take high dose folic acid supplements before becoming pregnant and during the first 12 weeks of pregnancy to minimise the risk of spina bifida.

High blood pressure (hypertension) is another medical problem which needs to be under good control when you are planning to become pregnant. The risk of developing pre-eclampsia (toxaemia) and severe problems with your blood pressure are greater if your blood pressure is high at the start of your pregnancy. Some of the anti-hypertensive drugs are not suitable for use in pregnancy, so please ensure that you have talked to your doctor about your plans to become pregnant well in advance, or as soon as the pregnancy test is positive. Asthma sufferers are another group who need to be carefully looked after before and during pregnancy. The aim is to reduce the amount of medication used without increasing the risk of an asthma attack.

Women with thyroid disease also need careful supervision during pregnancy. If you are taking drugs for your thyroid, the dosage required may alter during pregnancy. However, as we noted in Chapter 11, thyroid disease does not increase the risk of future miscarriage, although an under- or overactive thyroid may prevent you from falling pregnant.

Although acne cannot be classified as a serious medical disorder, I think it is important to remind the reader that some of the anti-acne drugs can cause serious abnormalities in the unborn baby. The vitamin A drugs which encourage the affected skin to peel off more quickly than usual are particularly dangerous and, as mentioned earlier in this book, the tetracycline antibiotics are contraindicated in pregnant women because the drug leaves deposits in the growing baby's teeth and bones and discolours them.

I meet an increasing number of women with renal disease requesting advice about pregnancy and miscarriage (see Chapter 9). Undoubtedly, one of the reasons for this is because the medical treatment of renal disease has improved so dramatically that some women who could never have risked a pregnancy before are now able to consider it as a distinct possibility. However, if you do suffer from renal disease, it is important that you consult with your renal doctors before attempting to become pregnant.

Is there a place for alternative medicine?

I am often asked for my views about alternative medicine by women who are trying to become pregnant after having suffered a miscarriage. My reply is always the same – until conventional medicine can sort out every problem faced by women wanting to achieve a successful pregnancy, I will remain open-minded about some alternative treatments. In fact, I positively encourage some women to look at alternative options such as acupuncture and homeopathy. My reason for this is simple. I do not understand how they work, or even if they do work, but I do recognise that trying to do something for oneself is a good way to tackle the impotence and frustration that so many miscarriage sufferers experience. Most of the women I talk to in the miscarriage clinic are distressed by the feeling that they are not in control of what is happening to them both physically and emotionally.

Having said all that, I do worry about the women I see in the clinic who are taking Chinese herbal remedies, since we know that these remedies can have potent effects on the endometrium or womb lining which could seriously interfere with successful implantation. When I ask them for the names of the herbs and what the herbs are meant to be doing, I invariably receive the answer that they are 'natural' and discover that the woman does not know the names of the herbs she has been prescribed and has been given no information about what effect they are meant to be having on her body.

I am genuinely puzzled by this blind acceptance of taking herbs and medicinal compounds without questioning what they are, what they do and whether they may cause her to experience side-effects. Particularly since so many of the women I see in the clinic are very concerned about whether conventional medicines may be having an adverse effect on their ability to get pregnancy or stay pregnant. The word 'natural' appears to be very powerful and hopefully this short section will mean that you can now assess the situation of whether you pursue alternative treatments with more confidence. One word of warning, however. Try not to become obsessed with alternative medicine. Cranky diets, worrying yourself silly that your hair analysis has suggested that you are deficient in zinc or magnesium, or taking so many vitamin tablets that you rattle when you jump up and down is not helpful. In fact, it is counter-productive because it causes further stress and anxiety.

Period problems

If your menstrual periods are irregular or infrequent, you may experience a delay in becoming pregnant. In young, healthy women the commonest cause of irregular periods is polycystic ovaries (discussed in detail in Chapter 11). However, it is important to remember that for many women who have just experienced a miscarriage, normal, regular periods do not return for a couple of months. There is nothing abnormal about this and the best remedy is not to worry about it. In many cases it reflects the emotional distress of the recent miscarriage. However, if you know that you have polycystic ovaries, it is sensible to talk to your doctor about undergoing some tests to see if you are ovulating. If you are not ovulating regularly, it may be appropriate to have treatment to help you produce and release an egg every month. This treatment needs to be carefully monitored to prevent complications.

Heavy periods are unpleasant for a woman, but they are not usually a cause of infertility. Nor do heavy periods increase the risk of miscarriage unless they are due to the presence of a fibroid or polyp in the womb which may interfere with successful implantation of the early embryo. An ultrasound scan can help to determine what is going on. Periods that are too frequent usually reflect a problem with ovulation.

Although an egg may be released, the next part of the menstrual cycle – the luteal phase – is too short and does not allow sufficient opportunity for a fertilised egg to implant properly. Light bleeding (spotting) in the middle of the menstrual cycle may be normal for some women, but it may also reflect hormonal imbalances or a physical problem such as a polyp in the womb or a raw area on the neck of the womb (cervix).

If you are experiencing period problems and you are preparing to become pregnant again, arrange to see your doctor. The likelihood is that nothing is seriously wrong but establishing this fact will give you much more confidence. And if your doctor suspects that you do have a problem, a prompt referral to a gynaecologist is likely to sort the problem out quickly.

How long should I wait before trying again?

I am frequently asked by women who have recently miscarried if there is a recommended period of time to wait until trying to become pregnant again. The answer is no – there are no black-and-white rules. Most women will not conceive again until they have had a normal period, but this is not always so. Certainly, waiting for a normal period to come is a good way to reassure yourself that your hormones are back to normal and it will make the doctor's job much simpler if the dates of the next pregnancy can be calculated easily.

However, there are no data to suggest that falling pregnant again soon after a miscarriage increases the risk of a further miscarriage. I suspect the old advice offered to women that they should wait for three months is based on the idea that after that time the woman is more likely to be emotionally ready for another pregnancy. My personal advice is simple and individual. The right time to embark on another pregnancy is when you feel ready for it. For some women this will be straight away. For others, particularly those who have suffered a late miscarriage, a longer period of time will be needed to make all the emotional adjustments for a new pregnancy. There are only very rarely medical reasons for delaying a future pregnancy. One example is when a woman has suffered a blood clot, or thrombosis, during her previous pregnancy. In this situation, it is usually necessary to give the woman anticoagulant drugs for a couple of months following the pregnancy, during which time it is not sensible to become pregnant again. Indeed, most thrombosis experts will probably advise that any future pregnancies are postponed for at least 12 months.

What contraception should I use?

I meet many women in the miscarriage clinic who find themselves pregnant unexpectedly. This can be a cause of enormous distress, particularly if the woman is in the middle of investigations into the cause of the previous pregnancy losses. Invariably, the interruption to the investigations brings fears that a possible cause may have been missed. Worse, that there is no time to start treatment which may have helped prevent a future miscarriage.

It is sensible to use an effective type of contraception until you are ready, both physically and emotionally, to embark on your next pregnancy. I know that there are many old wives' tales told about the dangers of the combined oral contraceptive pill in this situation. They are all untrue. There is no truth in the story that miscarriage is more common in women who conceive shortly after stopping the combined pill. If anything, the reverse is true. Several large prospective studies have shown that the risk of miscarriage may even be slightly lower in previous pill users.

Nor does the combined pill cause delays in becoming pregnant. In fact, there is some evidence suggesting that women with polycystic ovaries who have had ovulation problems, benefit from using the combined pill for several months before the next pregnancy. For some of these women, the pill appears to successfully correct the hormonal problems (most probably high LH levels) preventing regular ovulation, so that when they stop the pill they ovulate spontaneously for a short while and often conceive during the first or second month of trying. Hence, the widely quoted drug manufacturers' advice that women should avoid becoming pregnant for three months after stopping the combined pill (to allow time to clear the chemicals from her body) is both incorrect and unhelpful, but I am still asked this question by my patients on a very regular basis.

The situation with progestogen-only pills is not so clear cut. There is no evidence to suggest that they increase the risk of miscarriage. However, they do not offer the benefits of controlling ovulation and they do cause irregular bleeding in some women, which may cause alarm and confusion. However, for women who are not allowed to take the oestrogen in combined pills, they are very useful. All types of barrier methods can be used although these are not as effective in preventing pregnancy as hormonal contraception. The use of spermicide creams does not increase the risk of miscarriage, as has been suggested in the past.

The least suitable form of contraception for the miscarriage sufferer, in my opinion, is the intrauterine contraceptive device or 'coil'. I am always worried that they may cause infection in the uterus and pelvis, resulting in later infertility. Although the uncomplicated coil does not increase the risk of future miscarriage, if pregnancy occurs whilst the coil is in the uterus (IUCD failure), as many as 50% of the pregnancies will miscarry. In this situation, the best course of action is to have the coil removed as quickly as possible. The longer it remains in the uterus with the pregnancy, the more likely it is to cause bleeding, infection and miscarriage.

In summary, the best way to ensure that your next pregnancy occurs when you are physically and emotionally prepared for it, is to ensure that you use suitable contraception in the meantime. A combined oral contraceptive pill is probably the best method available for the majority of women, because it offers a low risk of failure, a low risk of future miscarriage and may even improve the chance of falling pregnant for some women when it is discontinued.

Your emotional health

Preparing yourself emotionally for the next pregnancy is often the most difficult task. What is more, every woman will have different needs. For some women, the only way to cope with the misery and disappointment of a miscarriage is to become pregnant again as soon as possible. The fear of 'losing valuable time' is one that is often expressed to me. This is very understandable but can sometimes lead to further anxieties and distress if pregnancy does not occur straight away. I often suggest to couples who are experiencing some delay in falling pregnant again that they try to go on a holiday and promise each other that they will stop talking and thinking about another pregnancy for a while. This is difficult to do, I know, but if the number of delighted post-holiday telephone calls we receive at the early pregnancy clinic is anything to go by, then it is certainly worthwhile trying!

For other women, the fear of losing another pregnancy prevents them from wanting to try to become pregnant again for a while. Although they desperately want a baby, the horror of reliving their worst nightmare is a very real one. In this situation, the only cure is time. Time for the fears to lessen and the drive to be pregnant to return. Hopefully, you will be able to talk about some of your fears with friends or close members of the family. However, I think there are some occasions when your partner, friends and family are too close to the problem to be able to offer you the help you need. Arranging to see a counsellor may be the answer in this situation. Certainly, some time spent talking to an individual who is able to remain more detached and objective can be of enormous value. Depending upon you and your lifestyle, this person may be your local doctor, health visitor, priest or a member of one of the voluntary bereavement organisations such as Cruse. I regularly have cause to feel very grateful to the two miscarriage counsellors who are attached to our clinic. They play an essential role in the healing process for some women, and their contribution is entirely different to that offered by the doctors, nurses or research fellows working with us. If you have difficulties in finding someone like this, try contacting the Miscarriage Association. They have a country-wide network of support volunteers, all of whom have experienced miscarriage themselves and so understand your need for support.

As I mentioned in an earlier chapter, one of the most important things to do when preparing for the next pregnancy is to collect as much information about your miscarriage as possible. Knowledge and understanding of your own problem is the best weapon you have for fighting the next battle. Even when there appear to be no answers to your questions, trying to help yourself is a positive course of action and will provide a measure of emotional comfort.

21

COPING WITH THE
NEXT PREGNANCY

Diet

Every pregnant woman needs to give some thought and attention to what she is eating and drinking. Much has been written about the dos and don'ts of diet during pregnancy. Some of the advice handed on down through the generations is useful. Some is wrong or simply unpalatable. For example, braised liver was considered a 'must' by my grandmother's generation. Liver is an excellent source of iron and folic acid, but we now know that the vitamin A content of liver can cause birth defects in the baby, such as facial, heart and brain abnormalities. Since the vitamin A content of fresh liver is variable, I think it is best to avoid it altogether when you are pregnant. If you hate spinach, there is little point in feeling guilty that you cannot stomach a kilogram of soggy greens every day. Furthermore, in our affluent society, I rarely meet vegetarians in my antenatal clinic who develop anaemia because of their vegetarian diet, although strict vegans are more likely to develop anaemia and other dietary deficiencies during pregnancy.

A well-balanced diet of regular meals including a mixture of protein, carbohydrate and fat is the optimum during pregnancy. This has been the received wisdom for many years and I do not argue with one bit of it. However, I think it is important to add that first and foremost your diet needs to be enjoyable and to suit your appetite and lifestyle. In the first three months of pregnancy, nausea often dictates what you can or cannot eat. In my own pregnancy, I remember vividly that during the first few months the only things that I really enjoyed were asparagus sandwiches, Marmite sandwiches and grapefruit juice! The smell of cooking meat made me actually retch and the taste of coffee, which I usually drink continuously throughout the day, was extremely unpleasant. These fads soon passed and by 16 weeks I was able to eat regular well-balanced meals.

Fish is a particularly good source of protein, and offers the advantage of containing special oils which are particularly good for the growth of the baby's brain. Any type of fish is beneficial but the best fatty acid content is found in oily fish such as tuna, mackerel, sardines and salmon. If you are a meat eater, choose lean meat and cut off the visible fat. Nuts, lentils, beans and peas can all be eaten as an alternative or an addition to meat or fish.

Dairy products provide good sources of proteins, fat and calcium and also offer great variety to your diet. Try to include one pint of fresh milk in your diet each day. Remember that skimmed milk is just as rich in calcium, but has a lower fat content. Many women find that a small pot of yoghurt is helpful in combating early nausea. Yoghurt is also very good towards the end of pregnancy if heartburn is troublesome. One word of warning about dairy products, however: avoid products made from unpasteurised milk which is found in some soft cheeses, such as Brie, camembert and some blue-veined varieties. The unpasteurised milk can harbour many different bacterial organisms, which can cause serious problems such as late miscarriage and intrauterine death during pregnancy. There is no need to stop eating all cheese, just look at the details on the packet. If the cheese is made with pasteurised milk it will state this fact. For the same reasons, avoid eating raw or soft cooked eggs and foods made from uncooked eggs (e.g. mousses and mayonnaise). Make sure that any meat or poultry you eat is well cooked and avoid pâtés, terrines, liver and liver sausage. Ensure that all fruits and vegetables are carefully washed.

Bread and cereals are important sources of energy, fibre, vitamins and minerals. Wholemeal bread, wholewheat pasta, rice and wholegrain breakfast cereals all offer a high fibre content which helps to prevent constipation and keeps the gut healthy. Make sure that you include at least two pieces of fruit per day in your diet and particularly citrus fruits such as oranges and grapefruits. It is also sensible to eat foods with a high folic acid content. Green leafy vegetables (which should not be overcooked) such as spinach, brussels sprouts, broccoli, cabbage and lettuce are all good sources, as are green beans, okra, parsnips, bean sprouts and pulses (for example, peas, cooked black-eyed beans and chickpeas). Fortified breakfast cereals, fortified bread and yeast extracts (such as Marmite) are all good ways to supplement your diet.

Make sure that you do not put on too much weight. The average weight gain during pregnancy is about 10 kilos (22 pounds). Many women find that they start having little snacks when they are pregnant. During the early months, frequent small meals may be the only way to cope with nausea. However, when the snacks contain lots of sugar and are later added to regular meals, there is no way that you will escape unnecessary weight gain. The problem will be made worse if you pretend to yourself that all of the weight you are putting on is the baby and that another few chocolate bars do not matter now because you can shed the weight easily after the baby is born. You will need to be as fit as possible for the birth of your baby and the demanding months afterwards, so try to avoid gaining more than the average. The old adage about 'eating for two' should be treated with a pinch of salt. You are not eating for two, you are eating sensibly for you and your tiny baby. Your baby will take everything that it needs from your diet and you do not need to eat vast quantities of food to ensure that your baby has enough. If you need further reassurance of this fact, remember that the birth weight of babies born in Third World countries is not significantly less than that of babies born in this country.

Vitamins

There is now clear evidence that folic acid and folates have a major role to play in the prevention and recurrence of neural tube defects (e.g. spina bifida). As a result, the Department of Health recommends that all women increase their intake of folic acid and folates by an additional 400 micrograms (0.4 milligrams) a day before pregnancy and during the first twelve weeks of pregnancy. There are three ways to increase your folate intake: eating more folate-rich foods; eating foods fortified with folate (see Diet, above) and taking supplements of folate in tablet form. A normal healthy diet already provides you with an average folate intake of about 200 micrograms per day. The recommended supplement of 400 microgram tablets is easily purchased over the counter at your chemist and will bring your total daily intake up to about 600 micrograms.

Many women I see in the miscarriage clinic like to take multivitamin preparations during pregnancy. However, it is important to remember that not all multivitamin tablets contain folic acid, nor in sufficient quantities. Furthermore, if you try to achieve the recommended dose of folic acid by taking several multivitamin pills, there is a risk that you will be taking an excess of the other vitamins, particularly vitamin A. For this reason, it is best to take the 400mcg folic acid tablets on their own. If you have not been taking folic acid before pregnancy and suspect that you might be pregnant, start taking supplements straight away and continue until the 12th week of pregnancy.

Iron tablets seem to be much beloved by patients and doctors alike. However, iron supplements are not needed routinely in pregnancy unless you are carrying twins or are already anaemic. Anaemia is definitely not a cause of miscarriage. I find that about a third of women taking iron tablets can take them without any complication, another third develop severe constipation, and the last third suffer from tummy upsets and diarrhoea as a result of the tablets. I think these are needlessly unpleasant complications to endure throughout your pregnancy if you are not actually anaemic. Your blood count will probably fall towards the end of pregnancy due to a dilution effect resulting from the increased amount of fluid in your blood. If, at this later stage of pregnancy, you are advised to take iron supplements and develop gastrointestinal symptoms, ask your doctor to prescribe another brand. There are many different preparations on the market and it is usually possible to find one that suits you better. Remember that there are many foods such as dried fruits (particularly apricots and raisins) and chocolate that are very good sources of extra iron and also very palatable! But do make sure that you keep a watchful eye on your calorie intake. A recent study in Australia has found that vitamin B3 can treat critical molecular deficiencies in pregnant women. The scientists used genetic sequencing on families suffering from miscarriages and birth defects and found gene mutations that affected production of the molecule, NAD (nicotinamide adenine dinucleotide). This supplement is vitamin B3, also known as niacin, which is found in various meats and green vegetables – as well as yeast extract spreads, such as marmite and its Australian equivalent, Vegemite. A single serving of this spread contains 36% of your recommended daily allowance of B3.

Constipation

Lots of pregnant women suffer from constipation. Undoubtedly, this is partly due to the high levels of progesterone hormone that are produced during pregnancy and which cause the smooth muscle of the gut to be much less active than usual. As mentioned earlier, some women taking iron tablets find that the iron makes the constipation significantly worse. If you find that you are becoming constipated, start eating extra fibre in your diet. Wholemeal bread, fresh fruits and vegetables, dried fruits (such as raisins and apricots) are all good sources of fibre. If this fails, daily tablespoons of real bran (the sawdust lookalike purchased in health food shops, not the breakfast cereal called bran flakes) usually does the trick, but is virtually inedible unless you mix it into some yoghurt, soup or gravy. If this does not resolve the problem, then it is sensible to use a bulk laxative such as Lactulose, Fybogel or Isogel. Remember that you will not cure your constipation unless you drink plenty of fluids to help the fibre along. Try and drink lots of water, fruit juice or unsweetened drinks rather than coffee, tea or soft fizzy drinks. Fortunately, I am able to reassure you firmly that however badly you may suffer from constipation, it will not cause you to miscarry.

On no account should you use Senna or any purgative laxative during pregnancy. Senna and its relatives causes irritation of the bowel which can, in some situations, irritate the uterus and even lead to the onset of premature labour. Moreover, the continued abuse of these purgative laxatives results in the destruction of the nerve-endings in the bowel and, as a result, in later years your bowel will become more constipated and more resistant to the use of bulk laxatives and dietary fibre.

Tobacco and alcohol

Smoking in pregnancy can lead to a reduction of the baby's supply of oxygen and nutrients and can produce smaller babies who are at increased risk of infection and may have developmental problems. Please try hard to stop smoking before becoming pregnant, and if this has not been successful, throw out your cigarettes the moment the pregnancy test is positive. I meet so many women who say, 'But I only smoke five cigarettes per day, doctor'. Any number of cigarettes per day is too many when you are pregnant. Think about the fact that five cigarettes a day during a 40-week pregnancy means that your baby will have been exposed to 1380 cigarettes before birth! If you are still not convinced, then please go back to Chapter 9 and read about all the adverse effects that cigarette smoking has on fertility and the growth and development of the fetus and placenta in pregnancy.

I have often reflected upon the fact that nature has some very clever ways of helping to ensure that women continue to produce healthy babies. What other explanation can there be for most women to hate the taste of alcohol in early pregnancy? Indeed, before the days of home pregnancy tests, becoming intolerant of alcohol was often considered one of the first symptoms of pregnancy. There are good reasons for this revulsion for alcohol, which fortunately (I think!) starts to fade later in pregnancy.

During the first three months of the baby's development, large quantities of alcohol can cause severe abnormalities. The fetal alcohol syndrome has been well described in the children of mothers who are alcoholic and details are included in Chapter 9 of this book. Some reports have also suggested that moderate regular drinking is also associated with miscarriage, milder fetal abnormalities and growth-restriction in the baby. However, there are no data that suggest that the occasional drink is harmful, particularly in later pregnancy. One or two glasses of wine during the week may be a very good way of increasing relaxation. I am reminded that in years gone by, an intravenous drip of alcohol was the only known method to quieten the uterus which was threatening to labour prematurely. I am not suggesting that you should hook yourself up to a bottle of scotch, but would suggest to you that after the first three months of pregnancy are completed, there is no need to deny yourself the odd drink if you fancy it.

Bed rest

The question that I am asked more than any other is: 'Doctor, should I bed rest during the first few weeks of my pregnancy?' I find this a very difficult question to answer medically, since I do not know of any data that suggests that resting in bed reduces the miscarriage rate in early pregnancy. If you have an episode of bleeding, then lying flat in bed may appear to stop the bleeding but this usually recurs when you get out of bed again, and particularly when going to the toilet. This is because the blood which has leaked from behind the placenta passes through the neck of the womb into the vagina in the upright position. Nonetheless, for many hundreds of years, doctors and midwives have advised women to rest in bed if they experience bleeding in early pregnancy. One of the reasons has always been that the more rest the pregnant woman has, the better the blood flow to the uterus, the placenta and therefore the baby, will be. This is certainly true in later pregnancy; indeed, plenty of rest during the last two months is the reason why maternity leave is a statutory right. However, in early pregnancy, there is no evidence that bed rest can affect the outcome of pregnancy.

Hence I think my response to the issue of bed rest in early pregnancy is that it depends on the woman. Her character and her past experience in pregnancy will be important factors to take into account. For the woman who has suffered repeated miscarriages in the past, resting in bed may provide her with the reassurance that she did everything she could to help the pregnancy continue, should anything go wrong in the future. For other women, resting in bed will lead to so much anxiety and distress that it is better for them to follow their usual day to day lifestyle including going to work. I suggest you ask yourself which of these two groups you fall into. If you are going to feel consumed with guilt and self-blame when some bleeding occurs whilst you are doing the shopping or are attending your yoga class, then stay in bed. On the other hand, if you need the distraction of domestic tasks or your job to help you cope with the fears and anxieties you have about this next pregnancy, then go to work. I really do not think it is necessary to wrap yourself in cotton wool in the first few weeks of a pregnancy. The reality is that a pregnancy that is going to miscarry is going to miscarry, and a pregnancy that is going to stick will stick.

Similarly, the value of a period of time spent in hospital which coincides with the time at which the previous miscarriages have occurred, is of no proven benefit. Some women will want to be hospitalised. Others will consider going into hospital to be the realisation of their worst nightmares. I am often asked to arrange admission to my hospital for patients with a history of miscarriage, particularly for those who have suffered late losses. I always manage to find a bed, however short they are reported to be, because I believe that a positive response to this request to be 'looked after' is extremely important emotionally. And since I cannot pretend that I understand all the reasons why some women miscarry repeatedly at the same time in pregnancy, perhaps it is helpful. I shall continue to advise this open-door policy unless someone persuades me that it is harmful.

One more point is worth mentioning on this subject. I meet many women who feel very pressurised by family and friends to retire to their bed if they have suffered a miscarriage in the past. I am sure the advice is meant well, but it can cause needless distress. Make up your own mind, with the help of your partner if possible, about what is the right thing for you to do. After all, it is your feelings that matter and only you know how best to cope with them.

Sex

It is usually quite safe to enjoy making love throughout pregnancy as long as you do not experience any pain or discomfort. I know that many doctors advise avoiding sex during the first 12 weeks of pregnancy, particularly if the woman has had a miscarriage in the past. There is no scientific basis for this viewpoint. I think the reason why this advice is offered is to protect the couple from feelings of guilt and self-blame if the woman should happen to have some bleeding after making love.

This is another situation in which it is important for the individual woman/couple to make their own decisions. I know of no data that could persuade me that sex is dangerous in early pregnancy, but if you are anxious about miscarriage and bleeding, I suggest you avoid sex until you feel more confident. Remember that it takes a big insult to disturb a healthy pregnancy!

Exercise and sport

Over the last few years I have received many more questions about the safety of exercise in pregnancy. So I feel that it is important to spend a bit of time at this point discussing the issues in more detail. Gentle regular exercise is a good thing in pregnancy. Current evidence points to the fact that exercise is safe and beneficial for the majority of pregnant women. Even if you have had several miscarriages in the past, there is no reason to stop the exercise that you are used to. And if you have not been taking regular exercise, start walking every day, or swim a couple of times per week. Daily exercise will help you to keep fit during pregnancy and is actually very relaxing.

If you are a keen sportswoman, you are probably quite fit anyway. Many female athletes now continue training programmes throughout their pregnancies and even go on to improve their sporting performances after childbirth. The reason for this is not entirely clear but it has been suggested that the increased blood volume and effort required to exercise at a greater body weight has long-term physiological benefits. An alternative explanation could be that there are important psychological benefits for a competitive sports-woman after enduring pregnancy, labour and motherhood!

Historically, women and their doctors have worried about the effect of exercise and sport on the unborn child, but this is really a bit misguided. The baby within the uterus is enclosed by the bony pelvic cage until 12 weeks of pregnancy. After this time the fetus is protected by thick, spongy layers of the uterine wall and at least a litre of amniotic fluid. As a result, damage to the baby because of maternal trauma or activity is very rare. On the other hand, because of the mother's increasingly lax ligaments, her shifting centre of gravity and changes in the curvature of her spine, she is at increased risk of trauma to herself towards the end of pregnancy. It is probably best to avoid contact sports such as field and court games during the last three months of pregnancy.

I think that much of the advice that strenuous exercise may put the baby at risk stems from animal studies which have suggested that the blood flow to the uterus is reduced. But there are just as many other studies that have demonstrated that even strenuous exercise is of no risk to the baby, certainly in the first half of pregnancy. It appears that some of the uterine blood flow is directed to the placenta during exercise and that the uterine circulation is able to increase the amount of oxygen it extracts from the mother's blood as a compensatory mechanism.

It is obviously very difficult to monitor the baby's response during exercise. Nonetheless, cardiotocography (fetal heart rate tracings) studies have been performed and usually show a short period of tachycardia (speeding up of the heart rate) after exercise, or alternatively that the baby's temperature increases slightly. Overall, the experts have concluded that maternal exercise up to 70% of maximal capacity does not interfere in any way with normal fetal growth and development. The only women whose babies appear to suffer are those who undertake daily endurance training near to the time of delivery and have poor weight gain – these babies are sometimes small for dates. Hence professional athletes need to be reminded to pay particular attention to good nutrition and should probably be advised to scale down their training schedules towards the end of pregnancy.

I recently had the pleasure of a medical sports expert as a patient. She provided me with a list of points to offer the pregnant athlete which I include here for you.

- Avoid exercising to exhaustion – you should be able to carry on talking normally during prolonged exercise
- Avoid exercising in the heat – especially in early pregnancy – and make sure you do not become dehydrated and that you drink sufficient fluids
- Begin and finish your exercise gradually – the message is warm up and warm down
- Always stop exercising if you experience any pain
- Exercise regularly to maintain fitness, rather than in fits and starts
- Aim to reduce your exercise programme in later pregnancy

Scuba diving is one sport that should not be undertaken during pregnancy because of the potential risk of bubbles (gas emboli) developing in the placental and fetal blood vessels as a result of the pressure changes in deep water. Parachute jumping should also be avoided and water-skiing enthusiasts are usually advised to wear a wet suit during pregnancy to avoid forceful vaginal douching.

Another very commonly asked question is 'Is it safe to take saunas while I am pregnant?' It is true that there was a single report in the 1970s which suggested that regular saunas may increase the risk of fetal malformations but this has never been confirmed. Reassuringly, there are more recent studies which have shown that maternal hyperthermia (overheating) during exercise does not result in fetal abnormalities. In summary, I don't believe that sport is harmful in early pregnancy. I suggest that you adopt a middle-of-the-road approach and if you enjoy sport, continue to play, but avoid very strenuous activity which tires you out. You will find it difficult not to blame yourself if you start miscarrying in the middle of a squash tournament.

Travel

Long-distance travel is one activity that I do think should be avoided if you have a history of miscarriage. Not because a transatlantic flight or a long car journey can cause a miscarriage, but because being a long way away from home and the doctor and hospital that you are familiar with, is bound to cause you even more distress if you start to miscarry again. Imagine what it feels like to stand in the casualty department of a hospital in a foreign country, when you cannot speak a word of the language and you are trying to explain to the doctor (they are tired and overworked overseas as well) that you want to have an ultrasound scan before anyone examines you or ships you off for a quick 'clear-out'.

You may have had the misfortune to have experienced going into a hospital before with a miscarriage, but did you have to fight to make yourself understood or have to worry about whether you have the correct insurance documents with you before anyone medical will pay you attention? No, I am not a reactionary British doctor who considers that the UK is the only country in the world capable of delivering good healthcare. Nor am I recounting a bitter personal experience. What I want to share with you is the misery that so many women have described to me, in graphic detail, when they have miscarried a long way from home. Fortunately, the chances of this happening to you are small, but it is possible to avoid the risk completely by not exposing yourself to it.

I think I need to make a few comments here about the safety of air travel in particular. I am struck by how many more questions I have been asked on this subject in the clinic recently. In theory, there are two potential areas of concern. The first is that spending a lot of time thousands of feet above the ground may lower the mother's oxygen levels because the pressure in most passenger cabins is lower than atmospheric pressure on the ground. The second is cosmic radiation – which simply means the radiation you receive from the sun – which of course is greater if you are nearer the sun, as is the case in an aeroplane.

I have scoured the literature in an attempt to answer the above questions, but there is really very little data to be found. One study from Finland reported that there may be a small increase in the risk of miscarriage among female flight attendants. Certainly most airlines offer their crews the option of switching to ground duties during pregnancy, but when I contacted the medical advisers to several airlines recently, they explained to me that this employment concession is not based on any firm evidence that flying regularly during pregnancy has any detrimental effect on pregnancy outcome.

Early pregnancy fears – what can I do to allay them?

If you have suffered previous miscarriages, it is entirely natural that you will have fears and anxieties in the next pregnancy. I think the best way of dealing with these worries is to try to ensure, before you become pregnant, that you know how to contact medical help promptly as soon as you get pregnant again. If you are able to obtain an appointment with your doctor, local hospital or early pregnancy clinic (if this is available in your area) quickly, many of your worries will probably be resolved very simply. Feeling that you are unable to access help and advice is certain to induce panic and distress if you are a miscarriage sufferer who has just become pregnant again. Fortunately, the value of early pregnancy clinics is becoming much better understood. More and more hospitals are introducing ultrasound services that are immediately accessible to women and their general practitioners. For anyone reading this book who has doubts about the importance and cost-effectiveness of such clinics – please read Chapter 21, which describes the proven benefits that such expertise and care can offer to women in early pregnancy.

If I was to recount all of the worries told to me in the early pregnancy clinic at St Mary's Hospital, this chapter would never be completed. However, I think it is useful to mention a few of the most frequently expressed concerns here.

By sheer weight of numbers, I have to conclude that the fear of bleeding is the commonest fear experienced by miscarriage sufferers. Try to remember that the majority of women who develop bleeding in early pregnancy will go on to have a normal pregnancy. If it is possible to have an ultrasound scan, this may provide some reassurance that the pregnancy is progressing and that there is no obvious cause for the bleeding. Some women are frightened of having a scan because it may confirm their worst fears – that the pregnancy is over. Although I understand the emotions involved here, I always strongly encourage women to establish what is happening as early as possible. It is only by making a diagnosis and obtaining as much information as possible, that you can move forwards. Burying your head in the sand will not help in the long term and may even prevent you and your doctor from obtaining useful information for the future.

Fears that the baby may be abnormal are also very common. This is always a difficult anxiety to allay because even the most sophisticated tests can only offer a degree of reassurance – it is never possible to promise a woman a 'normal' baby (see Chapter 7).

Another very common concern is that the woman has taken certain medical drugs before she realised that she was pregnant. In practice, these are usually antibiotics and fortunately only a few antibiotics cause abnormalities in early pregnancy. For example, tetracyclines (usually prescribed for acne or for infections caused by chlamydia) cause discoloration and deformity in the teeth and bones of the baby and chloramphenicol (rarely used nowadays) is responsible for the blue baby syndrome. Penicillin taken for a throat infection, a whitlow on your finger or an episode of cystitis has never been known to cause harm to the baby directly.

The nausea that invariably accompanies the early weeks of pregnancy can be very distressing and at least 50% of pregnant women also experience repeated episodes of vomiting. Despite the popular name of 'morning sickness' many women experience nausea throughout the day and for some women the symptoms continue way beyond 20 weeks of gestation. Some women may benefit from small doses of an anti-emetic (anti-sickness drug). However, the lessons learnt from the thalidomide disaster (thalidomide was prescribed for pregnancy nausea) have rightly resulted in doctors and patients being both wary and vigilant of all medications taken during pregnancy. I therefore think it is important that I do not sound too reassuring in this book about the use of drugs in early pregnancy and, instead, encourage all women who are planning to become pregnant and who are in early pregnancy, that they should take no drugs at all unless they are absolutely necessary.

I promise you that if your nausea is so severe that you become dehydrated, all doctors will recognise this problem (which is called hyperemesis gravidarum) and arrange for you to be admitted to hospital and treated with an intravenous drip to give you the fluids necessary to rehydrate you. I think it is important to remember that in the days when intravenous drips were not readily available, some pregnant women became very ill indeed as a result of the dehydration associated with hyperemesis. Fortunately, this is no longer the case. Although the intravenous drip obviously does not stop the woman feeling miserable because of her symptoms, it does prevent her getting into danger because of dehydration.

A wide variety of treatments have been tried to alleviate hyperemesis. Pyridoxine (vitamin B6) three times a day is probably the least likely to cause any side-effects. There is also a suggestion that powdered ginger may be helpful, although direct evidence is lacking and it can be difficult to eat sufficient quantities of dry powder. Acupuncture has also been reported as a successful alternative treatment. Steroids have been shown to be helpful but this treatment is usually reserved for very severe and unresponsive cases, in order to avoid the risks of steroid therapy in pregnancy.

It is interesting to note that there have been quite a few studies demonstrating that hospital admission, IV fluids and a small dose of an anxiolytic drug such as diazepam or lorazepam can be very effective. These drugs are probably very helpful and of no danger to mother or baby if used on a short-term basis. In my experience, some women suffering from hyperemesis gravidarum in early pregnancy are very anxious and emotionally distressed about how their pregnancy is progressing – particularly if they have had problems becoming pregnant or maintaining a pregnancy in the past.

Viral infections are very common during pregnancy, so it is not surprising that many women worry about the effects these illnesses may have upon their unborn child. Viral infections that cause specific abnormalities in the baby are discussed in Chapters 4 and 10. A bout of flu or a nasty headcold is much more common and considerably more difficult to give specific advice about. My impression is that these common respiratory viruses may cause miscarriage if they are severe enough, because they result in a major upset to the system, but they do not cause abnormalities in the baby. Similarly, an episode of food poisoning may be the cause of a sporadic miscarriage, but if the pregnancy continues, no fetal abnormalities are later recognised.

Should I ask my doctor for hormone treatment?

If only I had a pound for each time that I have been asked this question . . . My answer is always the same. Giving injections of progesterone or HCG (human chorionic gonadotrophin) during early pregnancy with the aim of reducing the miscarriage rate is worthless. There are several well-conducted treatment trials that have shown that these hormone treatments are not helpful. The only function they have is to postpone the inevitability of a miscarriage by a short interval.

The reason for this is simple. If the pregnancy hormones are low, this reflects the fact that the placenta has failed and cannot produce sufficient hormones to allow the pregnancy to continue. Injecting a small dose (compared to the amounts of hormone that the placenta should be producing, the dose is tiny) via a hypodermic syringe cannot make the placenta come alive again, although it may increase the levels of hormone circulating in the blood slightly. As a result, the bleeding and/or miscarriage that was scheduled to start today may be delayed for a short time. However, since the placenta is not functioning, it will not be long before the process of miscarriage continues.

So why, despite this knowledge, are some women still offered progesterone and HCG supplements in early pregnancy? I think the reason for continued differences of opinion on this subject can be explained by the emotional distress which accompanies so many miscarriages. These emotions are powerful and, if allowed, can override factual knowledge. The miscarriage patient wants to try anything that may help her hang on to her baby. She may have a friend or relative who has received hormone treatment in early pregnancy which appears to have resulted in a successful pregnancy. Not surprisingly, she exerts pressure on her doctor to do something. The doctor feels helpless because he or she has no magic solution to offer. It goes against the grain to do nothing and it is particularly difficult to be seen to 'deny' treatment that may just 'do the trick'. As a result, I think many prescriptions for hormone treatments in early pregnancy are written out because they make everyone concerned feel better that some action has been taken.

I have to confess here that there have been rare occasions when, faced with a distraught miscarriage patient, I have succumbed to the same pressures and prescribed hormones. I felt guilty afterwards, because this was the easy way out for me. I still feel guilty, because by allowing anecdotal reports to override my knowledge of the facts, I have contributed to the confusion and stood in the way of progress. Further confusion has arisen from the infertility world. Many of the assisted fertility treatments now include the use of drugs which shut down the ovary and are followed by further drugs which stimulate the ovary to produce multiple eggs. Because all natural ovarian hormone production has been turned off, it has become standard practice to give progesterone or HCG supplements after the eggs have been collected. This improves the chances of pregnancy by making the womb lining more favourable to the implanting embryo. The treatment is usually continued until about eight weeks into a successful pregnancy. Many infertility clinics have reported that the use of progesterone/HCG in this way improves the ongoing pregnancy rate. However, the reasoning behind this treatment is entirely different. It cannot be extrapolated to a patient who becomes pregnant spontaneously and then miscarries.

For the miscarriage patient, starting hormone injections after the pregnancy has already implanted is akin to shutting the stable door after the horse has bolted. If the placenta cannot produce sufficient progesterone or HCG to support the pregnancy during the first few weeks because it has implanted poorly, no amount of hormone treatment given as injections or pessaries can improve the quality of implantation, and the pregnancy will founder.

In the future it may be possible to use hormones to improve the quality of implantation. If this proves successful, I am sure that the treatment will need to be started long before the pregnancy test becomes positive.

Antenatal diagnostic tests

I meet many couples who are worried about the risks of miscarriage which are associated with invasive antenatal diagnostic tests such as amniocentesis and chorion villus sampling (see Chapter 7 for details). If you have suffered repeated miscarriages, you will feel particularly wary about undergoing any procedure that may put your pregnancy at risk. However, there may be very specific reasons why your doctor discusses these tests with you.

Your age may be an important factor – the risk of Down's syndrome increases steeply after the age of 35 years. Alternatively, it may be that one of your previous pregnancies is known to have miscarried because of a chromosomal abnormality, which does increase your risk of a future chromosome abnormality in the baby. If you or your partner carry a genetic abnormality such as a balanced translocation (see Chapter 7) there is a risk that the baby may inherit the unbalanced chromosome. In this latter situation, all doctors are agreed that, whatever the woman's pregnancy history, an amniocentesis should be performed to ensure that the baby is normal.

Of course the decision to have one of these tests is a very personal one. So, too, is the action that you may choose to take if you find out that your baby has an abnormality. There is no right or wrong way to deal with this difficult situation and it is important that any advice you seek from your doctors is individual to you and your pregnancy. There are only a few general points of guidance that I believe can be offered. The first is that you are not more likely to miscarry after an amniocentesis because you have suffered miscarriages in the past. The second is that amniocentesis is usually performed between 14 and 16 weeks. If your miscarriages have been after this date it is probably best to avoid an invasive test unless the results of detailed ultrasound scans and blood tests suggest that there is a specific problem. I have always found it impossible to reassure a woman who miscarries after an amniocentesis that the test was not the cause of the miscarriage – so if you have suffered late miscarriages, this is one potential source of self-blame which can be avoided.

22

THE IMPORTANCE OF JOINING A RESEARCH PROGRAMME

Recurrent miscarriage is an enormously distressing problem for both the sufferer and her doctor. It is common for both parties to experience feelings of helplessness and despair. One of the hardest issues to deal with, in my opinion, is that the emotions of everyone involved are so raw that it can be very difficult to look at the problem objectively. If you have just had another miscarriage, it is understandable that you will want to try anything that may help you to have a baby. You want the results of the test that has just been discovered to be abnormal. You want this test to lead to a new treatment option. At that moment you do not care if the treatment has not been subjected to the rigours of a controlled trial. You do not care that it has no logical basis. All you want to do is try it and hope that it will work for you.

Your doctor may well be having similar feelings. It is really quite difficult to look after recurrent miscarriage patients and resist falling into the trap of trying out some new treatment idea before it has been properly evaluated and tested. After the umpteenth miscarriage, your doctor has to look you in the eye and tell you that the only advice to be offered is to try again because he or she does not know why your miscarriage happened. This doctor will probably feel that he or she has let you down, because they have failed to give you an answer or solve your problem. After all, medicine in the twenty-first century is meant to have conquered most common medical disorders and, on many occasions in this book, we have noted just how common the problem of miscarriage is.

All of these emotional feelings encourage the use of treatments for miscarriage before they have been properly tried and tested. Once they have been introduced, it is almost impossible to then subject them to the rigours of a randomised controlled trial. Which patient wants to be in the 'no treatment' group of a trial when their underlying problem is recurrent miscarriage? Which doctor wants to be in the position of deciding who receives what treatment? It is not difficult to see why it has proven so difficult to conduct research in this field. As a result, fact and fiction become muddled and are difficult to separate.

Why are we still so ignorant about the causes and treatment of miscarriage? This is a conversation that I embark on very frequently in the clinic, and many patients have told me that they found it helpful in understanding the complexity of the problem. Some of the answers are contained in the paragraphs above. I do not pretend that I have any more answers hidden up my sleeve, but I do think that it would be useful for the reader to appreciate that in no other field of medicine do we have to try and treat the abnormal before understanding the normal.

This may sound a strange comment, but remember that we are still incredibly ignorant about how a tiny embryo manages to implant successfully in the womb lining. If we knew the answer to this, we would soon be able to achieve 100% pregnancy rates for women who were undergoing IVF treatment. Getting pregnant is the first hurdle, staying pregnant is the next. How does this barely visible embryo manage to cope with all the obstacles that it faces during the first few months of its life? If you have had early pregnancy scans you will, I am sure, have marvelled at the transformation that you have witnessed with your own eyes as the tiny blob on the screen turns into a comma and then into a recognisable fetus. If we understood all the mechanisms involved in this development, we would probably be able to prevent a large number of miscarriages, providing that the embryo was chromosomally normal.

The reality is that we know very little about these early stages of pregnancy and we have to glean our knowledge from the pregnancies that miscarry, since we cannot experiment on the pregnancies that are developing properly. Of course, we can watch the pregnancy develop on the scan and we can measure the baby's growth, blood flow and movements, but we are unable to find out what is causing all these changes at a molecular level unless we can examine the tissues of the fetus, placenta or the endometrial lining. We have to content ourselves with working backwards, looking at those pregnancies that went wrong and trying to deduce what should have happened. When you appreciate these difficulties, I think it is easier to understand why both you and I are often faced with the problem of 'not knowing why' the miscarriage occurred.

I do not want to give the reader the view that the outlook for the future is bleak. On the contrary, there are many research groups working in this field and using animal models, human blood samples and tissue biopsies (often obtained from pregnancies that have miscarried or been terminated) they are trying to unravel some of the mysteries using molecular biology techniques. Although progress is not fast, it is constant and I believe that we can look forward to great advances in our knowledge during the next few years. As the theories emerge, they will need to be carefully translated into practical treatment options. This is where the readers of this book will have their best opportunity to make a contribution and benefit from their efforts. We are all working towards the same goal – a live, take-home baby.

Europe's largest research centre focusing on preventing miscarriage has opened under the banner of Tommy's miscarriage centre. The centre is a partnership of three universities: the University of Birmingham, the University of Warwick and Imperial College London. Together they will allow 24,000 women every year to access treatment and support, and to take part in Tommy's cutting-edge clinical studies. Tommy's National Centre for Miscarriage Research focuses on four questions:

Why did it happen?

Will it happen again?

How can we prevent it?

How can we care for women emotionally?

Through their research, the team will help uncover what is going wrong in early miscarriage. They will save babies' lives by turning their discoveries into tests, treatments, and better care for women who are most at risk.

The best advice that I can give to couples who have miscarried repeatedly is to visit a clinic that is actively involved in research. You will find that the doctors running these clinics are interested in and knowledgeable about your problems. Ask them questions and make sure that all the treatment trials they are involved in have control groups. Remember that the only way to determine whether treatment A is superior to treatment B is to examine them carefully in a controlled trial. Try to resist the temptation to go and find a doctor elsewhere who will give you the new treatment without comparing it to anything else.

During the course of the treatment trials that I have described to you in this book, there were several occasions when patients from our clinic dropped out of the trial before their treatment had started. They thought that they should ensure that they received the new 'wonder treatment' rather than risk being in a control group. I understand their motives, but I believe that they were misguided.

Certainly, most of them returned to see us at a later date. Your future pregnancies are much too important to be looked after in isolation. What you need is evidence and the benefit of pooled knowledge with which you can give yourself the best opportunities for a successful outcome to your pregnancy. I should also mention here that control groups do not necessarily mean 'no treatment'. More usually they mean that the new treatment is being measured against the best available treatment known at the time that the trial was being performed.

When you join a controlled trial, you are not a guinea pig – you are doing the most useful thing that you possibly can to sort out your own problem. This is the time when you can get back into the driving seat. Now you can stop feeling lost and out of control and start to help yourself. It is impossible for me to emphasise this point strongly enough. I am absolutely convinced that the treatment trials that we have performed recently at the St Mary's clinic owe a part of their success to the fact that the couples participating have understood what the trial is trying to achieve and why. There is no doubt that being informed has a remarkable capacity to make people feel confident and optimistic. These important emotions are very valuable when you want to embark upon a new pregnancy.

There is one more important issue to mention about the importance of miscarriage research. It needs dedicated effort and money to push it forward. If you have benefited from being involved in a research project, remember that many patients before you contributed to the research without any promise of a happy outcome. Their efforts have helped you and your efforts will help the next group of miscarriers in their quest for a child. Encourage everyone you know with a miscarriage problem to seek help in centres that are actively involved in research. The only way to change the distress of repeated miscarriages into success stories is to ensure that every woman with this problem contributes her experience to the pool of knowledge.

And when you have succeeded and have a beautiful baby, please remember those women who are still waiting to experience this joy. There are many ways that you can help to raise money and campaign for research funding for miscarriage. Please explore them!

23

THE VALUE OF TENDER LOVING CARE IN EARLY PREGNANCY

A question that I am asked repeatedly: 'What happens to those miscarriage patients who undergo all the available tests and have completely normal results?' I have saved this account for the end because it is so important. Much of the work carried out in the miscarriage clinic at St Mary's is aimed at identifying the reasons why a woman miscarries repeatedly. Since we are a research unit, we are regularly assessing the benefits and the failings of new investigative tests and treatments.

Most of our miscarriage patients and their doctors hope that one of these tests will be abnormal and that, as a result, they will identify a definite cause for their miscarriages. Of course, they hope there is also a suitable treatment that is capable of curing the abnormality that has been identified. However, there are always some patients in whom all the test results are persistently normal. As a result, there is no known medical treatment available for them. Sadly, these patients are frequently offered a variety of treatments (hormones, antibiotics, aspirin, immuno-therapy – the list is a long one) in the hope that 'doing something' will help to resolve the miscarriage problem.

The reader will have noticed on several occasions in this book how important I believe it is to resist giving patients treatment for miscarriage when no cause can be identified. This is because I firmly believe that one of the most important reasons why our understanding of recurrent miscarriage is so incomplete is due to the use of 'empirical' treatments. Of course, every woman and her doctor wants to maximise the chances of her next pregnancy being successful. The trouble is that when a particular treatment is given empirically (given anyway) although no cause has been identified, the results of this treatment become impossible to assess. The waters are muddied and, most importantly, the true benefits of an individual treatment will remain a mystery.

Over the last ten years, we have identified several thousands of couples with recurrent miscarriage in whom we can find no obvious abnormalities. We refer to this group as having unexplained pregnancy losses, although we recognise that a substantial proportion of these unexplained miscarriages are probably cases of bad luck or sporadic pregnancy loss. I was particularly interested to know the outcome of future pregnancies in these women, since this is obviously valuable information for me to pass on to my miscarriage patients. Helped by my research fellows, the early pregnancy clinic was expanded to include these women. Alongside all the miscarriers who were undergoing trial treatments, we encouraged the 'unexplained' group to visit the early pregnancy clinic every week and undergo the ultrasound scans and receive tender loving care from the research fellows, clinic nurses and scanners.

We found that the unexplained group who received this supportive care were extremely successful in their next pregnancy. Nearly 80% of them had a live baby. From a scientific point of view, I would argue that this is not surprising, since these women have no evidence of any specific causes of miscarriage. However, convincing a distressed miscarriage sufferer of these facts can be very difficult, which is why I am so delighted that we have been able to demonstrate how very successful these women can be in their next pregnancy.

Even more remarkable is that this study of the future outcome of women with unexplained recurrent miscarriages also demonstrated that the tender loving care plays an important part in achieving a successful outcome. Among the unexplained miscarriage group was a subgroup of women who, for a variety of reasons, decided not to return to our early pregnancy clinic. Some of them felt disillusioned by the fact that we had been unable to identify an underlying cause for their miscarriages. Some of them felt that the geographical distances were too great to travel on a weekly basis. I should mention here that many of our patients travelled 400 miles to visit us each week, and I feel sure that this sort of dedicated attitude must have played a part in their success.

Among the women who did not attend the early pregnancy clinic, the live birth rate was much lower – only 50%. I cannot give you a scientific explanation for this, but I do recognise that tender loving care in early pregnancy improves the outcome for women who have experienced repeated, unexplained miscarriages. Perhaps the supportive care has a beneficial effect on the woman's hormones, or on the way in which her immune system responds to the pregnancy in those first few crucial weeks. Certainly, there are other workers in this field who confirm my opinion, which is why I feel it very important that as many units as possible set up early pregnancy clinics for their miscarriage patients.

Before closing this chapter, I should mention that some sceptical doctors have asked me why I bother to look for new tests and new treatments for women with recurrent miscarriages, when I can achieve a 70–80% live birth rate just through the policy of a little tender loving care. I hope that the readers of this book are now so well informed that they can answer the question themselves! If I was to treat women with phospholipid syndrome with supportive care alone, and no aspirin or heparin, the miscarriage rate would rise to 90% and the live birthrate would drop to 10%. If, on the other hand, I decided to give all women aspirin and heparin, even those with no identifiable causes for their miscarriages, it would not be long before some of them developed side-effects from the treatment.

Even more worrying is the likelihood that if I had given everyone with unexplained miscarriage the aspirin and heparin treatment, the success rate for this treatment for the phospholipid syndrome would have been much lower and the true benefit of this therapy would never have been established. Until we reach the point where we understand the underlying cause for every miscarriage we cannot afford to second guess and offer women empirical treatments. If we let ourselves fall into this trap we will never be able to identify new research tests and new successful treatment options.

I believe that the first role of a miscarriage clinic is to identify causes of recurrent miscarriage that we can treat and continue to look for further tests that will identify new causes that are amenable to treatment in the future. The second role is to offer early pregnancy care and support. If, after careful investigation, we can find no cause for your pregnancy losses, it is now possible to reassure you that your chances of a successful pregnancy are about 75% if you are looked after carefully in the early weeks. I know of no other type of treatment for miscarriage that can better these excellent results! At the end of the day, your chances of a healthy take-home baby are very high – so please do not give up.

A
FINAL WORD

In the introduction I explained that my aim in writing this book was to try and take the mystery and the fear out of the subject of miscarriage. I have attempted to describe the known causes and treatments of miscarriage in ways which my patients tell me they have found helpful. I hope that I have achieved what I set out to do, although I am conscious of the fact that, at the present time, there are still questions for which I cannot offer you an answer.

The answers will come if we continue to research them carefully. We must also resist the temptation to give miscarriage sufferers treatments until they have been shown to be of benefit in properly controlled trials, as the use of empirical treatment for women with unexplained miscarriages only serves to make this important subject more difficult to understand and conquer.

Happily, I can reassure you that the vast majority of women with a history of recurrent miscarriage eventually succeed in their aim of having a healthy child.

Good luck in your new pregnancy!

GLOSSARY

ACA: anticardiolipin antibodies – one of the family of antiphospholipid antibodies. The IgG, IgM and IgA variants are associated with miscarriage and placental insufficiency in later pregnancy.

adhesions, or synechiae: fibrous bands joining one tissue surface to another. When present inside the uterus, the walls of the uterus stick together, distorting the shape of the cavity.

allograft: a tissue or organ taken from one human and transplanted into another human being. Kidney transplants are allografts.

alloimmmune: immune reactions which occur between the tissues of different human beings.

amniocentesis: a procedure in which a fine needle is inserted into the amniotic sac via the mother's abdominal wall to obtain a sample of amniotic fluid for genetic or chemical analysis of the baby.

amniotic sac/fluid: two layers of membranes (the amnion and chorion) form the amniotic sac. The sac lies in the uterine cavity filled with amniotic fluid, which bathes the fetus.

aneuploidy: too many or too few chromosomes present in the cell. Normal cells contain 46 chromosomes arranged in 23 pairs.

anticoagulant: a substance that makes our blood less likely to form clots. Certain drugs can do this and normal blood contains natural anticoagulants.

anti-d: an injection of immunoglobulin (antibodies) capable of destroying rhesus positive (D) red blood cells. This is given to rhesus negative mothers after delivery of a rhesus positive baby to prevent them developing rhesus disease in a future pregnancy.

antiphospholipid syndrome: a condition in which antiphospholipid antibodies in the bloodstream lead to recurrent miscarriages and/or thrombosis.

APA: antiphospholipid antibodies – a family of autoantibodies, the most common of which are the lupus anticoagulant and anticardiolipin antobodies.

APCA: antipaternal cytotoxic antibody – an antibody which develops when the mother's immune system has recognised that the fetus contains cells from the father.

APCR: activated protein C resistance – an inherited type of blood clotting disorder which is found in some women with late miscarriages.

autoimmune: immune reactions caused by antibodies which are directed against our own tissues (anti-self). The reactions usually cause damage to our body tissues.

beta-2 glycoprotein 1: another antibody contributing to antiphospholipid syndrome.

bicornuate uterus: a congenital abnormality in which the two uterine horns do not fuse together but are joined by a single cervix.

biochemical pregnancy: a positive pregnancy test followed soon after by a menstrual period.

bromocryptine: a drug used to reduce high prolactin hormone levels.

brucella: bacterial organism causing brucellosis or undulant fever. An important cause of infertility and miscarriage in cattle. A rare cause of miscarriage among farm workers.

cell-free fetal DNA: fetal genetic material in maternal blood that allows the diagnosis of various genetic disorders in the fetus in early pregnancy.

cerclage: a stitch inserted into the cervix to close the cervical canal.

cervix: the muscular neck of the uterus (womb).

chlamydia: a sexually transmitted infective organism halfway between a bacterium and a virus. Common cause of damage to the fallopian tubes leading to infertility, and conjunctivitis in newborn babies. It does not cause miscarriage in humans.

chorion villus sampling: a procedure in which a sample of placenta is obtained for genetic or chemical analysis of the baby, using a special needle introduced through the mother's abdominal wall.

chromosome: rod-shaped bodies in the nucleus of cells which carry the genes that transmit inherited characteristics.

congenital: a structural or functional defect or malformation present at birth.

cordocentesis: a procedure used to sample the baby's blood in utero. A special needle is inserted into the umbilical cord under ultrasound control.

corpus luteum: 'yellow body' – formed in the ovary from an ovarian follicle which has released an egg. The corpus luteum produces progesterone hormone until the placenta takes over production.

CT: computerised tomography – a special imaging technique for body tissues.

cytogeneticist: a specialist in the genetic makeup of cells.

cytomegalovirus: a viral infection which may cause neurological problems in the baby.

D&C: dilatation and curettage – a minor operation in which tissue is removed from the lining of the uterus (a scrape).

de novo: an event that occurs out of the blue.

DNA: the chemical building blocks that genes are made of.

Doppler scan: measures the flow of blood through vessels and can be used to identify blood flow problems in the placenta and baby.

DRVVT: the dilute Russel's viper venom time test is the most accurate way to identify the presence of the lupus anticoagulant in blood.

ectopic pregnancy: a pregnancy that implants outside the uterus, usually in the fallopian tubes.

endocrine: hormones that are produced by a gland (e.g. pituitary, ovary) and carried in the bloodstream to act on another organ in the body (e.g. uterus).

endometritis: inflammation of the uterine lining, usually caused by infection.

endometrium: the uterine lining that is shed during each menstrual period and is the site for implantation of the embryo.

epidural: a local anaesthetic inserted into the back which numbs pain from the waist downwards.

ERPC: evacuation of retained products of conception – a surgical procedure to empty the uterus of pregnancy tissues that have not been expelled after the pregnancy has died.

factor v: one of the factors involved in the complex pathways which control the ability of our blood to coagulate (clot) and to dissolve these clots.

fetal pole: the term used to describe the tiny fetus before it has developed a recognisable form.

fetoscopy: a specialised test using a fine telescope inserted into the amniotic sac to visualise the fetus or baby and through which tissue samples can be taken.

fibroid: common non-malignant tumours that arise in the muscular wall of the uterus.

folic acid: one of the B vitamins. When it occurs naturally in foods it is known as folate.

follicle: the fluid-filled cysts in the ovary containing an egg surrounded by layers of cells.

formalin: a chemical which preserves tissues for histological analysis under the microscope.

FSH: this follicle-stimulating hormone is secreted by the pituitary gland and stimulates the growth of the ovarian follicles.

gene: a single unit of inheritance. Each chromosome is made up of thousands of genes which control the development and function of all the tissues of our body.

gnrh agonists: drugs which stop the secretion of FSH and LH from the pituitary gland when they are given for more than a few days.

gonadotropins: the collective term for FSH and LH hormones produced in the pituitary gland. These hormones can be used to induce multiple ovulation.

haematologist: a medical doctor who specialises in blood.

haematoma: a collection of blood (clot) inside the body tissues.

half life: the time taken for a drug or hormone level in the body to reduce by 50%.

HCG: human chorionic gonadotrophin. A hormone produced by the embryo which is measured in standard pregnancy tests.

heparin: an anticoagulant most commonly used to prevent or treat thrombosis.

HIV: human immunodeficiency virus which causes the AIDS disease.

hydatidiform mole: a tumour of the placental tissues (trophoblast).

hyperemesis gravidarum: extreme nausea and vomiting in pregnancy which can lead to severe dehydration.

hypothalamus: a control centre in the brain which plays a crucial role in the functioning of the pituitary gland.

hysterosalpingogram: HSG – a X-ray examination in which a special dye is injected through the cervix to visualise the cervical canal, the cavity of the uterus and the fallopian tubes.

hysteroscope: a fibre-optic telescope which is passed through the cervical canal into the uterus to visualise the uterine cavity.

ICSI: intracytoplasmic sperm injection. A recently developed fertility technique in which a sperm is injected into an egg to improve fertilisation, using specialised microscopic instruments.

incompetence (of the cervix): a cervix that starts to open during pregnancy due to weakness of the muscular wall.

IVF: in vitro fertilisation – infertility treatment involving the collection of eggs and sperm which are then fertilised in the laboratory. The resulting embryos are then replaced into the mother's uterus.

karyotype: a person's individual chromosome pattern. In women it is normally 46XX and in men 46XY.

LA: lupus anticoagulant – one of the antiphospholipid antibodies (APA) which have been strongly implicated as a cause of recurrent miscarriage.

laparoscopy: an operation during which a lighted telescope is introduced into the abdominal cavity to visualise the uterus, ovaries and fallopian tubes.

LH: luteinising hormone – secreted by the pituitary gland. The normal mid-cycle surge of LH triggers the process of ovulation. High levels of LH at other times in the cycle are associated with miscarriage and infertility.

listeria: bacteria present in animals and contaminated soil. If the mother becomes infected during pregnancy, listeria can cause late miscarriage.

manual vacuum aspiration: MVA – newly introduced technique to empty the uterus of pregnancy tissues that can be undertaken in the outpatient clinic with local anaesthetic.

meiosis: a special type of reduction cell division which only occurs in eggs and sperm. The numbers of chromosomes are halved to 23 in preparation for fertilisation.

mifipristone: an antiprogesterone (progesterone antagonist) which can be used to terminate early pregnancies without the need for surgery.

misoprostol: a prostaglandin drug that is used to empty pregnancy tissues from the uterus.

monosomies: the defect arising when one chromosome is lost. The most common example is Monosomy (45) X or Turner's syndrome.

mosaicism: two different cell lines in the same tissue or organ, made up of different chromosome numbers.

MRI: magnetic resonance imaging – a specialised three-dimensional scanning technique.

multiparous: a woman who has delivered babies in the past.

myomectomy: surgical procedure to remove a fibroid (myoma) from the uterus.

oestrogen: one of the female hormones produced by the ovary and placenta.

omnopon: a painkilling drug which also acts as a sedative.

partum, intra/post/ante: labour and delivery of the baby – hence intra (during), post (after) and ante (before) delivery.

parvovirus: a viral infection which only rarely causes miscarriage or intrauterine death. The baby may accumulate fluid in the abdomen, chest and brain 'hydrops'.

pethidine: a painkilling drug frequently used for women in labour.

pituitary gland: a small structure lying under the brain and behind the eyesockets. It controls the production and secretion of hormones from several other glands.

polycystic ovaries: ovaries in which the follicles are arranged around the outside of the gland in a 'pearl necklace pattern'. These ovaries tend to be larger than normal and may be associated with infertility and miscarriage.

polyploidies: the defect caused by the embryo receiving extra sets of 23 chromosomes; triploidy = 69XXY, tetraploidy = 92XXYY.

pre-eclampsia: a pregnancy disorder characterised by high blood pressure, swelling of the hands and feet and protein in the urine.

primigravida: a woman who is pregnant for the first time (gravid = heavy).

primiparous: a woman who has never delivered a baby before.

progesterone: one of the female hormones produced in increasing quantities by the ovary after ovulation and by the placenta during pregnancy.

prostaglandins: naturally occurring chemicals present in many tissues of the body. Some types cause the uterine muscles to contract, leading to labour.

reactive depression: depression which develops in response to major life events or crises.

resection: the paring away of a tissue (as opposed to complete removal) usually using telescopic instruments.

rhesus antibodies: antibodies produced by a rhesus negative mother in response to the presence of rhesus positive red blood cells entering her bloodstream from the baby.

SLE: systemic lupus erythematosis – the commonest autoimmune disease in women during the reproductive age. A woman who has lupus anticoagulant in her blood does not necessarily have or develop full-blown SLE.

spina bifida: a congenital abnormality in which the baby's delicate spinal cord is not covered by the bony spine. This is one type of neural tube defect.

subclinical: a very early pregnancy that is recognisable by biochemical tests but with no evidence of a pregnancy sac on the ultrasound scan.

subfertile: a delay or difficulty in becoming pregnant.

thrombosis: a blood clot which blocks the flow of blood in a blood vessel.

torch: the name of the infection screen that used to be advised for recurrent miscarriers. (T=toxoplasma, O=other, R=rubella, C=chlamydia and H=herpes).

toxaemia: another term for pre-eclampsia (see before).

toxoplasma: a parasitic infection which can cause miscarriage and congenital abnormalities. It is most often found in communities with lots of cats or where meat is undercooked.

translocations: when a piece of one chromosome becomes attached to the broken end of another.

trimester: pregnancy is divided into three trimesters of approximately three months.

trisomies: the presence of three copies of one chromosome instead of the normal two. The best known example is trisomy 21 – Down's syndrome.

ultrasound scan: high-frequency sound waves that are used to produce a grey-scale image of tissues in the body. Obstetric ultrasound has become extremely sophisticated and can now visualise tiny abnormalities in the baby.

unicornuate uterus: a single uterine horn usually accompanied by a redundant second horn which has failed to develop.

uterine septum: a dividing wall or curtain of tissue extending downwards from the top of the uterus.

uterus: the womb – consisting of a hollow muscular body and neck (the cervix). A canal through the cervix connects the body of the uterus to the vagina.

viability: the age at which a newborn baby is capable of survival outside the mother's womb.

TOMMY'S NATIONAL CENTRE FOR MISCARRIAGE RESEARCH

Tommy's National Centre for Miscarriage Research

The only national miscarriage centre was established in April 2016 bringing together three leading universities (Birmingham, Warwick and Imperial College, London), four major hospitals, the UK's leading scientific and clinical leaders and other research funders, to reduce miscarriage. The aim is to consider solutions from every angle, share patient samples and patient data, share learnings and ideas and work together to:

- Understand the basic science that underpins successful and unsuccessful early pregnancy – to identify potential avenues for clinical investigation
- What causes miscarriage – we want to give every parent a reason for their miscarriage
- Understand what healthy lifestyle advice we can give to parents to help them to have a successful pregnancy and persuade them to follow that advice
- Who is most at risk – to concentrate care on those who need it
- Find treatments that prevent miscarriage – so we can reduce the number of parents experiencing recurrent miscarriage
- Establish the best way to care for parents who have experienced a miscarriage – so they do not experience long-term mental health problems following miscarriage

- Ensure that wherever you live you can access the same high-quality standard of care and the latest treatments – by disseminating what we discover and ensuring that parents' voices are heard in both government and the NHS.

Our lifesaving research could not take place without the women who take part in our clinical trails. Getting involved in research also gives women the opportunity to benefit from new tests and treatments. So below you will find details of the trials that the Tommy's National Centre for Miscarriage are currently undertaking.

Tommy's research trials based at Imperial College London

PRECISE study

We are investigating if it is possible to look in detail at your baby's heart, brain, spinal cord, bones, kidneys and stomach before 18 weeks of pregnancy using new ultrasound techniques and 3D ultrasound scanning. We will perform two extra ultrasound scans of your baby between 12 and 18 weeks of pregnancy. To be eligible for the study participants must be aged over 18 years and more than seven weeks' pregnant. Please email: precise@imperial.ac.uk or ring: 07518 210 305 to register your interest in taking part in this research.

EPOS study

The early pregnancy period is critical for pregnancy success. We are investigating the impact of early pregnancy events such as pain and bleeding on the future risk of miscarriage and risk of long-term pregnancy complications such as pre-eclampsia and preterm labour. Women who are less than 14 weeks' pregnant, aged between 16 and 50 years, with or without the pregnancy events described, are eligible to participate in the study. Participants are seen up to six times during their pregnancy where ultrasound scans are performed, and samples collected to screen for differences between women who do and do not have adverse pregnancy outcomes. For more information about the study please email: ICHC-tr.epos@nhs.net or call the clinical research fellow on: 07934 920 180.

ASPIRE study

There is bacteria in all parts of our body and the work microbiome refers to the genetic material of these organisms. Currently, it is not known whether an imbalance of this bacteria or the presence of a certain type is linked to miscarriage. We are investigating whether there is a normal early pregnancy and endometrial microbiome, and whether this changes in miscarriage. We are also looking to identify a better way to see if someone has miscarried because of a chromosomal issue. Those undergoing management of the miscarriage will have the tissue analysed for chromosome abnormalities and are welcome to receive the results if they wish. Please email: aspire@imperial.ac.uk or ring: 0203 3035 131 if you would like to find out more information.

PIEPE study

In a recent pilot study published in BMJ Open we showed that women who have miscarried or had an ectopic pregnancy have high levels of post-traumatic stress disorder (PTSD) as well as anxiety and depression. We are currently analysing the data from the full study examining the psychological impact of early pregnancy events on both women and their partners. Our next study will be to examine the value of difference treatment strategies to help women deal with the psychological consequences of early pregnancy loss.

ABPEP

'PUL' (pregnancy of unknown location) is a phenomenon in early pregnancy where a woman has a positive pregnancy test but we cannot see where the pregnancy is with an ultrasound scan. The majority of women in this situation will sadly be undergoing a very early miscarriage but some will go on to have a healthy pregnancy. There is a period of uncertainty whilst the outcome of the pregnancy is determined. We are carrying out research that may help come to a diagnosis much earlier to better support women and their partners through what is an emotionally demanding time. If you would like more information, please contact: whrcenquiries@imperial.ac.uk.

CONCEIVE trial

We are investigating if maternal cardiovascular function prior to pregnancy and also an adaptation of the mum's heart and circulation to pregnancy impacts on pregnancy outcomes, specifically first trimester miscarriage, pre-eclampsia and fetal growth restriction. We have, therefore, been recruiting women pre-conception, and following them through pregnancy to the post-partum period with comprehensive cardiovascular investigations. This study is now closed for recruitment but for further information please email: conceive@nhs.net or visit our Facebook page: https://www.facebook.com/conceivestudy.

Tommy's research trials at Birmingham Women's Hospital

Cell-free fetal DNA study

This project is investigating whether analysis of cell-free fetal DNA could help us to ascertain genetic reasons for early miscarriages. Women with a diagnosis of recurrent miscarriage, threatened miscarriage, missed miscarriage or incomplete miscarriage are eligible to participate in the study. Please email: BWH-tr.tommysclinic@nhs.net to register your interest in taking part in this research at this hospital.

Sperm DNA fragmentation study

This project investigates whether miscarriage could be caused by sperm DNA damage in the male partner of couples having investigations for recurrent miscarriage. Please email: BWH-tr.tommysclinic@nhs.net to register your interest in taking part in this research at this hospital.

Immune phenotyping study

We are investigating whether adaptations of the maternal immune system could be implicated in patients with a history of recurrent miscarriage. Please email: BWH-tr.tommysclinic@nhs.net to register your interest in taking part in this research at this hospital.

MifeMiso trial

We are investigating whether a single drug treatment (misoprostol) or a combination of drug treatments (mifepristone plus misoprostol two days later) is best for the medical management of missed miscarriage. To be eligible for the study women must be diagnosed with a missed miscarriage by pelvic ultrasound scan in the first 13+6 weeks of pregnancy, be opting for medical management, be 16 years of age or over and be willing and able to give informed consent.

Please note, this trial is being conducted at several hospitals across the UK. Therefore, if you are not local to Birmingham, there might be a hospital close to where you live that is offering this trial. Please email: mifemiso@trials.bham.ac.uk to register your interest in taking part in this research.

Tommy's research trials at University Hospital Coventry

SiM trial

We are investigating whether scratching the lining of the womb could prevent miscarriage among women aged 18 to 42 years and with two or more previous miscarriages. Please telephone: 0247 6964 983 to speak to the clinic secretary about your interest in this research.

Tommy's research trials at multiple hospitals

Alife2 trial

This study is investigating whether anticoagulant (blood-thinning) treatment could reduce the risk of miscarriage in women aged 18 to 42 years, with two or more previous miscarriages and with inherited thrombophilia. Thrombophilia is when your blood has a tendency to clot more than normal. Please email: BWH-tr.tommysclinic@nhs.net to register your interest in taking part in this research at Birmingham Women's Hospital. To register your interest in taking part at University Hospital Coventry, please ring: 0247 6964, 983 to speak to the clinic secretary about your interest in this research. Your eligibility for the study will be assessed and if you are eligible you will be given further information about how to take part.

PRISM trial

We are investigating whether progesterone could prevent miscarriage in women with early pregnancy bleeding, a known sign of threatened miscarriage. To be eligible for the study participants must be aged 16 to 39 years; have an ongoing pregnancy; and have experienced recent early pregnancy bleeding within the last four days during the first 12 weeks of pregnancy.

Please note that this trial is being conducted at 48 hospitals across the UK. Therefore, if you are not local to Birmingham, there might be a hospital closer to where you live that is offering this trial. Please email: prism@trials.bham.ac.uk to register your interest in taking part in this research.

INDEX

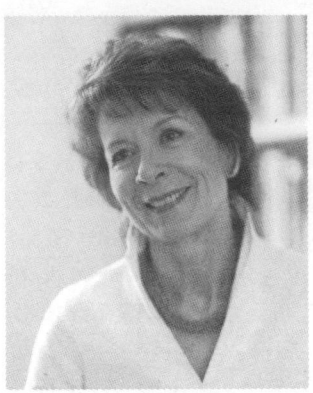

Professor Lesley Regan runs the recurrent miscarriage clinic at St Mary's Hospital, London, the largest referral unit of its kind in Europe. In addition to caring for women who are trying to find out why they have miscarried repeatedly, she has built a team of dedicated doctors and midwives who help her to look after these women throughout their future pregnancies. Lesley Regan is professor of Obstetrics and Gynaecology at Imperial College School of Medicine at St Mary's and director of the Women's Health Research Centre. She is a renowned teacher in the field of reproductive medicine, and has encouraged both her UK and overseas trainees to develop specialist expertise in the field of recurrent miscarriage and establish their own clinics.

Lesley Regan's contributions to research into the causes of and treatments for miscarriage are recognised internationally. She is an adviser to many national and international organisations and is in regular demand as a visiting lecturer. She is currently the president of the Royal College of Obstetricians and Gynaecologists, the first woman to be elected to this role in 65 years. She was recently elected to the prestigious US National Academy of Medicine – a rare honour for a UK clinician to receive. Her high-profile, extensive experience, expert knowledge and common-sense approach have resulted in her being in regular demand for both television and radio. Lesley Regan lives in central London with her twin daughters.

charm

There are a number of ways that you can help us to raise money for CHARM. Please tick any of the circles you can, fill in your details and send this form to the address below

☐ I would like to make a donation
(please see below for details)

☐ I might have a fundraising idea

☐ I would like to be on your mailing list for
information on future fundraising events

Name _____

Address _____

_____

_____

Tel _____

Email _____

Please make cheques payable to **CHARM Foundation UK**
and send with your form to **CHARM Foundation UK**,
**St Mary's Hospital, Department of Obstetrics and Gynaecology,
Ground Floor, Mint Wing, South Wharf Road,
London W2 1NY**

Registered Charity No1133659